# ANNUAL REVIEW OF NURSING RESEARCH

Volume 18, 2000

# ANNUAL REVIEW OF NURSING RESEARCH

## Volume 18, 2000

## Focus on Chronic Illness

Joyce J. Fitzpatrick, PhD, RN, FAAN
Series Editor

Jean Goeppinger, PhD, RN, FAAN
Volume Editor

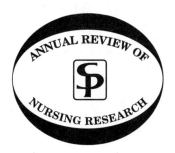

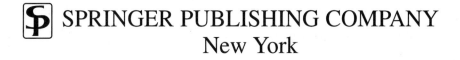

SPRINGER PUBLISHING COMPANY
New York

Order ANNUAL REVIEW OF NURSING RESEARCH, Volume 19, 2001, prior to publication and receive a 10% discount. An order coupon can be found at the back of this volume.

Springer Publishing Company, Inc.
536 Broadway
New York, NY 10012-3955

00 01 02 03 04 / 5 4 3 2 1

ISBN-0-8261-1328-1
ISSN-0739-6686

ANNUAL REVIEW OF NURSING RESEARCH is indexed in *Cumulative Index to Nursing and Allied Health Literature and Index Medicus.*

Printed in the United States of America

# Contents

**Part II: Milestones in Nursing Research**

# Preface

This is the 18th volume in the *Annual Review of Nursing Research* (ARNR) series. The course of nursing research is reflected in the eighteen-year time span between the volumes from 1983 through 2000. Nursing research has become targeted, particularly focused on clinical approaches to disease management, prevention of disease, and health promotion. Increasingly, nurse researchers have recognized the importance of the biobehavioral and health policy foundations of effective and efficient nursing intervention. Nursing research also has become more interdisciplinary. These changes are reflected in this volume of ARNR.

Volume 18 includes 10 chapters; the theme of the volume is chronic illness. Chronic illness in general and certain specific chronic diseases, such as heart disease, AIDS, and cancer, have attracted significant attention recently from researchers and policymakers. Common to all chapters in this volume of ARNR is a focus on chronic illness characterized by a prolonged and uncertain course, lack of easy resolution, rarity of complete cure, frequent unknown etiology, and multiple risk factors (Brownson, Remington, & Davis, 1998). The chapters reflect a variety of chronic illnesses; the full range of interventions, from intervention to management; samples diverse in age, race, and disease state; multiple intervention settings (school, hospital, community, home, clinic); and all types (educational, counseling/psychosocial, biobehavioral) and levels (individual, family, community, health care system) of intervention.

In chapter 1, Sally Thorne and Barbara Paterson review research describing the insider perspective on living with a chronic illness. In chapters 2 and 3, Joan Austin and David Dunn and Jacqueline Dunbar-Jacob and her colleagues at the University of Pittsburgh review research related to two critical issues in chronic illness: quality of life and adherence. In chapters 4 through 7, Debra Moser, Jeannie Pasacreta and Ruth McCorkle, Margaret Grey, and Jean Wyman review intervention studies examining patient outcomes in heart failure disease management programs; caregiver outcomes in cancer care; the disease knowledge, adjustment, and metabolic control of children with type 1 diabetes and parent–child conflict in their families; and urinary incontinence management among adult ambulatory care populations.

The final two chapters on chronic illness are centered on prevention. Carol Loveland-Cherry reviews research related to family interventions to prevent substance abuse and other chronic conditions resulting from it, and Janet C. Meininger reviews research on population-wide approaches to the school-based primary prevention of cardiovascular diseases. The final chapter in this volume is an analysis of nursing research from the perspective of scientific breakthroughs in the past 25 years. Sue Donaldson traces the history of "pathfinders" in nursing research, citing their contributions to the nursing and health literature. This is a feature that we plan to maintain in future volumes, requesting other key leaders in the nursing research community to evaluate the development of nursing science from their perspective.

This volume reflects the informed, energetic contributions of the chapter authors and the careful and systematic reviews of drafts by their peers. We thank them. In addition, we thank the researchers whose work the authors cite and the advisory board members for their contributions to the advancement of our discipline.

JEAN GOEPPINGER, PhD, RN, FAAN
Volume Editor

JOYCE J. FITZPATRICK, PhD, RN, FAAN
Series Editor

## REFERENCE

Brownson, R. C., Remington, P., & Davis, J. R. (1998). *Chronic disease epidemiology and control* (2nd ed.). Washington, DC: American Public Health Association.

# Contributors

**Joan K. Austin, DNS, RN, FAAN**
Distinguished Professor
School of Nursing
Indiana University

**Sue K. Donaldson, PhD**
Dean and Professor
School of Nursing
Professor, School of Medicine
Johns Hopkins University

**Willa M. Doswell, PhD, RN, FAAN**
Assistant Professor
Department of Health Promotion
  and Development
School of Nursing
University of Pittsburgh

**Jacqueline Dunbar-Jacob, PhD,
  RN, FAAN**
Professor, Schools of Nursing
  and Public Health
Director, Center for Research
  in Chronic Disorders,
  School of Nursing
University of Pittsburgh

**David W. Dunn, MD**
Associate Professor, Child
  Neurology and Psychiatry
Departments of Neurology
  and Psychiatry
School of Medicine
Indiana University

**Judith A. Erlen, PhD, RN**
Associate Professor, Center for
  Bioethics and Health Law
Associate Director, Center for
  Research in Chronic Disorders,
  School of Nursing
University of Pittsburgh

**Margaret Grey, DrPH, FAAN, CPNP**
Independence Foundation
  Professor of Nursing
Associate Dean for Research Affairs
School of Nursing
Yale University

**Carol J. Loveland-Cherry, PhD,
  RN, FAAN**
Professor and Associate Dean for
  Academic Affairs
School of Nursing
The University of Michigan

**Ruth McCorkle, PhD, RN, FAAN**
Professor and Director of Center
  on Chronic Illness
School of Nursing
Yale University

**Janet C. Meininger, PhD, RN,
  FAAN**
Lee and Joseph D. Jamail
  Distinguished Professor
School of Nursing
University of Texas at Houston

**Debra K. Moser, DNSc, RN**
Associate Professor
Department of Adult Health
  and Illness Nursing
College of Nursing
The Ohio State University

**Jeannie V. Pasacreta, PhD, RN (CS)**
Associate Professor and Specialty
  Director
Psychiatric Mental Health Nursing
School of Nursing
Yale University

**Barbara L. Paterson, PhD, RN**
Associate Professor
School of Nursing
University of British Columbia

**Christopher M. Ryan, PhD**
Associate Professor of Psychiatry,
  School of Medicine
Associate Professor of Health
  and Community Systems,
  School of Nursing
University of Pittsburgh

**Elizabeth A. Schlenk, PhD, RN**
Assistant Professor
School of Nursing
University of Pittsburgh

**Susan M. Sereika, PhD**
Assistant Professor, Nursing,
  Biostatistics, and Epidemiology
School of Public Health
University of Pittsburgh

**Sally E. Thorne, PhD, RN**
Professor
School of Nursing
University of British Columbia

**Jean F. Wyman, PhD, RN, CS,
  FAAN**
Professor and Cora Meidl Siehl
  Chair in Nursing Research
Director, Center for Nursing
  Research of Elders
School of Nursing
University of Minnesota

# PART I

## Research in Chronic Illness

Chapter 1

# Two Decades of Insider Research: What We Know and Don't Know About Chronic Illness Experience

SALLY E. THORNE AND BARBARA L. PATERSON

## ABSTRACT

Chronic illness in a general sense and certain chronic diseases in particular have attracted considerable attention from qualitative researchers in nursing as well as in other health and social sciences. This review critically examines the body of available research about the experience of living with a chronic illness from an "insider" perspective. From this foundation the authors interpret the manner in which this large body of writing both contributes to and complicates our theoretical understanding of what it is like to live with a chronic disease. In so doing they illuminate themes within the knowledge that can be gleaned from qualitative inquiry into the chronic illness experience, as well as inherent limitations that must be taken into consideration when applying such knowledge to practice.

**Key words: chronic illness, chronic illness experience, psychosocial impact of illness, qualitative health research**

The past 20 years of research in the field of chronic illness experience have witnessed a dramatic shift in methodological orientation from an exclusively "outsider" perspective toward a proliferation of what has been termed "insider" research, or the study of the experience of chronic illness from the perspective of the person with the disease (Conrad, 1990; Gerhardt, 1990; Thorne & Paterson, 1998). Building upon and extending the work of early social scientists such as Strauss (1975) and colleagues (Corbin & Strauss, 1988a, 1988b; Strauss et al., 1984), many nurse researchers have conceptualized chronic illness as a focus for their inquiry and have been drawn toward consideration of methods and approaches that allow for development of knowledge about what it means to live with a chronic illness (Thorne & Paterson, 1998; Wellard, 1998). Using a range of qualitative research methods to extend the kinds of knowledge that could be captured by more traditional descriptive and exploratory approaches, nurses have played a particularly prominent role in generating analyses of chronic illness that place the experience in a relational and social context. Such analyses represent persons with chronic illness as active agents within and analysts of their circumstances, and they challenge traditional biomedical and social science orientations of how we might understand and theorize about chronic illness.

In addition to the direct contribution it has made to theorizing about chronic illness, the body of qualitative research has created a context in which knowledge derived from quantitative research can be reconsidered in the light of insider perspectives (Casebeer & Verhoef, 1997). Although such studies will not be reviewed here, a number of health researchers have also combined strategies or developed programs of research in which evidence obtained using one methodology is challenged and tested by triangulated approaches. It seems that the very act of engaging in qualitative inquiry has created an attitudinal climate in which nurses and other health scientists critically deconstruct the foundations of what they think they know about illness phenomena and engage in an inquiry processes that include consumer criticism, social science, and biomedicine as equal partners in the development of new kinds of knowledge—knowledge that is respectful of diversity, socially responsible, applicable, and practical (Royer, 1998).

## SCOPE OF THE REVIEW

In this review we summarize some of the significant contributions that qualitative researchers have made to the project of theorizing chronic illness over the past two decades. We examine some of the major developments that have emerged and try to place them in a context of how the body of knowledge has taken shape as this extensive research initiative continues. In so doing, we attempt to critically interpret the current status of the field so as to be able to make recommendations for future research that will truly reflect the potential of what qualitative methods might offer, particularly for the practical science of health care.

Our own analysis has been informed, to a considerable extent, by our continued participation in a large metasynthesis project in which we have examined patterns and trends within the findings from qualitative research on individual adult experiences with various chronic diseases between the years 1980 and 1996 (Paterson, Thorne, & Dewis, 1998;

Thorne & Paterson, 1998, and work in progress). From the vantage point of this inquiry we have found it instructive not only to consider what has been learned from a generation of insider research into chronic illness but also to pose a number of relevant questions throughout our analytic process: Which chronic diseases have been studied, and which ignored? Which qualitative methods have been used to learn about illness experience, and how have their applications evolved over the two decades of development? How has the choice of research approaches influenced the way we now view chronic illness? Which disciplinary perspectives and theoretical orientations have shaped the research questions and directed the interpretations? Thus, our fascination has shifted over time from simply compiling what we know about chronic illness experience toward discovering the many ways in which our understanding remains confused and conflicted.

For the explicit purposes of this review, we used computer and hand searches of health research within the qualitative tradition from 1980 through 1998. Our computer searches relied on a number of databases, including CINAHL, PsychLIT, SocioFile, and MEDLINE, using such keywords as *chronic illness, chronic disease,* and *illness experience,* as well as selecting from among studies keyworded as *qualitative studies* in journals in nursing, medicine, psychology, sociology, medical anthropology, and rehabilitation sciences. While much of the research that has been published in this area derives from North American sources, we also searched among international English-language publications in various disciplines and located a number of studies deriving from Australia, New Zealand, Asia, the Scandinavian and other European countries, and the United Kingdom. Beyond sources that have been published in peer-reviewed scholarly journals, many of the particularly significant works within this body of research appear only in book, chapter, or dissertation format. Although such sources tend not to be as systematically accessible as are indexed journal articles, we have tried to locate as many as possible of those studies that the authors in this field themselves consider foundational.

There are a number of complexities inherent in this type of review that require explanation in order to put our inclusion criteria in some context. First, over the two decades in which qualitative research into chronic illness experience has flourished, the common understanding of what constitutes a chronic illness experience has changed considerably (Gerhardt, 1990). Some of the relevant research comes from an explicit conceptualization of chronicity (e.g., Curtin & Lubkin, 1990), but the vast majority of the research is conducted in the context of one or, at most, two disease categories. The frequency with which diseases appear in the research may have less to do with population prevalence than with matters of sampling convenience or theoretical simplicity. For example, as has been noted by Conrad (1990) and in our own metastudy research, diseases for which people attend ambulatory clinics seem to attract a considerable share of the research attention. Within a single disease category, individuals with more pronounced symptoms or limitations may consider themselves to have a chronic illness, whereas those who are less symptomatic may not. Some diseases previously conceptualized as acute, such as HIV/AIDS and some cancer illnesses, have come to be considered chronic because of the extended trajectory that medical advances have made possible (Bland, 1999). Other health conditions, such as chronic leg ulcer, are rarely acknowledged within the chronic illness literature, despite their conceptual similarity to many other recognized chronic diseases (Bland, 1999).

Although many clinicians and researchers have conceptually linked chronic illness and disability, consumer advocates often accentuate the experiential differences that make such comparison inappropriate (Gordon, Feldman, & Crose, 1998; Thorne, McCormick, & Carty, 1997). And although the individual is clearly the embodied source of a chronic disease, the illness experience it entails may be fully shared by significant others, particularly family caregivers (Robinson, 1998). Thus, any general review of chronic illness theory will inevitably reveal some rather arbitrary decisions as to what is and is not included.

Another major challenge in a review of this sort is to distinguish what constitutes qualitative as opposed to quantitative research. There are multiple traditions of inquiry and diverse standards of scholarship within the major disciplines involved in this inherently interdisciplinary effort. Because authors have shaped their research reports to match the constraints of the publishers as well as the ever-changing expectations of their audience, it becomes quite difficult to articulate quality criteria or baseline indicators that distinguish a study as explicitly qualitative.

A third challenge is to articulate a specifically nursing contribution to this body of developing knowledge. From our metasynthesis review we have determined that researchers with advanced nursing degrees have published an extraordinarily large volume of qualitative studies in many aspects of chronic illness experience. However, many nurse researchers have research training in the theoretical and methodological traditions of other social sciences, many work in interdisciplinary teams, and many publish their work in journals that are not nursing journals. Although some of the research published by nurses makes an explicit primary contribution to nursing knowledge, the vast majority of thoughtful nursing investigations are firmly grounded in and build upon the context of relevant research from other health and social sciences. Thus, for the purposes of this review, we have not distinguished nursing from nonnursing research in our analysis of the current state of the art.

The following review is therefore derived from published reports of research using some form of inductive analytic method to study some aspect of the subjective experience of individuals who have been diagnosed with a disease that is normally considered chronic. We estimate there to be well over a thousand such research reports published since 1980, and we cannot claim to have located them all. Studies from the explicit perspective of family members or caregivers have been excluded, although many of the studies of individuals also reflect perspectives of support network members as well as those who actually have the disease. For the most part, we have excluded studies focusing on children, although some studies of adolescents that extend their inquiry into the young adult stage have been included. Some studies of disability (such as spinal cord injury) have been included if the authors conceptualize them in the context of chronic illness experience literature. Other disabilities not so conceptualized (such as blindness) have been excluded. Finally, we have not included research explicitly directed toward chronic mental illness for the simple reason that most of the literature continues to reflect a sharp distinction between diseases of the body and diseases of the mind. In acknowledging those bodies of thought that we have excluded, we recognize that our analysis will represent only a fragment of all that has been studied and all that can be known.

## COMMONALITIES AND VARIATIONS IN CHRONIC ILLNESS EXPERIENCE

Researchers interested in how chronic illness is experienced have tended to investigate either the experience of living with a specific disease or the themes associated with a wide variety of diseases in a singular research study (Conrad, 1990). Those who have chosen the latter approach have assumed that chronic illness experience is generic, that its unique distinctions from acute or episodic illness will be similar among chronic diseases. For example, researchers have investigated general aspects of chronic illness experience by interviewing persons with such chronic illnesses as terminal cancer, acquired immune deficiency syndrome (AIDS), psoriasis, multiple sclerosis (MS), rheumatoid arthritis (RA), or chronic obstructive pulmonary disease (COPD). Uncovering common themes within the accounts of individual perceptions of what it is like to live with each particular disease creates the context for an understanding of patterns applicable to the more general notion of chronic illness experience.

Examples indicative of commonalities within chronic illness experience abound. For example, where there is profound fatigue, it tends to become a pervasive and prominent feature of the chronic illness experience, whether the disease is cancer (Glaus, Crow, & Hammond, 1996; Graydon, 1994), diabetes (Shah, 1989), or systemic lupus erythematosis (SLE) (Wagenaar, 1995). Pain and suffering are similar in their capacity to profoundly shape the lived experience, regardless of whether the origin of the pain is associated with fibromyalgia (Henriksson, 1995), advanced cancer (McGregor, 1994), chronic low back pain (Bowman, 1991), RA (Ailinger & Schweitzer, 1993; Dildy, 1996), or chronic venous leg ulcer (Bland, 1999; Walshe, 1995). Chronic diseases that force dramatic changes in biographical course, especially in terms of roles and responsibilities, inevitably challenge identity or self-concept. This has been reported in spinal cord injury (Carpenter, 1994; Yoshida, 1993), HIV infection (Tewksbury, 1995), cancer (Coyler, 1996), coronary artery disease (Newman & Moch, 1991), and Type I diabetes mellitus (Hernandez, 1996). Thus, despite the fact that some chronic diseases do not induce fatigue, cause pain, or trigger identity changes, it may be useful to generate understandings of common patterns within chronic illness experience according to our understanding of relevant physical symptomatology, adjustment patterns, and social contexts. In this way, our usable knowledge can expand on that which has been obtained in relation to particular diseases and contribute to more individualized and relevant health care initiatives.

However, when findings about chronic illness that have been derived from studies of distinct chronic diseases are compared, it is also possible to detect evidence of a range of experiential features peculiar to certain disease conditions that cannot be adequately captured by a generic orientation to the phenomenon. For example, Brydolf and Segesten's (1996) inductive inquiry into the experience of 28 young Swedish adults with ulcerative colitis revealed that the nature of living conditions and the amount of personal space to which these individuals had access were of paramount significance, taking precedence over other elements more commonly associated with quality of life. In contrast, Clayton and Chubon's (1994) study of 100 individuals with long-term spinal cord injuries revealed that those persons consider employment status and social activities to be the most critical determinants of the quality of life they are able to attain. Disorders that produce profound visible differences tend to engender serious challenges for social relationships, as Lennon, Link, Marback, and Dohrenwend (1989) learned in their study of women with temporomandibular disorders. In contrast, it can be difficult to come to terms with the reality that one has a serious chronic condition when the disorder is invisible to others, as was reported by Parker (1994), who used grounded theory methodology to study Native Americans' experiences with Type II diabetes.

In the case of those with differing trajectories and prognoses, for example, it has been well established that the experience of life-threatening chronic illness is unique and cannot be readily compared to that of individuals with an illness that is chronic but not terminal (Gullickson, 1993; Thoman-Touet, 1992). Some chronic illnesses, such as inflammatory bowel disease (IBD) or asthma, are characterized by periods of acuity or unpredictability; others, such as MS or Type II diabetes, may be considerably more gradual in their progression or even somewhat stable over time. Diseases that are traditionally discredited, such as epilepsy (Iphofen, 1990; Scambler & Hopkins, 1986), seem to represent profoundly different social experiences than do those for which there are no particular stigmatizing assumptions, such as RA. Similarly, chronic illnesses that are considered common and well understood, such as diabetes or heart disease, engender responses from others within the social network that are quite different from responses to diseases for which there is no currently accepted biological basis, such as fibromyalgia or chronic fatigue syndrome (CFS), or which are considered rare, such as scleroderma (Thorne, 1993).

In addition, there are important categorical differences between various kinds of chronic diseases. A number of research-derived models of illness experience imply a trajectory that is initiated with the inevitable grief and loss associated with being diagnosed with a chronic disease (e.g., Charmaz, 1991; Corbin & Strauss, 1988b; Morse, 1997; Morse & Johnson, 1991). According to such models, coming to terms with the disease involves a process of mastery and normalization, and many persons remain in sorrow about their illness. However, some insider research has challenged these assumptions in relation to certain diseases. For example, Schaefer (1995a, 1995b), in phenomenological studies of women with various chronic diseases, including fibromyalgia; Stewart and Sullivan (1982), in a generic qualitative study of men and women with MS in the United States; and Woodward, Broom, and Legge (1995), in a longitudinal study of individuals diagnosed with chronic fatigue syndrome in Australia, all report feelings of relief at being diagnosed with a disorder, because the diagnosis validated extended periods of unexplained suffering and therefore marked the beginning of a process of healing.

The commonalities and variations within chronic illness experience make it apparent that neither a disease-specific nor a generic approach alone creates an understanding of the phenomenon of what it is like to live with a chronic condition sufficient to guide decision making in clinical practice or health service delivery. Within the broad rubric of chronic illness, it is important to compare and contrast experiences of living with specific chronic diseases in order to identify the distinctive features and attributes of diseases and the variables by which they may most usefully be categorized. In turn, this process creates an analysis that helps us to identify with more precision and insight the mechanisms by which the personal, medical, and social constructions associated with chronicity shape the way an individual experiences those diseases we consider chronic.

Because of this dynamic tension between general chronic illness knowledge and the dimensions of it that emerge in the examination of specific disease experiences, some researchers are more recently turning to explicit comparative studies involving selected chronic conditions representing a range of specific theoretical variables. One such example is the work of

Russell, Geraci, Hooper, Shull, and Gregory (1998), who used naturalistic inquiry methods to compare the explanatory models of 30 individuals with cardiac disease against those of another 30 individuals with exacerbations of COPD. Despite the fact that both conditions are chronic and progressive, these authors found that individuals with heart failure tended to view their disease as beyond their personal control, whereas those with COPD viewed themselves as largely responsible for the self-management of the disease. Thus, the researchers concluded that the two conditions were "separate and distinct disease processes" that are experienced quite differently from one another (p. 182). Another example is the work of Price (1993b), who compared experiential knowledge revealed in daily diaries of 9 patients with MS and another 9 with asthma against earlier findings from 18 individuals with diabetes. Her studies, representing three distinct variations in symptom predictability, made it possible to learn more about body listening as a general chronic illness coping strategy. Such studies differ from those that involve multiple patient populations as a matter of convenience or because of presumed similarities between certain disease experiences. In capitalizing upon the variation between different chronic illnesses according to strategically selected theoretical variables, they create a means whereby our understanding of the complexities within chronic illness experience in a more general sense becomes possible.

## FRAME OF ANALYSIS

Another layer in the complexity of chronic illness experience knowledge becomes apparent when we examine the analytic perspective from which various researchers have generated their interpretive conclusions. Because of the interactive nature of qualitative research, it is easier and in most cases more effective to conduct research if the participant is articulate, reflective, and willing to speak about his or her experiences (Erlandson, Harris, Skipper, & Allen, 1993; Gilchrist, 1992). Consequently, the vast majority of insider research in chronic illness has included participants who are able to talk coherently, who are well educated, and who are not in crisis.

Most commonly, the participants in such research are recounting elements of illness experience that have occurred in the past. Whereas retrospective accounts afford the participant the advantage of sufficient distance and perspective to present a clear picture of the experience in context, we know that reflective processes may have reframed some aspects of the experience in predictable ways, making that form of knowledge slightly different from the knowledge that is needed to apprehend direct embedded experience (Altheide & Johnson, 1994; Sandelowski, 1999). Retrospective memory can be selective, and there is much about the everyday world of chronic illness that is taken for granted. What is viewed as mundane is unlikely to be reported in retrospective reports. Therefore, retrospective accounts guide us in generating an understanding of many aspects of chronic illness experience, but they render other equally relevant aspects invisible.

A related gap in the available knowledge emerges when we consider that there are some kinds of chronic illness experiences that tend not to appear in the qualitative research literature because of the challenges they pose to the research process. For example, as Folden (1994) reported in a grounded theory study of 20 stroke survivors, stroke experience has been investigated primarily as retrospective accounting by persons who have since recovered from its devastating effects. The experiences of those who have trouble communicating, who have a limited attention span, who are cognitively impaired, or who are in crisis are not easily accessible to researchers. Similarly, recovered patients whose adaptive strategies make them unwilling to focus on the illness within their lives may be reluctant to volunteer for research participation. Thus, our theoretical conclusions about the insider experience of a chronic condition such as stroke may be shaped by the selective analysis of those who self-identify as having overcome adversity and those with the fewest permanent impairments.

Another powerful factor shaping the interpretations that can be derived from the body of insider chronic illness research is the larger context in which it has been generated. There is no question that political, economic, and social trends over the past 20 years have influenced the way researchers and clinicians have viewed chronic illness and articulated the health care needs of persons with chronic illness (Thorne & Paterson, 1998). Yet the historical construction of chronic illness and the discourses of researchers and clients in relation to it has largely been ignored within this body of research. As May, Doyle, and Chew-Graham (1998) explain, examination of the changes in this discourse over time is instructive, not only in revealing the origins of problems now faced by clients and practitioners but also in illuminating the directions that open up for future changes in this regard. Their analysis of how chronic low back pain has been variously conceptualized over the past century by medical researchers, psychosocial researchers, and theorists, as well as by individuals with back pain is an excellent example of this form of critical reinterpretation.

Among the more important frames of analysis that may shape research findings is the lack of conceptual clarity regarding the relationship between the mind and the body as it is manifested in chronic illness experience. Many people with chronic physical illness experience challenges to their mental health as an outcome of pathophysiological processes, just as those with mental illness can experience physical manifestations of their conditions. In many instances, whether the physical or mental elements of the imbalance become the focus may be simply a matter of chance and circumstance (Janes, 1990). However, the degree to which a particular disease is understood to be physical or mental in origin at any particular time can profoundly shape the way it is socially and psychologically experienced. The phenomenon of chronic pain illustrates the problem inherent in a dualistic interpretation of mind/body relationship in chronic illness. Pain is generally conceptualized in this manner when there is no known physical cause and there is insufficient evidence of an entirely psychological basis (May et al., 1998; O'Loughlin, 1999). Researchers exploring the experience of chronic pain document suffering that is discredited and invalidated by others, who cannot understand it as "real" in the absence of an established cause, as Bowman's (1991) phenomenological study of persons with chronic low back pain revealed. Thus, the adherence to mind/body dualism in our illness causation models becomes a powerful influencing factor shaping the way such an illness is experienced (Bates, Rankin-Hill, & Sanchez-Ayendez, 1997; Price, 1996).

Another particularly prominent discourse shaping many of the qualitative investigations in chronic illness experience is the conceptualization of compliance (Wellard, 1998). Although representations from numerous qualitative inquiries suggest that people with chronic illnesses tend to become expert self-care managers and in fact know their bodily responses better than do their professional health care practitioners (LeMone, 1993; Maclean & Oram, 1988; Madsen, 1992; Price, 1993a, 1993b; Wikblad, 1991), the assumption underlying much of the writing in the field of noncompliance is that if we understood why people fail to adhere to prescribed regimens we would be able to control and reconfigure such behavior (Thorne, 1990; Trostle, 1988). However, findings from several studies over the past decade, such as Roberson's (1992) ethnographic study of African Americans with a variety of chronic conditions, Ford's (1989) phenomenological inquiry into persons recovering from myocardial infarction (MI), and Hernandez's (1995, 1996) grounded theory studies of adults with insulin-dependent diabetes, reveal that decisions regarding medical compliance reflect a wide range of thoughtful and legitimate coping strategies or self-care management initiatives. These authors conclude that there is an urgent need for a shift in focus within chronic illness theory from a compliance model toward a mechanism for shared decision making.

As has been noted in a metaanalysis of qualitative research regarding the experience of living with diabetes (Paterson, Thorne, & Dewis, 1998), persons with that condition may consciously choose not to comply in an overly rigid manner with prescribed regimens because to do so would jeopardize their health and well-being or because they have different interpretations from those of health care professionals as to what is important in living with the disease. When one considers that the existing research consistently reports noncompliance rates of between one-half and one-third, this persistent loyalty to the compliance myth demonstrates that the assumption of a correlation between compliance and health, well-being, or quality of life has remained largely unchallenged (Morris & Schulz, 1992; Trostle, 1988).

Where traditional compliance assumptions have been contested, a competing discourse arises within the research literature with regard to shared decision making. Among some researchers it is accepted that persons with chronic illness should actively participate in decisions about their care (Donovan, 1995). However, health care professionals are often skeptical or disbelieving of accounts of illness experiences that cannot be proved by the use of objective evidence (Jackson, 1992; Stewart & Sullivan, 1982). For example, persons with chronic pain frequently report encounters with health care professionals who doubt the legitimacy of their illness, as Jackson (1992) revealed in a participant observation study of patients and staff in a chronic pain treatment center and Howell (1994) reported on the basis of a grounded theory study of women with chronic pain. If such individuals believe that they are labeled as hypochondriacs or difficult patients, the development of equal partnerships in disease management decision making is clearly precluded (Charmaz, 1991).

Despite the consistency of such claims, there has been surprisingly little qualitative research aimed at learning more about how people with chronic illness experience share decision making in relation to everyday self-care issues or how they learn to assume a partnership role with clinicians. Thus, much of the writing that recognizes the competence of patients to make decisions about their own care takes on an adversarial stance in health care relationships, oversimplifying the issue into an analysis of power imbalances. Adopted uncritically, such interpretations ignore the perspective of those who, for various reasons, prefer to defer all health-related decision making to their professional care providers. As has been reported by Kirk (1993), on the basis of her phenomenological study of health care perceptions among persons with rheumatic disorders, some individuals with chronic illness are unwilling or unable to assume a decision-making role in relation to disease management, especially during times of crisis. For such persons, the health care professional in a parent-surrogate role may become the ideal. Thus, the discourse about appropriate strategies for health care relationships in chronic illness becomes complicated with overgeneralized claims made from particularized and essentialized perspectives (Thorne & Paterson, 1998).

Finally, there is also a confusing and elusive body of work deriving from insider research in chronic illness experience that draws on related concepts such as hope, control, spirituality, courage, and transformation as characteristic of chronic illness. The degree to which such interpretations reflect wishful thinking or efforts to avoid negative conclusions has been challenged, because such concepts seem to have replaced a focus on loss, burden, and suffering in an earlier decade of inquiry (Thorne & Paterson, 1998). Whether chronic illness produces such phenomena or they represent the precursor to adapting to and accepting chronic illness is variously assumed by different researchers. On the basis of interviews with 38 persons with cancer, Fife (1994), for example, concludes that a person with chronic illness attempts to find meaning in the experience and that this search culminates in being able to come to terms with his or her illness. In contrast, Ragsdale, Kotarba, and Morrow (1994), on the basis of their interviews with persons with HIV/AIDS, describe spirituality and mysticism as a result of trying to cope with the disease. Further research that explicates the interrelationships between these concepts and chronic illness experiences is clearly needed (Benzein & Saveman, 1998; Lindsey, 1996), but additional narrative analysis without some shared understandings of conceptual linkages may further confuse the issue.

Examination of the frame of analysis underlying the interpretations that are made of qualitative research findings in chronic illness reveal a number of competing theoretical and conceptual challenges that complicate simple aggregation of the research findings into coherent theories of what chronic illness experience is all about and how we ought to understand it. It seems apparent, from an analysis of which questions have been asked and which individuals within theoretical populations have found their way into our research projects, that our concern for methodological integrity and conceptual purity may have led us toward certain kinds of conclusions and away from others.

Despite the demands on qualitative researchers to reflect critically upon their role as instruments of the research, a wide-angled analysis of the field suggests that the body of work may have been influenced by a number of implicit theoretical assumptions and sociopolitical commitments (Thorne & Paterson, 1998). Clearly, there will be a need in the future to create sufficient methodological flexibility to study those persons and illness situations that are less accessible by using our current popular approaches and to locate our interpretations more firmly in the context of how they extend or compete with both dominant and marginalized theoretical opinions.

## CONTEXTUAL AND MEDIATING FACTORS IN ILLNESS EXPERIENCE

From a broad analysis of the range and diversity of findings within the insider research on chronic illness experience it becomes apparent that the way chronic illness shapes a life will be influenced by a number of factors associated with unique life circumstances, individually and in interaction. Although we may be able to make generalizations about a few of the more prominent contextual and mediating factors, such as age, gender, and ethnicity (Bates et al., 1997), many equally powerful influences on how life is lived become less visible when the researcher's gaze is focused on general and transferable interpretations. Examples of what we do know about the influence of those factors that have been addressed in the research serve to illustrate the potential impact of those that have as yet been unstudied.

Despite the common agreement that age and stage of life will inevitably influence a person's response to chronic illness (Dimond & Jones, 1983; Felton & Revenson, 1987), the specific ways in which age shapes chronic illness experience have typically been ignored by most researchers. Generally, researchers have recruited sample populations they term "adults," whose ages may range from 16 to 94. Rarely are distinctions in illness experience conceptually linked to issues of living at particular developmental stages within adulthood (McWilliam et al., 1997). Even when age has been a focus of inquiry, there may still be conceptual problems within the available knowledge. For example, although Finfgeld (1995) and Young (1993) have investigated concepts such as courage and spirituality among chronically ill older adults, they have explored singular aspects of the chronic illness experience, tending to ignore the implications of such critical factors as comorbidity, social context, and life experience. Thus, knowledge as to the way in which age influences the experience that individuals might have with a particular illness or the way in which those chronic diseases typically associated with advancing age are variously treated within our social and health care context is not accessible from the current research literature.

In contrast, insider research has contributed considerably to a delineation of the differences that exist in chronic illness experience as a product of gender. For example, Ablon (1996) analyzed gender differences in the perceptions of social response to pain and appearance by comparing the narratives of 14 men and 14 women with neurofibromatosis. Whereas this disease was found to be equally problematic for both genders, Ablon was able to document that men and women often had different perceptions about the degree to which it was disabling, depending on their priorities for normalization. Charmaz (1995) conducted a grounded theory study of 20 men with chronic illness and was able to compare their accounts with data from prior studies involving women. She concluded that reluctance to assume the public identity of the ill person may be a reflection of cultural expectations of a man's role in society and the family. Interestingly, in contrast to the identified deficits in studies of women's health issues in a more general sense, the vast majority of chronic illness insider research has been dominated by studies specifically investigating the experiences of women or involving samples consisting of mostly women (exceptions to this generalization include the study of AIDS, testicular cancer, and spinal cord injury in young adults).

Among the studies of illness experience in relation to a number of chronic diseases, the ratio of female to male research participants seems considerably higher than would be anticipated from the gender distribution of the illness. For example, review of the samples in studies of the experience of renal failure and MS reveals that they include mostly women despite an equal or greater prevalence of those diseases in men. A clue to interpreting this observation may be found in Charmaz's (1995) work with men with chronic illness. She postulates that men may be reluctant to place their illness front and center because the masculine role in Western society precludes an image of weakness and vulnerability. If this is indeed so, it is possible that men are less likely than women to volunteer for research studies that ask them to disclose those aspects of the illness experience that emphasize their dependence and vulnerability. Thus, not only does gender influence the experience of having a chronic illness, but it also may explain some aspects of the way we have come to understand it through our qualitative research approaches.

Another major factor that may be implicated in chronic illness experience can be generally described as social location. Analysis of the sample populations reported by researchers explicating chronic illness experiences reveals that those dimensions of the phenomenon that have been well represented in the literature have come to us primarily through the voices of those who are privileged, middle-class, and of European descent (Anderson, Elfert, & Lai, 1989; Loewe, Schwartzman, Freeman, Quinn, & Zuckerman, 1998). There has been very little research into the chronic illness experience of those who cannot read and write, who are poor, and who are members of a visible or invisible minority.

When we do explicitly study the chronic illness experience of culturally or ethnically diverse groups, we tend to report and analyze their accounts as differing from what we understand as the dominant or normal view (Wellard, 1998). Because of this, it seems self-evident that certain ideals of this subgroup within the population have predominated the conclusions deriving from this body of research. According to Miewald (1997), such ideals include self-control, autonomy, and individualism. Wellard (1998) concurs, noting that the emphasis on individualism within this body of research has created a discourse that supposes that people with chronic illness are responsible for their disease. As Paterson and Sloan (1994) discovered, in their phenomenological study of nine Canadian individuals with diabetes, unexplained blood glucose elevations resulted in accusations that they were "cheating" on their diet, even when they had followed the prescribed regimen.

Similarly, when qualitative chronic illness researchers consider such concepts as compliance and self-care, for example, they typically reveal an underlying assumption that the valuation of shared participatory decision making between patients and health care practitioners is universal. There is little consideration of the cultural and personal factors that might make such a concept foreign and unacceptable to many individuals with chronic illness. Exceptions, such as the exploratory descriptive study by Hunt, Arar, and Larme (1998) of 51 people with type II diabetes and 35 practitioners, reveal that the notion of compliance and partnership in decision making with health care professionals may be ludicrous when patients are too poor to afford the prescribed diets and have insufficient social power to effectively negotiate the health care system. Similarly, in an extended fieldwork study involving persons with sickle cell anemia in a low-income African American community clinic and their health care providers, Ragins (1995) concluded that the ideal of self-care promoted by practitioners may actually interfere with their ability to meet their clients' need for supportive interaction.

Another limitation of this body of research is that, where any of these contextual variables is explicitly addressed in the research, it is almost always studied in isolation from other sociocultural factors that might impact on and shape the individual life circumstances. An exception is the work of Anderson (1991), who used phenomenological methods to study the experience of 15 women with diabetes who were first-generation immigrants to Canada from Hong Kong and mainland China. Her analysis considered their chronic illness in relation to their ethnicity and gender but also took account of their socioeconomic status as factory workers. On the basis of analysis of these complex factors in interaction, she was able to interpret their reluctance to defy employer's policies by eating at times other than scheduled breaks as a reflection of their perceptions of a woman's role, their fear of losing employment, and their tenuous status as immigrants rather than as a specific act of noncompliance with prescribed management strategies. Such findings illustrate the kind of embedded complexity that may be uncovered when research methods permit analysis of various coexisting factors in interaction rather than in isolation.

In our own metasynthesis of insider research, we have come to the conclusion that living with a chronic illness is typically experienced as an uneven trajectory in which the individual learns to put the disease focus (e.g., burden, loss, unbearable symptoms) into the background of consciousness some of the time but also experiences times during which the overwhelming significance of the sickness dominates living with the disease. Shifts from one perspective to the other can be precipitated by personal and sociocultural factors unrelated to the disease. For example, losing a job might precipitate a shift to an illness orientation, and having to attend to a family crisis might force illness management to the background of consciousness. The foreground/background perspective of chronic illness may explain many of the contradictory conclusions reported by qualitative researchers with regard to how people respond to the disease, themselves, their caregivers, and their health care professionals.

Such an understanding of chronic illness experience requires that we account for the larger sociocultural and psychological context in which an illness is experienced before we can begin to understand its impact on the individual.

Thus, it seems clear that much of what we think we know about chronic illness experience cannot, at this point in our inquiry process, be entirely decontextualized from what we do not yet know about the ways in which various lives are lived. Although we have some tentative understandings of the implications of such discrete factors as age, gender, and ethnicity, for example, our interpretations are embryonic and therefore must be understood as insufficient for our collective purposes. Studies that explicitly examine the influence of such factors, alone and in isolation, will contribute considerably to our general understanding of how diseases shape life experience. In addition, critical reflection on what we see when we conduct research may reveal an infinite number of additional variables and factors that play an equally important role in the way one lives with chronic illness. As our research develops, the questions we pose must expand to include inquiries that tease out new dimensions that might be of critical importance in understanding variations within chronic illness experience, such as whether or not we accept a higher power, whether our natural attitude is one of optimism or pessimism, whether our social circles feed or are fed by our energy, and whether our worldview is shattered or confirmed by the diagnosis of an illness that cannot be cured.

## IMPLICATIONS FOR FUTURE DIRECTIONS IN CHRONIC ILLNESS RESEARCH

From the analysis provided in this discussion, a number of issues emerge as important for the continuing development of insider knowledge into chronic illness experience. Clarity as to the theoretical significance of major commonalities and variations within those diseases and conditions we categorize as chronic will make an important contribution to the available knowledge in this field. As we become more effective and explicit about comparing and contrasting the influence of selected theoretical variables, we will be able to develop strategies for appropriate generalization and for translating findings to the practice context. Similarly, it seems important for chronic illness researchers to become increasingly sophisticated in their ability to use critical interpretive approaches toward understanding their studies in context. As is evident from the review above, useful knowledge in this field will not come from increasingly narrow and focused studies but rather from the efforts of researchers to make sense of the frame of analysis that their contributions represent and interpreting that frame in a wider context. Further, it seems clear that a stronger analysis of the influence of contextual and mediating factors will be important in sifting through the findings that have already been reported, in sorting out which factors seem most relevant to which disease contexts, and in making wise decisions as to which variables will be of most importance to ongoing inquiry in this field. Rather than basing their analysis on those variables commonly employed by quantitative researchers to distinguish subgroups within populations, qualitative researchers may find that they have access to many more abstract and compelling options.

Although the potential value of longitudinal studies in this field is widely acknowledged, much of what we currently know about chronic illness experience is based on studies composed of a single interview with each research participant. As our body of work develops, it will be imperative to tackle such questions as how people's response to chronic illness changes in the context of disease-related complications, exacerbations of the disease, new developments in treatment, or changing popular beliefs, none of which can be tracked in an approach to understanding based on a single moment in time (Russell et al., 1998).

Beyond the retrospective interpretations of illness experience currently accessible to us in our research literature, we must also begin to account for the temporal aspects of our data collection and resultant conclusions (Sandelowski, 1999). Although retrospective accounts permit rich description based on reflection upon meaning that may be possible only at some distance from immediate experience, there is also an important place for prospective interviews in which researchers attempt to uncover the taken-for-granted and difficult-to-articulate aspects of living with a chronic illness on an everyday basis. As self-care practices and everyday routines become more familiar and established, they may become submerged in other aspects of the experience and rendered inaccessible to inquiry. However, for qualitative research to contribute usefully to practice science, many of these immediate and embodied aspects of chronic illness experience may be the most important for us to know about.

The way in which various researchers define the concept of chronic illness is often implicit rather than fully articulated. As the body of research-based knowledge evolves, however, it will be increasingly important to come to some conceptual agreement as to which diseases and situations are usefully depicted in this manner. One critical issue requiring widespread consideration will be the theoretical and pragmatic distinctions between chronic illness and disability, and the conditions under which it might be advisable for their sociopolitical agendas to be separated or brought into alignment. Another important dialogue will be the utility of distinguishing diseases understood as mental from those considered physical in our chronic illness work. Although a mind/body dualism has been challenged in many health disciplines as misguided and inappropriate, it continues to dominate the literature concerning chronic illness.

Although qualitative inquiries from a range of perspectives and about a range of diseases will build additional confidence in what we think we know and what we still don't understand, an analysis of the existing insider research makes apparent the advantage of strategic progress in building a coherent and usable body of knowledge. In general, we must find ways to support studies that are longitudinal in scope, more thoughtful in their recruitment and sample-inclusion strategies, more reflective in their data-gathering processes, and more critical in their interpretive analyses. Furthermore, we clearly require advances in methodological approaches to synthesizing knowledge on the basis of a body of discrete but related qualitative studies. Although there is much that we think we have come to know about how persons afflicted by a chronic illness make sense of their diagnosis, adjust their daily lives and life plans, interact with the existing health care system structures, and engage in a socially complex world, our inquiries into insider experience make it clear that we must continue to struggle with how we can best understand both the unique and particular as well as the common and generalizable as they combine in some exquisitely complicated formula to create the phenomenon we call chronic illness experience.

## REFERENCES

Ablon, J. (1996). Gender response to neurofibromatosis. *Social Science and Medicine, 42,* 99–109.

Ailinger, R. L., & Schweitzer, E. (1993). Patients' explanations of rheumatoid arthritis. *Western Journal of Nursing Research, 15,* 340–351.

Altheide, D. L., & Johnson, J. M. (1994). Criteria for assessing interpretive validity in qualitative research. In N. K. Denzin & Y. S. Lincoln (Eds.), *Handbook of qualitative research* (pp. 485–499). Thousand Oaks, CA: Sage.

Anderson, J. M. (1991). Immigrant women speak of chronic illness: The social construction of the devalued self. *Journal of Advanced Nursing, 16,* 710–717.

Anderson, J. M., Elfert, H., & Lai, M. (1989). Ideology in the clinical context: Chronic illness, ethnicity and the discourse of normalisation. *Sociology of Health and Illness, 11,* 253–278.

Bates, M. A., Rankin-Hill, L., & Sanchez-Ayendez, M. (1997). The effects of cultural context on health care on treatment of and response to chronic pain and illness. *Social Science and Medicine, 45,* 1433–1447.

Benzein, E., & Saveman, B. I. (1998). One step towards the understanding of hope: A concept analysis. *International Journal of Nursing Studies, 35,* 322–329.

Bland, M. (1999). On living with chronic leg ulcers. In I. Madjar & J. A. Walton (Eds.), *Nursing and the experience of illness: Phenomenology in practice* (pp. 36–56). St. Leonards, NSW: Allen & Unwin.

Bowman, J. M. (1991). The meaning of chronic low back pain. *AAOHN Journal, 39,* 381–384.

Brydolf, M., & Segesten, K. (1996). Living with ulcerative colitis: Experiences of adolescents and young adults. *Journal of Advanced Nursing, 23,* 39–47.

Carpenter, C. (1994). The experience of spinal cord injury: The individual's perspective—implications for rehabilitation practice. *Physical Therapy, 74,* 614–629.

Casebeer, A. L., & Verhoef, M. J. (1997). Combining qualitative and quantitative research methods: Considering the possibilities for enhancing the study of chronic diseases. *Chronic Diseases in Canada, 18,* 130–135.

Charmaz, K. (1991). *The self, control, illness and time.* New Brunswick, NJ: Rutgers University Press.

Charmaz, K. (1995). Identity dilemmas for chronically ill men. In D. Sabo & D. F. Gordon (Eds.), *Men's health and illness: Gender, power and the body* (pp. 266–291). Thousand Oaks, CA: Sage.

Clayton, K. S., & Chubon, R. A. (1994). Factors associated with the quality of life of long term spinal cord injured persons. *Archives of Physical Medical Rehabilitation, 75,* 633–638.

Conrad, P. (1990). Qualitative research on chronic illness: A commentary on method and conceptual development. *Social Science and Medicine, 30,* 1257–1263.

Corbin, J. M., & Strauss, A. L. (1988a). Shaping a new health care system: The explosion of chronic illness as a catalyst for change. San Francisco: Jossey-Bass.

Corbin, J. M., & Strauss, A. L. (1988b). *Unending work and care: Managing chronic illness at home.* San Francisco, CA: Jossey-Bass.

Coyler, H. (1996). Women's experience of living with cancer. *Journal of Advanced Nursing, 23,* 496–501.

Curtin, M., & Lubkin, I. M. (1990). What is chronicity? In I. M. Lubkin (Ed.), *Chronic illness: Impact and interventions,* 2nd ed. (pp. 2–20). Boston: Jones & Bartlett.

Dildy, S. M. P. (1996). Suffering in people with rheumatoid arthritis. *Applied Nursing Research, 9,* 177–183.

Dimond, M., & Jones, S. L. (1983). *Chronic illness across the lifespan.* Norwalk, CT: Appleton-Century-Crofts.

Donovan, J. L. (1995). Patient decision making: The missing ingredient in compliance research. *International Journal of Technology Assessment in Health Care, 11,* 443–455.

Erlandson, D. A., Harris, E. L., Skipper, B. C., & Allen, S.D. (1993). *Doing naturalistic inquiry: A guide to methods.* Newbury Park, CA: Sage.

Felton, B. J., & Revenson, T. A. (1987). Age differences in coping with chronic illness. *Psychology and Aging, 2,* 164–170.

Fife, B. L. (1994). The conceptualization of meaning in illness. *Social Science and Medicine, 38,* 309–316.

Finfgeld, D. L. (1995). Becoming and being courageous in the chronically ill elderly. *Issues in Mental Health Nursing, 16,* 1–11.

Folden, S. L. (1994). Managing the effects of a stroke: The first months. *Rehabilitation Nursing Research, 3,* 79–85.

Ford, J. S. (1989). Living with a history of a heart attack: A human science investigation. *Journal of Advanced Nursing, 14,* 173–179.

Gerhardt, U. (1990). Qualitative research on chronic illness: The issue and the story. *Social Science and Medicine, 30,* 1149–1159.

Gilchrist, V. J. (1992). Key informant interviews. In B. F. Crabtree & W. L. Miller (Eds.), *Doing qualitative research* (pp. 70–89). Newbury Park, CA: Sage.

Glaus, A., Crow, R., & Hammond, S. (1996). A qualitative study to explore the concept of fatigue/tiredness in cancer patients and in healthy individuals. *Supportive Care in Cancer, 4,* 82–96.

Gordon, P. A., Feldman, D., & Crose, R. (1998). The meaning of disability: How women with chronic illness view their experiences. *Journal of Rehabilitation, 64*(3), 5–11.

Graydon, J. E. (1994) Women with breast cancer: Their quality of life following a course of radiation therapy. *Journal of Advanced Nursing, 19,* 617–622.

Gullickson, C. (1993). My death nearing its future: A Heideggerian hermeneutical analysis of the lived experience of persons with chronic illness. *Journal of Advanced Nursing, 18,* 1386–1392.

Henriksson, C. M. (1995). Living with continuous muscular pain—patient perspectives: Part 1: Encounters and consequences. *Scandinavian Journal of Caring Sciences, 9,* 67–76.

Hernandez, C. A. (1995). The experience of living with insulin-dependent diabetes: Lessons for the diabetes educator. *Diabetes Educator, 21,* 33–3.

Hernandez, C. A. (1996). Integration: The experience of living with insulin dependent (Type I) diabetes mellitus. *Canadian Journal of Nursing Research, 28,* 37–56.

Howell, S. L. (1994). Natural/alternative health care practices used by women with chronic pain: Findings from a grounded theory research study. *Nurse Practitioner Forum, 5,* 98–105.

Hunt, L. M., Arar, N. H., & Larme, A. C. (1998). Contrasting patient and practitioner perspectives in Type 2 diabetes management. *Western Journal of Nursing Research, 20,* 656–682.

Iphofen, R. (1990). Coping with a "perforated life": A case study in managing the stigma of petit mal epilepsy. *Sociology, 24,* 447–463.

Jackson, J. E. (1992). "After a while no one believes you": Real and unreal pain. In M. D. Good, P. E. Brodwin, B. J. Good, & A. Kleinman (Eds.), *Pain as a human experience: An anthropological perspective* (pp. 138–168). Berkeley, CA: University of California Press.

Janes, G. (1990). A better life than before: Quality of life in people with renal failure. *Professional Nurse, 6*(1), 26–28.

Kirk, K. (1993). Chronically ill patients' perceptions of nursing care. *Rehabilitation Nursing, 18,* 99–104.

LeMone, P. (1993). Human sexuality in adults with insulin-dependent diabetes mellitus. *Image: The Journal of Nursing Scholarship, 25,* 101–105.

Lennon, M. C., Link, B., Marback, J., & Dohrenwend, B. (1989). The stigma of chronic facial pain and its impact on social relationships. *Social Problems, 36,* 117–134.

Lindsey, E. (1996). Health within illness: Experiences of chronically ill/disabled people. *Journal of Advanced Nursing, 24,* 465–472.

Loewe, R., Schwartzman, J., Freeman, J., Quinn, L., & Zuckerman, S. (1998). Doctor talk and diabetes: Toward an analysis of the clinical construction of chronic illness. *Social Science and Medicine, 47,* 1267–1276.

Maclean, H., & Oram, B. (1988). *Living with diabetes.* Toronto: University of Toronto Press.

Madsen, W. C. (1992). Problematic treatment: Interaction of patient, spouse, and physician beliefs in medical noncompliance. *Family Systems Medicine, 10,* 365–383.

May, C., Doyle, H., & Chew-Graham, C. (1998). Medical knowledge and the intractable patient: The case of chronic low back pain. *Social Science and Medicine, 48,* 523–534.

McGregor, S. (1994) Quality of life in advanced cancer. *Journal of Cancer Care, 3,* 144–152.

McWilliam, C. L., Stewart, M., Brown, J. B., McNair, S., Desai, K., Patterson, M. L., Del Maestro, N., & Pittman, B. J. (1997). Creating empowering meaning: An interactive process of promoting health within chronically ill older Canadians. *Health Promotion International, 12,* 111–123.

Miewald, C. E. (1997). Is awareness enough?: The contradictions of self-care in a chronic disease clinic. *Human Organization, 56,* 353–363.

Morris, L. S., & Schulz, R. M. (1992). Patient compliance: An overview. *Journal of Clinical Pharmacy and Therapeutics, 17,* 283–295.

Morse, J. M. (1997). Responding to threats to integrity of self. *Advances in Nursing Science, 19*(4), 21–36.

Morse, J. M., & Johnson, J. L. (1991). *The illness experience: Dimensions of suffering.* Newbury Park, CA: Sage.

Newman, M. A., & Moch, S. D. (1991). Life patterns of persons with coronary heart disease. *Nursing Science Quarterly, 4,* 161–167.

O'Loughlin, A. (1999). On living with chronic pain. In I. Madjar & J. A. Walton (Eds.), *Nursing and the experience of illness: Phenomenology in practice* (pp. 123–144). St. Leonards, NSW: Allen & Unwin.

Parker, J. G. (1994). The lived experience of native Americans with diabetes within a transcultural nursing perspective. *Journal of Transcultural Nursing, 6,* 5–11.

Paterson, B. L., & Sloan, J. (1994). A phenomenological study of the decision-making experience of individuals with long-standing diabetes. *Canadian Journal of Diabetes Care, 18,* 10–19.

Paterson, B., Thorne, S., & Dewis, M. (1998) Adapting to and managing diabetes. *Image: Journal for Nursing Scholarship, 30,* 57–62.

Price, M. (1993a). An experiential model of learning diabetes self-management. *Qualitative Health Research, 3,* 29–54.

Price, M. (1993b). Exploration of body listening: Health and physical self-awareness in chronic illness. *Advances in Nursing Science, 15*(4), 37–52.

Price, B. (1996). Illness careers: The chronic illness experience. *Journal of Advanced Nursing, 24,* 275–279.

Ragins, A. I. (1995). Why self-care fails: Implementing policy at a low-income sickle cell clinic. *Qualitative Sociology, 18,* 331–356.

Ragsdale, D., Kotarba, J. A., & Morrow, J. R., Jr. (1994). How HIV+ persons manage everyday life in the hospital and at home. *Qualitative Health Research, 4*(4), 431–443.

Roberson, M. H. B. (1992). The meaning of compliance: Patient perspectives. *Qualitative Health Research, 2,* 7–26.

Robinson, C. A. (1998). Women, families, chronic illness, and nursing interventions: From burden to burden. *Journal of Family Nursing, 4,* 271–290.

Royer, A. (1998). *Life with chronic illness: Social and psychological dimensions.* Westport, CT: Praeger.

Russell, C. K., Geraci, T., Hooper, A., Shull, L., & Gregory, D. M. (1998). Patients' explanatory models for heart failure and COPD exacerbations. *Clinical Nursing Research, 7,* 164–188.

Sandelowski. M. (1999). Time and qualitative research. *Research in Nursing and Health, 22,* 79–88.

Scambler, G., & Hopkins, A. (1986). Being epileptic: Coming to terms with stigma. *Sociology of Health and Illness, 8,* 26–43.

Schaefer, K. M. (1995a). Struggling to maintain balance: A study of women living with fibromyalgia. *Journal of Advanced Nursing, 21,* 95–102

Schaefer, K. M. (1995b). Women living in paradox: Loss and discovery in chronic illness. *Holistic Nursing Practice, 9,* 63–74.

Shah, H. S. (1989). *Psychosocial adjustment, self-concept, and sexual satisfaction of women with diabetes.* Unpublished doctoral dissertation, Boston University.

Stewart, D. C., & Sullivan, T. J. (1982). Illness behavior and the sick role in chronic disease: The case of multiple sclerosis. *Social Science and Medicine, 16,* 1397–1404.

Strauss, A. L. (1975). *Chronic illness and the quality of life.* St. Louis: Mosby.

Strauss, A. L., Corbin, J., Fagerhaugh, S., Glaser, B. G., Maines, D., Suczek, B., & Weiner, C. L. (1984). *Chronic illness and the quality of life* (2nd ed.). St. Louis: Mosby.

Tewksbury, R. (1995). Sexual adaptations among gay men with HIV. In D. Sabo & D. F. Gordon (Eds.), *Men's health and illness: Gender, power and the body* (pp. 222–245). Thousand Oaks, CA: Sage.

Thoman-Touet, S. K. (1992). *A qualitative study of the effect of chronic illness on marital quality.* Unpublished doctoral dissertation, Iowa State University, Ames, Iowa.

Thorne, S. E. (1990). Constructive noncompliance in chronic illness. *Holistic Nursing Practice, 5*(1), 62–69.

Thorne, S. (1993). *Negotiating health care: The social context of chronic illness.* Newbury Park, CA: Sage.

Thorne, S., McCormick, S., & Carty, E. (1997). Deconstructing the gender neutrality of chronic illness and disability. *Health Care for Women International, 18,* 1–16.

Thorne, S., & Paterson, B. (1998). Shifting images of chronic illness. *Image: Journal for Nursing Scholarship, 30,* 173–178.

Trostle, J. A. (1988). Medical compliance as an ideology. *Social Science and Medicine, 27,* 1299–1308.

Wagenaar, H. (1995). *An exploratory descriptive study of fatigue in women with systemic lupus erythematosus.* Unpublished master's thesis, Dalhousie University, Halifax, Nova Scotia, Canada.

Walshe, C. (1995). Living with a venous leg ulcer: A descriptive study of patients' experiences. *Journal of Advanced Nursing, 22,* 1092–1100.

Wellard, S. (1998). Constructions of chronic illness. *International Journal of Nursing Studies, 35,* 49–55.

Wikblad, K. F. (1991). Patient perspectives of diabetes care and education. *Journal of Advanced Nursing, 16,* 837–844.

Woodward, R. V., Broom, D. H., & Legge, D. G. (1995). Diagnosis in chronic illness: Disabling or enabling—the case of chronic fatigue syndrome. *Journal of the Royal Society of Medicine, 88,* 325–329.

Yoshida, K. K. (1993). Reshaping of self: A pendular reconstruction of self and identity among adults with traumatic spinal cord injury. *Sociology of Health and Illness, 15,* 217–245.

Young, C. (1993). Spirituality and the chronically ill Christian elderly. *Geriatric Nursing, 14,* 298–303.

Chapter 2

# Children with Epilepsy: Quality of Life and Psychosocial Needs

JOAN K. AUSTIN AND DAVID W. DUNN

## ABSTRACT

In this chapter, research related to quality of life in children with epilepsy and their psychosocial needs is reviewed. Nursing and nonnursing research reports and descriptions of instruments developed between January 1994 and February 1999 are included. Most research reports described quality-of-life problems, especially psychological functioning in school-age children. Less attention was devoted to psychosocial needs. Major gaps included intervention studies and research on infants and young children. Conclusions include recommendations for future research.

Key words: children, adolescents, epilepsy, quality of life, psychosocial care

Epilepsy, which is defined as recurrent unprovoked seizures, is one of the most common neurological conditions in childhood. Seizures are episodic neurological events that are caused by a sudden paroxysmal electrical discharge that spreads from a group of epileptigenic cells to adjacent cerebral tissue. Between 4% and 10% of all children will have a seizure before adulthood. By age 20, however, only about 1% will have a diagnosis of epilepsy (W. A. Hauser, 1994). The estimated cost of seizures and epilepsy in children in the United States in 1990 was more than $800 million (Annegers & Begley, in press). The federal government estimates that the economic costs associated with epilepsy in adulthood are $3.5 billion annually (Begley, Annegers, Lairson, Reynolds, & Hauser, 1994).

There is much diversity in how epilepsy is manifested. Epilepsy is classified by both seizure type and epileptic syndrome. The most widely accepted classification of seizure type is the International Classification of Epileptic

Seizures (Commission on Classification and Terminology of the International League Against Epilepsy, 1981). Seizures are divided into generalized and partial types. Generalized seizures affect the entire brain and result in loss of consciousness. In contrast, only one portion of the brain is affected in partial seizures. Partial seizures are further divided into simple and complex types. Consciousness is not affected in simple partial seizures but is impaired in complex partial seizures. Epileptic syndromes also are classified by the International League Against Epilepsy (Commission on Classification and Terminology of the International League Against Epilepsy, 1989). Syndromes are categorized into primary and secondary, with primary syndromes being idiopathic or having a presumed genetic etiology and secondary syndromes having a cause such as a brain abnormality or acquired central nervous system damage. Depending on the origin of the epileptigenic discharge each of these syndromes is then further divided into generalized or partial. For example, a child with idiopathic seizures and a single originating epileptic focus would be classified as having a primary partial epileptic syndrome.

With treatment, the prognosis for epilepsy is relatively good. Approximately 90% of children achieve a 1-year remission and about half have a remission of seizures that lasts 5 years or more (Cockerell, Johnson, Sander, & Shorvon, 1997; E. Hauser, Freilinger, Seidl, & Groh, 1995). Seizure control is often obtained by using two first-line antiepileptic drugs (AEDs): carbamazepine and valproic acid. Phenytoin, ethosuximide, and phenobarbital also are well established AEDs. In addition, gabapentin, lamotrigine, topiramate, tiagabine, and vigabtrin are new AEDs that have been proven efficacious. For the approximately 20% of children whose seizures are not controlled on AEDs (W. A. Hauser & Hesdorffer, 1990), there are other treatments. Epilepsy surgery, in which epileptigenic tissue is removed, has a significant role in the treatment of children with intractable partial seizures. Other treatment modalities for children include the ketogenic diet and vagus nerve simulation. The major goal of treatment for epilepsy is the elimination or reduction of seizures while maintaining a reasonable quality of life for the child and the family.

## OVERVIEW

### Purpose

The purpose of this chapter is to describe the state of research related to quality of life in children with epilepsy. Because quality-of-life outcomes are related to psychosocial needs, research on psychosocial needs of children with epilepsy also is included. There is no universally accepted operational definition of quality of life in children (Levi & Drotar, 1998), but dimensions commonly included are physical, psychological, social, and school functioning. In childhood epilepsy, physical functioning is rarely affected except during seizures. In contrast, other quality-of-life dimensions can be negatively affected in children with epilepsy. Epidemiological studies indicate that children with epilepsy are over 4½ times more likely to have quality-of-life problems than are children in the general population (McDermott, Mani, & Krishaswami, 1995; Rutter, Graham, & Yule, 1970). Furthermore, such problems are more common in childhood epilepsy than in other chronic childhood physical conditions, especially those without brain involvement (Breslau, 1985; Rutter et al., 1970). Therefore, a review of the state of the quality-of-life research in childhood epilepsy is especially important to the development of future research in the area.

## Search Strategies

Various strategies were used to identify relevant research studies published from January 1994 to February 1999. An on-line computer search using Ovid Technologies was carried out on English-language publications using the following key words: *children, adolescents, epilepsy, quality of life, adaptation, social adjustment, cognitive, academic achievement, chronic illness, psychological or mental disorders,* and *psychosocial needs.* An additional strategy included the ancestry approach in which searches were made of references from recently published articles. Finally, the authors conducted a search of articles sent to them by other behavioral scientists. Articles were included if they described the development of instruments to measure aspects of quality of life or if they reported research findings related to quality of life in children with epilepsy. Articles were considered to be research if the sample was described, purposive data collection was carried out, data were analyzed, and results were reported.

## Selected Articles

Of the 41 articles selected for the final review, over half ($n = 24$) were from four journals: *Epilepsia* ($n = 8$), *Developmental Medicine and Child Neurology* ($n = 7$), *Seizure* ($n = 5$), and *Journal of Neuroscience Nursing* ($n = 4$). About half ($n = 20$) of the articles were found in either medical or behavioral science pediatric journals. The majority of the articles had multiple authors, and approximately one fourth had a nurse as first author.

Only 5 of the 41 articles described the development of instruments that measured concepts related to either quality of life or psychosocial care needs. One of these articles also contained results of the use of that scale in a research study. There was a total of 37 articles in which authors reported findings from their research. In 29 of these studies the focus was primarily on quality-of-life findings. Only 8 were reports of studies addressing psychosocial care, needs, or concerns of children with epilepsy or their family members. For ease of presentation the 37 research reports are grouped into five categories: studies of adults who had childhood epilepsy (*n* = 4), comprehensive quality-of-life studies (*n* = 4), psychosocial functioning studies (*n* = 14), cognitive/academic functioning studies (*n* = 7), and studies of psychosocial care, needs, and concerns (*n* = 8). In each category studies are briefly described, major findings are presented, and the studies are briefly critiqued. The chapter concludes with an evaluation of the whole body of literature and with recommendations for future research.

## INSTRUMENT DEVELOPMENT STUDIES

### Quality-of-Life Scales

Four groups of authors developed scales to measure quality of life in children with epilepsy and their families. Three authors (Apajaslo et al., 1996; Cramer et al., 1999; Wildrick, Parker-Fisher, & Morales, 1996) developed scales for the child or adolescent to complete, and one group of authors (Hoare & Russell, 1995) developed a scale for the parent to complete. The child-completed scales are described first, followed by a description of the parent-completed scale. Two of the child-completed scales are specific to adolescents with epilepsy (Cramer et al., 1999; Wildrick et al., 1996), and one (Apajaslo et al., 1996) is generic for adolescents with a chronic health condition.

Cramer and colleagues (1999) developed a 48-item scale for measuring quality of life in adolescents with epilepsy (QOLIE-AD-48) across eight dimensions: epilepsy impact, memory/concentration, attitudes, physical functioning, stigma, social support, school, and health perceptions. When the scale was administered to 197 adolescents, it was found to have strong psychometric properties, including internal construct validity, external validity, internal consistency reliability, and test-retest reliability. Wildrick, Parker-Fisher, and Morales (1996) developed a 25-item scale to measure five dimensions of quality of life: self-concept, home life, school life, social activities, and medicine. The target population was school-age youth (8–18 years) with mild epilepsy. No data were provided on the psychometric properties of this scale. A description of sources for the items (i.e., the literature, the first author's clinical experience, and a quality-of-life scale for adults with epilepsy), however, provided some support for its content validity. Results from the study in which the scale was administered to 60 children are reported later under major findings.

The final child-completed scale was developed by Apajaslo et al. (1996) for adolescents (12–15 years) with a chronic health condition. Questions measured functioning related to mobility, vision, hearing, breathing, sleeping, eating, elimination, speech, mental functioning, discomfort and symptoms, school and hobbies, friends, physical appearance, depression, distress, and vitality. The scale was administered to four groups of early adolescents: 239 healthy controls, 5 children waiting for an organ transplant, 19 children with genetic skeletal dysplasia, and 32 children with epilepsy. The scale was found to have adequate content validity and test-retest reliability. Support also was found for its construct validity, with healthy controls receiving higher scores (showing fewer problems) than did children with health problems in the areas of mobility, friends, and school and hobbies.

The parent-completed scale developed by Hoare and Russell (1995) was a modification of a previous scale developed by Hoare (1993). The 1993 scale had 29 items that measured three areas: epilepsy and its treatment, child's adjustment and development, and effects on family life. The 1995 scale, entitled Impact of Childhood Illness Scale, is a 30-item scale that measures the impact of epilepsy across four dimensions: epilepsy and its treatment, impact on the child's development and adjustment, impact on the parent, and impact on the family. On this scale parents respond to items with both frequency and importance ratings. The scale was administered to parents of 21 children with epilepsy between the ages of 6 and 17 years. Support for construct validity was found when children with poorly controlled seizures were found to have consistently higher scores (poorer quality of life) than those with well-controlled seizures across all subscales.

## Psychosocial Needs Scales

Only one group of authors developed scales to measure psychosocial needs. Austin, Dunn, Huster, and Rose (1998) developed two scales, one for children and one for parents. Both scales were designed to measure satisfaction with care received, perceptions of unmet needs for care (information and support), and concerns/fears related to seizures. Prior to piloting the scales, both were found to have content validity by four clinical nurse specialists with expertise in pediatric epilepsy. The scales were administered to 117 parents and 43 children. Each of the four sections was found to have adequate internal consistency reliability (alpha > .70). Support also was found for the construct validity. Parent information needs, support needs, and concerns were positively correlated with parents' perceptions of stigma and negatively correlated with parents' ratings of their positive mood. Support for the child scale was found when the child's attitude toward having seizures was negatively correlated with information needs, support needs, and concerns/fears related to having seizures.

## Critique

There were several strengths noted in the articles reporting on instrument development. First, there is a moderate amount of activity in an area in which most previous instrument development in quality of life has focused on adults with epilepsy. The fact that instruments are being developed to measure these constructs in children shows an increase in interest in assessment of their quality of life and psychosocial care needs. Another strength is that, with the exception of the scale developed by Wildrick and colleagues (1996), authors provided information on the psychometric properties of the scales. It also is desirable that instruments were developed for both parents and children to complete. Having both parent and child scales available provides an opportunity for researchers to obtain both objective and subjective data on older children and adolescents. A final asset of instrument development during this period is that investigators developed both general and specific quality-of-life scales. Both are needed for a comprehensive assessment of quality of life in clinical research (Shumaker et al., 1990).

Despite these strengths, there are still gaps and limitations in this area. First, a major gap is that there has been no scale development for infants and young children with epilepsy. This is particularly unfortunate because the early childhood period is when the greatest number of seizure conditions have their onset (Hauser, 1994). Clearly, future instrument development should focus on scales for this population. Another limitation is that none of the scales has been used in more than one study, and all are in need of further development to establish their reliability and validity for use in future research. The fact that no scales have been used, however, is most likely because they have all been very recently developed, and there has not been time for more testing.

## STUDIES OF ADULTS WHO HAD CHILDHOOD EPILEPSY

### Design and Sampling

Four groups of authors (Jalava, Sillanpaa, Camfield, & Camfield, 1997; Kokkonen, Kokkonen, & Saukkonen, 1998; Sillanpaa, Jalava, Kaleva, & Shinnar, 1998; Wirrell et al., 1997) assessed quality of life outcomes in three studies of adults who had epilepsy during childhood. All of the studies compared outcomes of the adults with childhood epilepsy to either healthy controls (Jalava et al., 1997; Sillanpaa et al., 1998) or to other chronic illness samples (Kokkonen et al., 1998; Wirrell et al., 1997). All of the studies addressed several quality-of-life domains. Epilepsy samples were relatively large, ranging from 56 to 220. Ages ranged from 22 to 36 years. Three of the studies (Jalava et al., 1997; Kokkonen et al., 1998; Sillanpaa et al., 1998) were conducted in Finland and one (Wirrell et al., 1997) was completed in Nova Scotia.

## Major Findings

Authors of two studies (Jalava et al., 1997; Sillanpaa et al., 1998) reported on the same population-based cohort of children in Finland who were entered into a prospective study prior to age 16 and followed for an average of 35 years. These authors compared quality-of-life outcomes in this population to that in two control groups (community and employed). Subjects with epilepsy in adulthood had no other neurological problems. When compared to controls, those with uncomplicated epilepsy had less success in education, employment, and marriage. Moreover, those with epilepsy were four times more likely than employee controls to report that they had limited control of their lives. Compared to employee controls, persons with epilepsy who were receiving more than one antiepileptic medication (i.e., polypharmacy) and those with continuing seizures were significantly less satisfied with their present life.

Wirrell and colleagues (1997) evaluated outcomes in young adults ($M =$ 23 years) who had epilepsy during childhood and compared them to a similar sample of those who had juvenile RA. They found subjects with childhood epilepsy to have had more academic and behavioral problems than did subjects with arthritis even though more of those with epilepsy had experienced a remission of their condition. In the academic domain, those with seizures (compared to those with arthritis) were more likely to have repeated a grade, required special help, or failed to graduate from high school or to attend a college or university. Other quality-of-life areas in which those with childhood epilepsy fared worse than those with juvenile RA included more emotional difficulties, more unplanned pregnancies, fewer planned social outings, and more impaired relationships with siblings. In this study, adverse outcomes were not predicted by any of the seizure variables assessed.

The Kokkonen, Kokkonen, and Saukkonen (1998) study of quality-of-life outcomes in young adults who had childhood epilepsy was one of the few studies that included physical symptoms as a part of the measurement of quality of life. In this prospective study young adults (19 to 25 years) who had had either childhood epilepsy ($n = 81$) or motor disability since childhood ($n = 52$) were compared to age-matched population controls. Mental health disorders were found in 37% of those with motor disabilities, in 18% of those with epilepsy, and in 22% of controls. Most of these differences were accounted for by different rates of depressive syndromes; however, few other differences in mental health problems were found across the three samples.

## Critique

Major strengths of these studies were the prospective designs and relatively strong retention rates over several years or even decades. Other strengths were the relatively large samples and the use of comparison groups. In addition, all of the studies measured several quality-of-life domains. These studies also provided important information on outcomes of children who developed epilepsy during childhood. In relation to limitations, however, only one of the four studies (Kokkonen et al., 1998) used previously developed standardized measurements. Moreover, none reported on the reliability or validity of the measurements. Also, findings of these studies might not generalize to children currently being treated for epilepsy because of improvements in the treatment of epilepsy over the past two decades.

## COMPREHENSIVE QUALITY-OF-LIFE STUDIES

### Design and Sampling

Four studies (Austin, Huster, Dunn, & Risinger, 1996; Austin, Smith, Risinger, & McNelis, 1994; Mandelbaum & Burack, 1997; Weglage, Demsky, Pietsch, & Kurlemann, 1997) investigated several quality-of-life domains in children with epilepsy. All of these studies investigated the psychological and cognitive/academic domains. With the exception of the study by Mandelbaum and Burack (1997), the studies employed comparison samples. Austin and colleagues (1994, 1996) used children with asthma as a comparison sample. Weglage et al. (1997) used a healthy control sample matched to the epilepsy sample in age, sex, and socioeconomic status. Finally, in two of the studies (Austin et al., 1996; Weglage et al., 1997), analysis was carried out to identify differences in quality of life within the epilepsy sample.

### Major Findings

Austin et al. (1994, 1996) assessed physical, psychological, social, and school domains in children with epilepsy and children with asthma. Parents rated their children's behavior on a well-developed behavioral rating scale (Child Behavior Checklist [CBCL; Achenbach, 1991]) and participated in structured interviews about seizures, medication, physical problems, and school progress. Children completed self-concept, attitude, and family scales. Teachers completed the teacher's version of the CBCL, and a neurologist reviewed clinical records and parent interviews of seizure descriptions to classify seizures and determine seizure severity. In their first study, Austin et al. (1994) found that children with asthma had relatively more physical problems, including frequency of episodes, school absences, and medication side effects. In contrast, children with epilepsy were more impaired in the psychological, social, and school domains. Compared to the children with asthma, the children with epilepsy had more internalizing and externalizing behavior disturbance, less satisfaction with family relationships, poorer peer relations, and decreased academic progress and achievement.

The second study (Austin et al., 1996) assessed the same children 4 years later. Approximately half the epilepsy sample and one fifth of the asthma sample were inactive (i.e., off medication and having no episodes of seizures or asthma). Differences between children with epilepsy and those with asthma remained apparent: children with epilepsy had more internalizing and attention problems, poorer social relations, and more of both behavior and learning difficulties in school. An assessment of subgroups of children with epilepsy showed that the children with active epilepsy (i.e., treatment with medication and recent seizures) had more problems than did the children with inactive epilepsy. When compared to children with inactive asthma, however, children with inactive epilepsy had more internalizing problems and worse school progress, achievement, and intellectual self-concept.

Mandelbaum and Burack (1997) used multiple measures of cognitive function and the CBCL to measure behavior. The sample of children with newly diagnosed seizures was evaluated prior to starting antiepileptic drugs, and 6 and 12 months afterward. Children were assessed for intelligence, motor ability, learning, and behavior problems. Of the 43 children with epilepsy who began the study, 26 remained at 6 months, and only 12 remained at 1 year. Differences in quality-of-life dimensions were explored among four different seizure types: simple partial, complex partial, generalized nonconvulsive, and generalized convulsive. Few significant differences were found. At baseline, children with nonconvulsive seizures did more poorly on cognitive measures than those with either partial or generalized convulsive seizure types. At follow-up, subjects with generalized nonconvulsive seizures had more internalizing behavior problems than did those with either generalized nonconvulsive or simple partial seizures. No deterioration in functioning was found in any group.

Weglage et al. (1997) found that their group of children with centrotemporal spikes had both more cognitive and more behavioral problems than controls had. The children were assessed for intelligence, language, motor performance, attention, learning, and behavior (CBCL). Children with centrotemporal spikes did worse than controls on IQ, visual perception, short-term memory, and fine motor performance tasks. On the CBCL, the children with spikes had higher total behavior scores, as well as higher scores on social problems, delinquent problems, and thought problems subscales. Cognitive deficits correlated with frequency of spikes on the EEG but not with frequency of seizures.

## Critique

A major strength of these studies was the use of well-developed and standardized scales to measure several dimensions of quality of life. Other strengths included the incorporation of comparison groups into the design and the use of multiple data sources. For example, Austin and colleagues (1994, 1996) collected data from children, parents, and schoolteachers. Findings also provided information about factors associated with different quality-of-life outcomes. Finally, with the exception of one study (Mandelbaum & Burack, 1997), samples of children with epilepsy were relatively large, ranging from 80 to 117. Despite these many strengths, however, there were some limitations. First, all of the studies used samples from clinics so it is not known how generalizable these results are to community samples. Children with more severe epilepsy would most likely be overrepresented in clinic samples. There also was a gap in populations studied—not one study investigated infants or children under the age of 4 years. Finally, the only prospective study (Mandelbaum & Burack,1997) had several limitations (e.g., a very wide age range, a large number of subjects lost to follow-up, and small cell sizes [$n = 2$]) that made conclusions most tentative.

## PSYCHOSOCIAL FUNCTIONING STUDIES

### Design and Sampling

In 13 studies, psychosocial functioning was the primary quality-of-life dimension investigated. Only one of these studies (Rossi, Bonfiglio, Veggiotti, & Lanz, 1997) tested an intervention that attempted to improve the psychological functioning of adolescents with epilepsy. The remaining studies either described the child's psychosocial functioning or identified factors that were related to the child's functioning in this area. Seven studies addressed the general question of the prevalence of behavioral problems. The scale used most commonly to measure behavior problems was the CBCL, which was employed in four studies (Dunn, Austin, & Huster, 1997; Hoare & Mann, 1994; Mitchell, Scheier, & Baker, 1994; Pianta & Lothman, 1994). Several studies used a control group, including one with chronic illness controls (Hoare & Mann, 1994) and five with controls from the general population (Caplan et al., 1997, 1998; Carlton-Ford, Miller, Brown, Nealeigh, & Jennings, 1995; Sikic, Buljan-Fander, Marcelja, & Mejaski-Bosnjak, 1995; Stores, Wiggs, & Campling, 1998). Factors related to behavior problems were investigated in four studies (Carlton-Ford, Miller, Nealeigh, & Sanchez, 1997; Ettinger et al., 1998; Pianta & Lothman, 1994; Stores et al., 1998). Data on intelligence were available in five studies (Caplan et al., 1997, 1998; Mitchell et al., 1994; Pianta & Lothman, 1994; Steffenburg, Gillberg, & Steffenburg, 1996).

### Major Findings

In all of these studies, results indicated impairment in psychosocial functioning in children with epilepsy. Hoare and Mann (1994) compared CBCL scores for behavior problems in children with epilepsy and in children with diabetes mellitus. Children with epilepsy had higher mean scores on total and individual problem subscales. Carlton-Ford et al. (1995), using data from a national health survey, found that children with epilepsy had worse adjustment than did children with no history of seizures and that children with inactive epilepsy had the same level of adjustment problems as did children with active seizures. Dunn, Austin, and Huster (1997) evaluated children with new-onset seizures and found that 24% had elevated CBCL scores in the 6 months prior to the first recognized seizure. These authors hypothesized that neurological dysfunction was related to behavior problems. Caplan et al. (1998) found two to three times more children with psychiatric diagnoses in the epilepsy sample when compared to controls. Most frequent were the disruptive behavior disorders, which were found in one fourth of children with epilepsy. In this study, behavioral problems were predicted by lower IQ but not by seizure type. Sikic et al. (1995) analyzed personality traits and found children with epilepsy to be more introverted than were healthy controls. Only one study (Steffenburg et al., 1996) focused exclusively on children with mental retardation. Of the 98 children with both mental retardation and epilepsy, 30 were too impaired for classification, and 53 had at least one psychiatric diagnosis, including 24 with autistic disorder and 10 with an autistic-like conditions.

Four studies evaluated children with epilepsy for psychological functioning other than behavior problems. Hoare and Mann (1994) found that children with epilepsy had lower self-esteem than did children with diabetes mellitus. Caplan et al. (1997) studied thought processing and found that the children with complex partial seizures had more illogical thinking than did either children with generalized seizures or children with no seizures. Ettinger et al. (1998) found an increased rate of depression in children with epilepsy. Stores, Wiggs, and Campling (1998) discovered that children with seizures had more sleep disturbances than did a control group. Specifically, they found an association between behavioral problems and poor sleep in children aged 5–11 years with epilepsy.

In three studies, family or social factors were associated with psychosocial functioning. Mitchell, Scheier, and Baker (1994) found that low acculturation (defined as lower maternal education, fewer years residence in the United States, and English as a second language) predicted both negative attitudes of the parent and behavioral problems in the child with epilepsy. Pianta and Lothman (1994) found ratings of mother-child interaction to be associated with child behavior problems in 51 children with epilepsy. The parent-child relationship was related to behavioral problems even when controlling for seizure-related variables.

The relationship between perceptions of stigma and psychosocial functioning was evaluated by Carlton-Ford, Miller, Nealeigh, and Sanchez (1997). They found that behavioral problems in the child with seizures were associated with parental expectations of stigmatization and limitations from seizures and also with children's reports that their parents were overcontrolling. Findings on the effect of IQ and seizure severity on psychosocial functioning were inconsistent. Low IQ was associated with more behavioral problems in three studies (Caplan et al., 1997, 1998; Steffenburg et al., 1996), and seizure severity was related to behavior problems in three studies (Carlton-Ford et al., 1997; Dunn et al., 1997; Hoare & Mann, 1994). In contrast, Mitchell et al. (1994) found no association between behavior problems and cognitive function or seizure severity.

The lone intervention study used qualitative methods to describe changes in a group of seven adolescents with epilepsy. The intervention, which used psychoanalytic methods to improve their understanding and acceptance of the epilepsy, lasted for 2 years. Although no formal data were collected, the authors had the impression that the group process was beneficial, for example, in helping the adolescents become more compliant with their AED regimens.

## Critique

A major strength of these studies is the large number of authors who are focusing their research on a common quality-of-life problem for children with epilepsy-impaired psychosocial functioning. A general strength of these studies is that authors took advantage of the large number of well-developed scales in this area. Moreover, with the exception of the one intervention study, samples were relatively large, and differences based on seizure variables were explored. The number of subjects ranged from 37 to 120. Although most authors used clinic samples, two (Carlton-Ford et al., 1995; Steffenburg et al., 1996) used an epidemiological approach. A final strength of these studies was the large number that used comparison groups. There were areas, however, that were less strong. None of the studies included children under the age of 4 in the sample, which might be because there are fewer scales available to reliably and validly measure psychosocial functioning in young children. Another limitation was that the large majority of the studies had cross-sectional designs, making it difficult to identify predictors of psychosocial functioning problems. Moreover, the one study with a longitudinal design (Mitchell et al., 1994) had a high attrition rate that made conclusions from that study tentative.

## COGNITIVE/ACADEMIC FUNCTIONING STUDIES

### Design and Sampling

Seven studies assessed the effect of epilepsy on cognitive or academic dimensions of quality of life. Sample sizes ranged from 33 to 117. Three studies focused primarily on academic achievement (Austin, Huberty, Huster, & Dunn, 1998, 1999; Sturniolo & Galletti, 1994), and four studies primarily investigated cognitive functioning (Aldenkamp et al., 1998; McCarthy, Richman, & Yarbrough, 1995; Semrud-Clikeman & Wical, 1999; Williams, Griebel, & Dykman, 1998). Five of the studies used comparison samples. Two groups of authors (Aldenkamp et al., 1998; Sturniolo & Galletti, 1994) used controls from the general population, Austin, Huberty, and colleagues (1998, 1999) selected children with asthma as controls, and Semrud-Clikeman and Wical (1999) used normal children and children with attention deficit hyperactive disorder (ADHD) as controls. Of the two studies that did not have comparison samples, one (Williams, Griebel, & Dykman, 1998) used normative test data for comparison purposes. In the final study (McCarthy et al., 1995), the authors made comparisons within the sample on the basis of seizure type and the presence or absence of school problems.

## Major Findings

A consistent finding across the three studies focusing primarily on academic achievement was the adverse effect of epilepsy on academic function. Sturniolo and Galletti (1994) found academic underachievement in 61% of a sample of elementary school-age children with idiopathic epilepsy attending ordinary schools. The children with academic underachievement also were noted to have behavioral disturbances, whereas the behavior of children with good academic functioning did not differ from controls. Both studies by Austin, Huberty, and colleagues (1998, 1999) focused on the same sample of children. In the 1998 study the sample was 117 children with chronic seizures and 108 children with asthma. Children with seizures had significantly lower scores on group-administered academic achievement tests than did the children with asthma. Boys with severe epilepsy were at the highest risk for underachievement. This study also documented associations between negative child attitudes toward their health condition and both poorer adaptive function and decreased academic achievement. In the 1999 study the sample size was 98 children with epilepsy, including half with inactive epilepsy, and 96 children with asthma. There had been no change in academic achievement scores, even in those adolescents who had a remission of their seizures. In that study, adolescents with seizures continued to have scores lower than those of the children with asthma in all areas of academic achievement.

Other studies have assessed particular cognitive skills. Williams, Griebel, and Dykman (1998) did extensive neuropsychological evaluations on 79 children with epilepsy. Excluded were children with IQs below 70 and those with a history of neurosurgical procedures, neurodegenerative disorders, head trauma, or motor handicaps. They found normal neurocognitive functioning, with the exception of impaired verbal and visual attention. Attentional problems also were identified by parental report. Scores on attention were significantly below those expected on the basis of normative data. Semrud-Clikeman and Wical (1999) used a computer-administered test of attention and found that children with complex partial seizures and ADHD had the poorest performance, and those with complex partial seizures without ADHD were just as impaired as those with ADHD without epilepsy.

In contrast, McCarthy, Richman, and Yarbrough (1995) found no difference in attention in children with epilepsy, compared to normative data. Children with seizures in this study, however, did have lower scores on tests of memory compared to norms. When the children with epilepsy were separated into those with and without school problems, there was a significant association between memory problems and poor school function. Neither seizure type nor medication was associated with cognitive difficulties. Aldenkamp et al. (1998) assessed the effect of AEDs on cognitive function by evaluating children before and after tapering off medication. Children reported significantly less tiredness when off medication, and their parents noted better alertness and concentration and less tiredness, drowsiness, and memory problems in their children. A control group showed no change over time.

## Critique

The design was a strength in many of the studies. Not only did the authors show that children with epilepsy have high rates of learning problems, they identified factors related to such problems. Although the samples were small in some of the studies, the selection of specific groups and comparisons allowed research questions to be answered. A final strength was that standardized instruments were employed. Limitations included the relatively small number of studies, considering the importance of cognitive and academic functioning in the life of a child. Despite the high number of children who are doing poorly at school, only two of the studies (Austin, Huberty, et al., 1998; Sturniolo & Galletti, 1994) included data from teachers. Other studies were very limited in scope. For example, McCarthy et al. (1995) used only two tests of memory and one of attention. Finally, only one study (Aldenkamp et al., 1998) included data from both parents and children.

# PYSCHOSOCIAL CARE, NEEDS, AND CONCERNS STUDIES

## Design and Sampling

Psychosocial aspects of care were addressed in eight studies. The majority of these studies sought to evaluate psychosocial care and focused on caregivers of children with epilepsy. One study (McNelis, Musick, Austin, Dunn, & Creasy, 1998) focused exclusively on children. Five studies (Brown, 1994; Hanai, 1996; Suurmeijer, 1994; Webb, Coleman, Fielder, & Kennedy, 1998; Williams et al., 1998) used mailed surveys and had large samples. Most of the studies used questionnaires developed by the authors. Two studies (McNelis et al., 1998; Shore et al., 1998) reported on results from the administration of the psychosocial care scales (Austin, Dunn, et al., 1998) described previously in this chapter. One study (Mims, 1997) collected data from siblings of children with epilepsy about their concerns and fears.

## Major Findings

Two studies investigated several aspects of psychosocial care. Shore et al. (1998) used the Parent Report of Psychosocial Care Scale (Austin, Dunn, et al., 1998) to assess both satisfaction with care and worries and concerns of parents of children with new-onset seizures. They found that approximately a third of the mothers and a fifth of the fathers were less than satisfied with the information they received about seizures, medication effects, problems to report, or handling future seizures. Half of the mothers of children with new-onset seizures reported being less than satisfied with the information they received on handling seizures at school. When questioned 6 months after the initial seizure, approximately two thirds of mothers felt some to strong need for information or support. At the same time, half the fathers expressed a need for information, and one third expressed a need for support. The percentage of parents who were somewhat to very worried changed little between 3 months and 6 months after the first seizure. At 6 months 30%–40% of mothers and 20%–30% of fathers were worried about the potential of death, brain damage or loss of intelligence, the possible presence of a brain tumor, or addiction to antiepileptic medication. Hanai (1996) sent questionnaires concerning seizures, medication, behavior, school, and future prospects to both parents and teachers. He found that parents were worried about seizures and the future, and a fifth reported that their children were having difficulties keeping up in academic situations. In this study, two thirds of teachers wanted more information about seizures.

Satisfaction with care was addressed in several studies. In each case, communication with health care personnel was the major variable associated with satisfaction with care for the child with epilepsy. Suurmeijer (1994) defined quality of life in terms of structure, primarily the accessibility of care; process was defined by the communication and relationship between patient or family and the providers of health care; and outcome by the patient and family's satisfaction with care. He further conceived of outcome as a measure of the match between care provided and needs of the patient and family. He found that a third of the parents or partners of individuals with epilepsy believed there was inadequate access and/or communication and were not satisfied with the care given.

Williams et al. (1995) used a mailed questionnaire to look for predictors of satisfaction with care. They found that 95 of 136 respondents rated the quality of care as excellent and noted that information given and the staff attitude were the best predictors of satisfaction with care received. The number of clinic visits was not associated with satisfaction with care. Webb et al. (1998) made a general assessment of care for children with epilepsy. The first parts of their study was an audit of correspondence, prescription of medication, and laboratory use. They also mailed a 13-item questionnaire measuring parental satisfaction with epilepsy care, with specific questions about courtesy, communication, and the process of the clinic visit. Results indicated that parents were satisfied with the clinic visits and courtesy of staff, but only half were mostly or very satisfied with the explanation of epilepsy, information given, or questions answered.

McNelis et al. (1998) and Brown (1994) both questioned children with seizures. McNelis et al. studied children with first seizures and found that, at 6 months after the onset of seizures, 20%–40% were less than satisfied with the information they had received and 50%–75% wanted more information. They found that 38% of children with seizures felt they were not told how antiepileptic medication worked, and a similar number were not given the opportunity to talk about fears and worries. In their group, 74% of children with new-onset seizures wanted information on handling future seizures; 70%, information on preventing injuries; and 65%, information on the etiology of their seizures. Brown (1994) sent questionnaires to children with seizures. A third of the children said their physicians never explained the seizures, and half of the group whose physicians had talked to them said they did not understand what the doctor said. Approximately two thirds described fatigue from the AED, and half described feeling helpless, scared, or different from others.

Mims (1997) studied siblings of children with either frequent or infrequent seizures, matched to a control group with no chronic illness. No statistical difference in self-esteem, behavior, or concerns was found between groups. There was a trend for the siblings of the children with frequent seizures to have more concerns about their sibling's epilepsy and more externalizing behavior than was seen in the siblings of children with infrequent seizures. Mims also found that significantly more stress was experienced in the families of children with intractable seizures.

### Critique

A strength of most of these studies was the use of relatively large, diverse samples. The age ranges of the children being served were quite large. The study by Williams et al. (1995) included children as young as 2 months.

Data on the psychometric properties of the scales were available in four of the studies (McNelis et al., 1998; Shore et al., 1998; Suurmeijer, 1994; Williams et al., 1995) but were not provided for two other studies (Brown, 1994; Hanai, 1996). A limitation of the study by Williams et al. (1995) was the 22% response rate. Webb et al. (1998) had response rates of 64% and 61%, and Hanai (1996) had a 78% return rate. Brown (1994) and Suurmeijer (1994) described the results of mailed questionnaires but did not provide information on the number of persons to whom the questionnaires were sent. Finally, none of the authors of surveys explored differences between responders and nonresponders.

## RECOMMENDATIONS FOR FUTURE RESEARCH

The ultimate goal of providing care to children with epilepsy is to control seizures while facilitating an optimal quality of life for the child as well as the family. In this section two questions are addressed. What are the overall strengths and weaknesses of the research in relation to meeting this goal? What are recommendations for future research?

The majority of research has been descriptive in nature and has documented the extent to which children with epilepsy were experiencing quality-of-life problems. Findings have clearly indicated that at least some of these children are at risk for impaired functioning, compared to either general population controls or to other chronic illness groups such as asthma, diabetes, and juvenile RA. Descriptive research is still needed, however, on the extent to which problems exist across the entire population of children with epilepsy. Most research has focused on school-age children who attend regular schools. In contrast, infants and preschool children are understudied, as are children with both epilepsy and mental retardation. The only study on children with both mental retardation and epilepsy showed that the prevalence of quality-of-life problems was extremely high in this subgroup (Steffenburg et al., 1996). Most past research has investigated children from clinic populations, which most likely has resulted in overrepresentation of children with more-difficult-to-control seizures. In contrast, few authors have studied children who are cared for by primary care physicians. More research is needed to describe quality of life in these understudied populations.

Past research also has been uneven in scope, some domains being studied more frequently than others. In this review, only four studies were comprehensive and addressed several quality-of-life domains. Most studies focused on psychological functioning, especially behavioral problems; few authors investigated academic and social functioning domains. In addition, few past studies have investigated the impact of childhood epilepsy on other family members. Research on how family environment variables are related to quality-of-life problems also is understudied. The one study of siblings in this review showed that they were in need of psychosocial care. Moreover, the psychosocial needs studies also documented that families were in need of interventions to help them cope with epilepsy in their child. Future research should be more comprehensive in scope and should describe a broad range of quality-of-life functioning in these understudied groups to identify children and families who are most in the need of interventions.

Research also is needed to identify intervenable factors that are causally related to quality of life, to provide a foundation for the development of interventions to facilitate optimal outcomes in both children and their families. Such research will be difficult to design because of the vast diversity in how epilepsy is manifested in children. Epilepsy is a heterogeneous disorder varying by seizure type, epileptic syndrome, seizure severity, seizure frequency, and the presence of other conditions (e.g., mental retardation). Each subtype of epilepsy may influence disorder prognosis as well as outcomes. A weakness of much of the past research is that children with epilepsy were viewed as a homogeneous group, and differences based on these variables were not explored. The few studies that did investigate differences in quality of life on the basis of seizure variables have found that such differences do exist. Research in this area is complicated by the large number of variables that can potentially affect quality of life, such as child variables (e.g., age, age of onset, gender, developmental stage), demographic variables (e.g., socioeconomic status, culture), and family variables (e.g., coping responses). Few of these variables have been fully explored in past studies. Finally, research testing interventions aimed at improving quality of life in children with epilepsy and their families is greatly needed to provide a foundation for practice with this population.

## ACKNOWLEDGMENTS

The authors acknowledge support from the National Institute for Neurological Disorders and Stroke (NS22416) and the National Institute of Nursing Research (NR04536) in preparation of this chapter. The authors also acknowledge Deborah Anzalone for conducting the literature search, Janet Kain for technical assistance in reviewing the literature, and Phyllis Dexter for editorial assistance.

## REFERENCES

Achenbach, T. M. (1991). *Manual for the Child Behavior Checklist/4-18 and 1991 Profile*. Burlington: University of Vermont, Department of Psychiatry.

Aldenkamp, A. P., Alpherts, W. C. J., Blennow, G., Elmqvist, D., Heijbel, J., Nilsson, H. L., Tonnby, B., Wahlander, L., & Woose, E. (1998). Antiepileptic drug-related cognitive complaints in seizure-free children with epilepsy before and after drug discontinuation. *Epilepsia, 39,* 1070–1074.

Annegers, J. F., & Begley, C. E. (in press). Costs of pediatric epilepsy. In W. E. Dodson, J. M. Pellock, & B. Bourgeois (Eds.), *Pediatric epilepsy: Diagnoses and therapy* (2nd ed.). New York: Demos Vermande.

Apajaslo, M., Sintonen, H., Holmberg, C., Sinkkonen, J., Aalberg, V., Pihko, H., Siimes, M. A., Kaitila, I., Makela, A., Rantakari, K., Anttila, R., & Rautonen, J. (1996). Quality of life in early adolescence: A sixteen-dimensional health-related measure (16D). *Quality of Life Research, 5,* 205–211.

Austin, J. K., Dunn, D., Huster, G., & Rose, D. (1998). Development of scales to measure psychosocial care needs of children with seizures and their parents. *Journal of Neuroscience Nursing, 30,* 155–160.

Austin, J. K., Huberty, T. J, Huster, G. A., & Dunn, D. W. (1998). Academic achievement in children with epilepsy or asthma. *Developmental Medicine and Child Neurology, 40,* 248–255.

Austin, J. K., Huberty, T. J., Huster, G. A., & Dunn, D. W. (1999). Does academic achievement in children with epilepsy change over time? *Developmental Medicine and Child Neurology, 41,* 473–479.

Austin, J. K., Huster, G., Dunn, D., & Risinger, M. (1996). Adolescents with active or inactive epilepsy or asthma: A comparison of quality of life. *Epilepsia, 37,* 1228–1238.

Austin, J. K., Smith, S., Risinger, M., & McNelis, A. (1994). Childhood epilepsy and asthma: Comparison of quality of life. *Epilepsia, 35,* 608–615.

Begley, C. E., Annegers, J. F., Lairson, D. R., Reynolds, T. F., & Hauler, W. A. (1994). Cost of epilepsy in the United States: A model based on incidence and prognosis. *Epilepsia, 35,* 1230–1243.

Breslau, N. (1985). Psychiatric disorder in children with physical disabilities. *Journal of the American Academy of Child Psychiatry, 24,* 87–94.

Brown, S. W. (1994). Quality of life: A view from the playground. *Seizure, 3,* 11–15.

Caplan, R., Arbelle, S., Guthrie, D., Komo, S., Shields, D., Hansen, R., & Chayasirisobhon, S. (1997). Formal thought disorder and psychopathology in pediatric primary generalized and complex partial epilepsy. *Journal of the American Academy of Child and Adolescent Psychiatry, 36,* 1286–1294.

Caplan, R., Arbelle, S., Magharious, W., Guthrie, D., Komo, S., Shields, W. D., Chayasirisobhon, S., & Hansen, R. (1998). Psychopathology in pediatric complex partial and primary generalized epilepsy. *Developmental Medicine and Child Neurology, 40,* 805–811.

Carlton-Ford, S., Miller, R., Brown, M., Nealeigh, N., & Jennings, P. (1995). Epilepsy and children's social and psychological adjustment. *Journal of Health and Social Behavior, 36,* 285–301.

Carlton-Ford, S., Miller, R., Nealeigh, N., & Sanchez, N. (1997). The effect of perceived stigma and psychological over-control on the behavioral problems of children with epilepsy. *Seizure, 6,* 383–391.

Cockerell, O. C., Johnson, A. L., Sander, J. W., & Shorvon, S. D. (1997). Prognosis of epilepsy: A review and further analysis of the first nine years of the British national general practice study of epilepsy, a prospective population-based study. *Epilepsia, 38,* 31–46.

Commission on Classification and Terminology of the International League Against Epilepsy. (1981). Proposal for revised clinical and electroencephalographic classification of epileptic seizures. *Epilepsia, 22,* 489–501.

Commission on Classification and Terminology of the International League Against epilepsy. (1989). Proposal for revised classification of epilepsies and epileptic syndromes. *Epilepsia, 30,* 389–399.

Cramer, J. A., Westbrook, L. E., Devinsky, O., Perrine, K., Glassman, M. B., & Camfield, C. (1999). Development of the quality of life in epilepsy inventory for adolescents: The QOLIE-AD-48. *Epilepsia, 40,* 1114–1121.

Dunn, D. W., Austin, J. K., & Huster, G. A. (1997). Behavior problems in children with new-onset epilepsy. *Seizure, 6,* 283–287.

Ettinger, A. B., Weisbrot, D. M., Nolan, E. E., Gadow, K. D.,Vitale, S. A., Andriola, M. R., Lenn, N. J., Novak, G. P., & Hermann, B. P. (1998). Symptoms of depression and anxiety in pediatric epilepsy patients. *Epilepsia, 39,* 595–599.

Hanai, T. (1996). Quality of life in children with epilepsy. *Epilepsia, 37,* 28–32.

Hauser, E., Freilinger, M., Seidl, R., & Groh, C. (1995). Prognosis of childhood epilepsy in newly referred patients. *Journal of Child Neurology, 11,* 201–204.

Hauser, W. A. (1994). The prevalence and incidence of convulsive disorders in children. *Epilepsia, 25,* (Suppl.2), s1–s6.

Hauser, W. A., & Hesdorffer, D. C. (1990). *Epilepsy: Frequency, causes, and consequences.* New York: Demos Publications.

Hoare, P. (1993). The quality of life of children with chronic epilepsy and their families. *Seizure, 2,* 269–275.

Hoare, P., & Mann, H. (1994). Self-esteem and behavioral adjustment in children with epilepsy and children with diabetes. *Journal of Psychosomatic Research, 38,* 859–869.

Hoare, P., & Russell, M. (1995). The quality of life of children with chronic epilepsy and their families: Preliminary findings with a new assessment measure. *Developmental Medicine and Child Neurology, 37,* 689–696.

Jalava, M., Sillanpaa, M., Camfield, C., & Camfield, P. (1997). Social adjustment and competence 35 years after onset of childhood epilepsy: A prospective controlled study. *Epilepsia, 38,* 708–715.

Kokkonen, E. R., Kokkonen, J., & Saukkonen, A. L. (1998). Do neurological disorders in childhood pose a risk for mental health in young adulthood? *Developmental Medicine and Child Neurology, 40,* 364–368.

Levi, R., & Drotar, D. (1998). Critical issues and needs in health-related quality of life assessment of children and adolescents with chronic health conditions. In *Measuring health-related quality of life in children and adolescents.* Mahwah, NJ: Lawrence Erlbaum.

Mandelbaum, D. E., & Burack, G. (1997). The effect of seizure type and medication on cognitive and behavioral functioning in children with idiopathic epilepsy. *Developmental Medicine and Child Neurology, 39,* 731–735.

McCarthy, A. M., Richman, L. C., & Yarbrough, D. (1995). Memory, attention and school problems in children with seizure disorders. *Developmental Neuropsychology, 11,* 71–86.

McDermott, S., Mani, S., & Krishnaswami, S. (1995). A population-based analysis of specific behavior problems associated with childhood seizures. *Journal of Epilepsy, 8,* 110–118.

McNelis, A., Musick, B., Austin, J., Dunn, D., & Creasy, K. (1998). Psychosocial care needs of children with new-onset seizures. *Journal of Neuroscience Nursing, 30,* 161–165.

Mims, J. (1997). Self-esteem, behavior and concerns surrounding epilepsy in siblings of children with epilepsy. *Journal of Child Neurology, 12,* 187–192.

Mitchell, W. G., Scheier, L. M., & Baker, S. A. (1994). Psychosocial, behavioral and medical outcomes in children with epilepsy: A developmental risk factor model using longitudinal data. *Pediatrics, 94,* 471–477.

Pianta, R. C., & Lothman, D. J. (1994). Predicting behavior problems in children with epilepsy: Child factors, disease factors, family stress, and child-mother interaction. *Child Development, 65,* 1415–1428.

Rossi, G., Bonfiglio, S., Veggiotti, P., & Lanz, G. (1997). Epilepsy: A study of adolescence and groups. *Seizure, 6,* 289–296.

Rutter, M., Graham, P., & Yule, W. (1970). A neuropsychiatric study in childhood. *Clinics in Developmental Medicine, 35/36,* 1–265.

Semrud-Clikeman, M., & Wical, B. (1999). Components of attention in children with complex partial seizures with and without ADHD. *Epilepsia, 40,* 211–215.

Shore, C., Austin, J., Musick, B., Dunn, D., McBride, A., & Creasy, K. (1998). Psychosocial care needs of parents of children with new-onset seizures. *Journal of Neuroscience Nursing, 30,* 169–174.

Shumaker, S. A., Moinpour, C. M., Aaronson, N. K., Gand, P.A., Lang., M. H., & Kane, R. L. (1990). Design and implementation issues. In National Institutes of Health (Eds.), *Quality of life assessment: Practice, problems and promise* (pp. 27–45). Washington, D.C.: U.S. Department of Health and Human Services, Public Health Service.

Sikic, N., Buljan-Fander, G., Marcelja, A., & Mejaski-Bosnjak, V. (1995). Personality traits in school children with epilepsy. *Acta Medica Croatica, 49,* 121–126.

Sillanpaa, M., Jalava, M., Kaleva, O., & Shinnar, S. (1998). Long-term prognosis of seizures with onset in childhood. *New England Journal of Medicine, 338,* 1715–1722.

Steffenburg, S., Gillberg, C., & Steffenburg, U. (1996). Psychiatric disorders in children and adolescents with mental retardation and active epilepsy. *Archives of Neurology, 53,* 904–912.

Stores, G., Wiggs, L., & Campling, G. (1998). Sleep disorders and their relationship to psychological disturbance in children with epilepsy. *Child: Care, Health and Development, 24,* 5–19.

Sturniolo, M. G., & Galletti, F. (1994). Idiopathic epilepsy and school achievement. *Archives of Disease in Childhood, 70,* 424–428.

Suurmeijer, T. P. B. M. (1994). Quality of care and quality of life from the perspective of patients and parents. *International Journal of Adolescent Medicine and Health, 7,* 289–302.

Webb, D. W., Coleman, H., Fielder, A., & Kennedy, C. R. (1998). An audit of pediatric epilepsy care. *Archives of Diseases of Childhood, 79,* 145–148.

Weglage, J., Demsky, A., Pietsch, M., & Kurlemann, G. (1997). Neuropsychological, intellectual, and behavioral findings in patients with centrotemporal spikes with and without seizures. *Developmental Medicine and Child Neurology, 39,* 646–651.

Wildrick, D., Parker-Fisher, S., & Morales, A. (1996). Quality of life in children with well-controlled epilepsy. *Journal of Neuroscience Nursing, 28,* 192–198.

Williams, J., Griebel, M. L., & Dykman, R. A. (1998). Neuropsychological patterns in pediatric epilepsy. *Seizure, 7,* 223–228.

Williams, J., Sharp, G. B., Griebel, M. L., Knabe, M. D., Spence, G. T., Weinberger, N., Hendon, A., & Rickert, V. (1995). Outcome findings from a multidisciplinary clinic for children with epilepsy. *Children's Health Care, 24,* 235–244.

Wirrell, E. C., Camfield, C. S., Camfield, P. R., Dooley, J. M., Gordon, K. E., & Smith, B. (1997). Long-term psychosocial outcome in typical absence epilepsy. *Archives of Pediatric and Adolescent Medicine, 151,* 152–158.

# Chapter 3

# Adherence in Chronic Disease

JACQUELINE DUNBAR-JACOB, JUDITH A. ERLEN,
ELIZABETH A. SCHLENK, CHRISTOPHER M. RYAN,
SUSAN M. SEREIKA, AND WILLA M. DOSWELL

## ABSTRACT

Nonadherence to treatment regimen is a prevalent problem of patients with chronic disorders. Approximately half of the patients with a chronic disease have problems following their prescribed regimen to the extent that they are unable to obtain optimum clinical benefit. This chapter reviews the state of knowledge regarding adherence to chronic disease regimens across the life span and demonstrates that the extent and nature of the adherence problems are similar across diseases, across regimens, and across age groups. Adherence to the commonly prescribed regimens is addressed, including pharmacological therapies, therapeutic diets, and therapeutic exercise. Randomized, controlled studies focusing on various educational, behavioral, cognitive, and affective interventions to improve adherence are included. Based on this review, further work is needed to better understand and improve adherence. New strategies for analysis and measurement will support these needed advances in the field of adherence.

**Key words: patient compliance, chronic disease, medications, diet, exercise**

Poor adherence to therapeutic regimen is a pervasive and costly problem in the care of patients with chronic disorders. Estimates are that approximately one-half of patients have adherence problems to the extent that optimum clinical benefit is not obtained. This poses a significant challenge to patient education and to ongoing management of the patient with chronic disease.

This chapter reviews the state of knowledge regarding adherence to chronic disease regimens. The focus is across the life span. Adherence to the commonly prescribed regimens is addressed, including pharmacological therapies, therapeutic diets, and therapeutic exercise. As will be seen, the extent and nature of the adherence problems are similar across diseases, across regimens, and across age groups.

A systematic search strategy was used for this overview of adherence in chronic disorders. The following seven databases were searched from 1995 to 1999, using the terms *compliance, adherence, diet, medication,* and *exercise:* Medline, PsychINFO, International Pharmaceutical Abstracts, Aidsline, CancerLit, CINAHL, and Current Index to Statistics. The search was limited to humans, English language, and references with abstracts. A total of 2,814 abstracts were reviewed to eliminate duplicate references as well as references that were not applicable owing to discussion of adherence to acute conditions or adherence by health care providers to practice guidelines. The authors selected from among the 1,166 remaining references for the review that follows. In addition, classical articles in the area of patient adherence are cited, as are selected recent published abstracts.

## EXTENT OF THE PROBLEM

### Magnitude of Poor Adherence Across Disorders

*Medication Taking.*    Rates of poor adherence to medication are remarkably similar for various chronic disorders; many studies reported nonadherence rates near 50%. Some differences in rates may be seen between settings and measurement methods. For example, nonadherence to a medication regimen for tuberculosis was 69% in a symptomatic HIV cohort (Cosler, Markson, Fanning, & Turner, 1996), 48% in the absence of public health adherence intervention (Pablos-Mendez, Knirsch, Barr, Lerner, & Frieden, 1997), and only 18% in patients receiving outpatient directly observed therapy (Burman et al., 1997). Similarly, adherence rates in clinical trials can exceed those found in clinical settings (Andrade et al., 1995; Atwood et al., 1996; Bergeron et al., 1998; Heinasmaki et al., 1998).

There is some suggestion that persons with life-threatening disorders may adhere somewhat better that others. But in these disorders, for example, AIDS (Flexner et al., 1998; Frick, Gal, Lane, & Sewell, 1998; Kastrissios et al., 1998), cancer (C. R. Lee, Nicholson, Ledermann, & Rustin, 1996), and transplantation (De Geest et al., 1998; Dew, Roth, Thompson, Kormos, & Griffith, 1996; Grady, Jalowiec, & White-Williams, 1998; Hilbrands, Hoitsma, & Koene, 1995; Siegal & Greenstein, 1997), there is a beginning literature to suggest that even moderate alterations have significant clinical impact (Bangsberg, Robertson, et al., 1998; De Geest et al., 1998).

Nonadherence to medication among the more common chronic disorders, however, falls near or significantly below the 50% level. For example,

using electronic monitoring of medication adherence, rates under
50% have been reported for hypertension (J. Y. Lee, Kusek, et al., 1996;
Mounier-Vehier et al., 1998), heart disease (Carney, Freedland, Eisen,
Rich, & Jaffe, 1995; Carney et al., 1998; Cheng, Rozenfeld, Pflomm,
Singh, & Bazil, 1998; Straka, Fish, Benson, & Suh, 1997), asthma (Apter,
Reisine, Affleck, Barrows, & ZuWallack, 1998; Bender, Milgrom, Rand, &
Ackerson, 1998; Berg, Dunbar-Jacob, & Rohay, 1998; Bosley, Fosbury, &
Cochrane, 1995; Gibson, Ferguson, Aitchison, & Paton, 1995), diabetes
mellitus (Mason, Matsuyama, & Jue, 1995), epilepsy (Cramer, Vachon,
Desforges, & Sussman, 1995), ankylosing spondylitis (de Klerk & van der
Linden, 1996), rheumatoid arthritis (Dunbar-Jacob et al., 1995), depres-
sion (Demyttenaere et al., 1998; Hylan, Dunn, Tepner, & Meurgey, 1998),
and schizophrenia (Duncan & Rogers, 1998; Favre, Huguelet, Vogel, &
Gonzalez, 1997; Razali & Yahya, 1997).

*Dietary Adherence.*    Dietary recommendations frequently accompany
medication prescriptions for chronic disorder regimens. Nonadherence
with low-fat, low-cholesterol diets ranges from 15% to 88% (Franklin,
Kolasa, Griffin, Mayo, & Badenhop, 1995; D. L. Katz et al., 1998; Knopp et
al., 1997; Van Horn, Dolecek, Grandits, & Skweres, 1997), whereas nonadherence with weight-reducing diets is greater than 50%, with few persons
maintaining the weight loss (Lyon, Di Vetta, Milon, Jequier, & Schutz,
1995; Wadden, Vogt, Foster, & Anderson, 1998; Wing & Anglin, 1996).

*Exercise Adherence.*    Adherence to therapeutic exercise is also a problem
in chronic disorder populations, with 50% dropping out of exercise during the first 3 to 6 months, leveling off to a dropout rate between 55% and
75% at 12 months (Dew et al., 1996; Ecclestone, Myers, & Paterson, 1998;
J. Y. Lee, Jensen, et al., 1996; Moore, Ruland, Pashkow, & Blackburn, 1998).

*Appointment Keeping.*    Follow-up is a critical component of most chronic
disorder regimens. Yet nonadherence rates for appointment keeping have
ranged from 8.5% to 63.4% (Catz & McClure, 1998; Dooley, Kunik, &
Molinari, 1998; Dyer, Lloyd, Lancashire, Bain, & Barnett, 1998; Frank,
1996; Habib, Sanchez, Pervez, & Devanand, 1998; Ibach, 1995; Ifudu et
al., 1996; Kissinger et al., 1995; Leggat et al., 1998; Nadra, Knight, Lee, &
Meehan, 1995).

*Other Regimens.*    Nonadherence to a variety of other regimens has been
reported in the literature. Rates less than 50% have been reported for neb-
ulizer therapy (Corden, Bosley, Rees, & Cochrane, 1997; J. Turner, Wright,
Mendella, & Anthonisen, 1995), peak flow monitoring (Murata, Kapsner,
Lium, & Busby, 1998), and continuous positive airway pressure (Fleury,
Rakotonanahary, Hausser-Hauw, Lebeau, & Guilleminault, 1996; Weaver

et al., 1997), as well as dialysis (Amici et al., 1996; Bernardini & Piraino, 1998) and sports injury rehabilitation (Taylor & May, 1996).

## Temporal Trends in Adherence

Nonadherence varies over the course of treatment of chronic disorders; problems in adoption of the treatment regimen are fairly significant. There are some data to suggest that as many as 30% of persons fail to fill medication prescriptions (Watts, McLennan, Bassham, & el-Saadi, 1997). Discontinuation of treatment rates are relatively high within the first several months in treatment (Flack, Novikov, & Ferrario, 1996; Jones, Gorden, Lian, Staffa, & Fletcher, 1995; Lin, VonKorff, Katon, & Bush, 1995; Moore et al., 1998). For those who remain on treatment, adherence rates tend to decline for medication (Ailinger & Dear, 1998; Rand, Nides, Cowles, Wise, & Connett, 1995), appointment keeping (Ailinger & Dear, 1998), exercise (Ecclestone et al., 1998), and diet (Lipid Research Clinics Program, 1984a, 1984b; Van Horn et al., 1997), as well as peak flow monitoring (Cote, Cartier, Malo, Rouleau, & Boulet, 1998). In addition to these long-term declines, adherence also has been shown to decline between clinic visits (Cramer, Scheyer, & Mattson, 1990; Simmons, Nides, Rand, Wise, & Tashkin, 1996). For example, Cramer et al., (1990) reported mean adherence rates of 88% at 5 days before the clinic visit, 86% at 5 days after, and 67% during a 5-day period 1 month later.

## Pediatric and Adolescent Populations

The prevalence of adherence problems in pediatric and adolescent populations has been detailed in recent reviews of adherence research over the past decade (Burkhart & Dunbar-Jacob, in press; Rapoff, 1998). Specifically, adherence research in pediatric and adolescent populations over the past 5 years has focused primarily on the chronic disorders of asthma (Eggelston et al., 1998; Van Sciver, D'Angelo, Rappaport, & Woolf, 1995; Wamboldt, Wamboldt, Gavin, & Roesler, 1995), insulin-dependent diabetes mellitus (Gowers, Jones, Kiana, & North, 1995; Kyngas, Hentinen, Koivukangas, & Ohinmaa, 1996; LaGreca et al., 1995; Palardy, Greening, Ott, Holderby, & Atchison, 1998; Schlundt et al., 1996), and immunizations (Lopreiato & Ottolini, 1996; Moore-Caldwell, Werner, Powell, & Greene, 1997; Schlenker, Sukhan, & Swenson, 1998).

To a lesser extent some studies have examined contraceptive use (Brill, 1997; Harel, Biro, Kollar, & Rauh, 1996; Rainey, Parsons, Kenney, & Krowchuk, 1995), adherence with psychiatric therapy (King, Hovey, Brand, & Gooziuddin, 1997; Piacentini et al., 1995; Rotheram-Borus et al., 1996), sickle cell disease (Berkovitch et al., 1998; Olivieri & Vichinsky, 1998), and rheumatoid arthritis (Gallo & Knafl, 1998; Thompson, Dahlquist, Koenning, & Bartholomew, 1995). It is fair to say that the adherence rates among children and adolescents are no better than those seen in adults.

## Summary

Thus, the rates of poor adherence in chronic disorders are of a significant magnitude, with fewer than half of patients following their treatments adequately. This is the case for both pediatric and adult populations and is consistent across diseases and regimen. Dropout rates are high early in treatment, whereas poor adherence rates tend to increase with time on treatment. Thus, attention must be directed toward both the adoption of treatment and long-term maintenance.

# IMPACT OF POOR ADHERENCE

## Costs of Poor Adherence

Estimates of the costs of poor adherence to pharmacological regimen are as high as $100 billion annually (Lewis, 1997). These costs are based on, among other factors, unnecessary hospitalizations and emergency room visits. Unclaimed prescriptions are one reason for hospital and emergency room admissions (Achusim, Caselnova, & Cosgrove, 1998; Agi et al., 1996). Over half of hospital admissions (Nelson & Talbert, 1996), drug related visits to the emergency room (Toh, Low, & Goh, 1998), and asthma ER visits (Schmaling, Afari, & Blume, 1998) have been found to be related to nonadherence to medication. Conversely, patients who do adhere to treatment have demonstrated fewer emergency visits (Laumann & Bjornson, 1997), fewer psychiatric hospitalizations (Conte, Ferrari, Guarneri, Calzeroni, & Sacchetti, 1996; Daley, Salloum, Zuckoff, Kirisci, & Thase, 1998) and hospitalization days (DeProspero & Riffle, 1997), fewer health care services used (Bentsen, Lindgarde, & Manthorpe, 1997), and less sick leave (Bentsen et al., 1997).

## Clinical Outcome and Poor Adherence

An association exists between poor adherence and multiple adverse clinical outcomes. Research with ambulatory care patients treated for hypertensive urgencies or emergencies showed that two-thirds were nonadherent with medications (Adarmes & Sunahara, 1997). Other studies of patients with hypertension also show that nonadherence to antihypertensive medications is related to blood pressure control (Morrell, Park, Kidder, & Martin, 1997). Patients who adhered to a program of nondrug therapies, including diet, exercise, and weight control, were able to use these means to help control their hypertension (Gearhart, Stowers, & Hope, 1997).

Much of the work on adverse outcomes and patients with AIDS has not been published; however, abstracts of papers presented at recent meetings report that nonadherence to highly active antiretroviral therapy (HAART) leads to failed therapy and a worsening of viral load due to nonadherence (Abel, Sobesky, Cabie, Conlan-Nayaud, & Durocher, 1998; Acurcio & Guimares, 1998; Esch, Shelton, Esch, Morse, & Hewitt, 1998; Vanhove, Schapiro, Winters, Merigan, & Blaschke, 1996; Woodward, Wareham, Grohskopf, Madigan, & Hooton, 1998). When HAART is initiated early and there is good adherence, there is a virologic benefit and a low rate of drug resistance (Bangsberg, Zolopa, et al., 1998; Hecht, Colfax, Swanson, & Chesney, 1998).

Adherence to diabetic regimen continues to receive attention. This research shows that diabetic patients who are more adherent with blood glucose monitoring (Anderson, Ho, Brackett, Finkelstein, & Laffel, 1997) and with insulin doses (Morris et al., 1997) have better diabetes control.

Studies among transplant populations show that nonadherence accounts for as many as 25% of failed grafts (Schweizer et al., 1990). In the heart transplant population in particular, even modest failures at regular adherence have been shown to contribute to adverse outcomes (De Geest et al., 1998).

The findings of studies addressing the impact of adherence in patients who have chronic mental illnesses are not unlike the findings of studies using patients with chronic physical illnesses. Patients with schizophrenia who do not take neuroleptic drugs as prescribed are more likely to have an exacerbation and require hospitalization (Ayuso-Gutierrez & del Rio Vega, 1997). Discontinuing antidepressant medications greatly increased the risk of relapse of depression in adults with this diagnosis (Melfi et al., 1998), and discontinuing lithium was associated with increased suicide in a group of 100 persons who were placed on lithium following a suicide attempt (Bocchetta et al., 1998). Homebound mentally ill who were adherent to follow-up with a primary care physician or a psychiatrist showed significantly greater improvement (Habib et al., 1998). Drug abstinence has been found to be positively associated with consistent attendance at an outpatient perinatal addiction program (Nardi, 1997).

Adherence to nonpharmacological interventions contributes to improved outcomes. Adherence to diet has shown better outcomes for children with phenylketonuria (Agostoni et al., 1998), persons at risk for cardiovascular disease (Metz et al., 1997), overweight women (Lyon et al., 1995), and men and women with hypercholesterolemia (M. H. Davidson, Kong, Drennan, Story, & Anderson, 1996; Geil, Anderson, & Gustafson, 1995). Interestingly, patients in India with or at risk for coronary artery disease, who adhered to both dietary and exercise recommendations, were found to have a greater reduction in obesity, cardiac events, and mortality, compared with those who were advised only to follow a fat-modified diet (Singh, Rastogi, Rastogi, Niaz, & Beegom, 1996).

Studies examining the effects of exercise on clinical outcomes show that there is improved sensorimotor function in elderly women who exercise and potentially a reduction in the frequency of falls (Lord, Ward, Williams, & Strundwick, 1995). Shumway-Cook et al. (Shumway-Cook, Gruber, Baldwin, & Liao, 1997) found improved balance and mobility and a greater reduction in fall risk to be associated with exercise in community-dwelling elderly who had a history of falling. Women had a lowering of their blood pressure when they participated in a lower intensity exercise program (Cox et al., 1996). Those adults who were high adherers to an exercise program were found to have a more significant reduction in systolic blood pressure than did low adherers (Taylor, Doust, & Webborn, 1998). Nonadherence with peritoneal dialysis was found to contribute to increased risk for peritonitis, hospitalization (Bernardini & Piraino, 1998), anemia (Ifudu et al., 1996), and graft loss posttransplantation (Douglas, Blixen, & Bartucci, 1996).

## Quality of Life and Poor Adherence

Researchers are beginning to examine the association between adherence and quality of life. Improved therapies that have increased the lifespan have heightened the interest in quality of life. Quality of life is considered a significant and desirable outcome for persons with chronic disorders, where the goals of treatment often are to prevent or retard disease progression and maintain function. Quality of life may reinforce adherence through the increased efficacy of treatment but also may impair adherence when side effects and a complex regimen accompany treatment. Indeed, the limited research in this area supports both positive (Baier, Murray, North, Lato, & Eskew, 1996; Corden et al., 1997; Erlen & Mellors, 1999; Jeng & Braun, 1997; Meslier et al., 1998) and negative (Hallert et al., 1998) effects of adherence on quality of life. Studies finding no effect have been reported as well (Erikson, Slaughter, & Halapy, 1997; R. C. Katz et al., 1998; N. Singh et al., 1996).

The research that has been conducted in this area has focused on adults. Few data are available on children and adolescents. And indeed, few measures are available to assess quality of life in youth.

In the limited number of studies reported in the literature, quality of life is defined and measured in various ways. These definitions lead to difficulties in making comparisons across studies. However, quality of life should be considered in efforts to improve adherence (Hedge & Petrak, 1998).

## Summary

Poor adherence has a substantial impact on costs in the health care arena, on clinical outcomes, and on quality of life. Regardless of the patient population, research examining the association between adherence and outcomes generally shows improved clinical outcomes and reduced cost with greater adherence. The data for quality of life are more variable. Despite the amount of work that has been done in this area, further research is needed to address ways to increase adherence to diet, exercise, and medication regimens in order to sustain the positive outcomes of treatment.

## PREDICTORS OF POOR ADHERENCE

Given the magnitude of the problem of poor adherence and the significance of its impact, there is considerable interest in identifying individuals at risk for poor adherence, with the objective of designing preventive strategies. Earlier studies emphasized theory-based investigations (e.g., Health Belief Model, Theory of Reasoned Action, and other such motivational models). More recent studies have tended to be empirically based.

### Regimen Management

The most commonly reported reason for poor adherence, particularly to medication regimen, is "forgetting" (Arabe et al., 1998; Chang, Chan, Chan, Raymond, & Critchley, 1998; Cline, Foster, Lee, & Pait, 1998; Conway, Pond, Hamnett, & Watson, 1996; Gir, Pratt, Bunch, & Holzemer, 1998; Hales, Mitchell, Smith, & Kippex, 1998; Khalil & Elzubier, 1997; Lorenzen et al., 1998; Simon, Morse, & Besch, 1995). Conflicts with the usual routine also play a significant role (Besch, Morse, Simon, Hodges, & Franchino, 1997; Gifford, Shively, Bormann, Timberlake, & Bozzette, 1998; Hales et al., 1998; Simon et al., 1995). Difficulties with the regimen itself also pose problems (Battegay et al., 1998; Chizzola, Mansur, da Luz, & Bellotti, 1996; Gallant & Block, 1998; Lloyd, Paisley, & Mela, 1995; Swift, Armstrong, Campbell, Beerman, & Pond-Smith, 1997).

### Cognitive Motivation

A variety of motivational constructs have also been examined in light of adherence. The personal model of illness (Glasgow, Hampson, Strycker, & Ruggiero, 1997), perceived benefits of treatment (Aversa & Kimberlin, 1996; Balestra et al., 1996; Buck, Jacoby, Baker, & Chadwick, 1997; Caserta & Gillett, 1998; Muma, Ross, Parcel, & Pollard, 1995; Siegal & Greenstein, 1997), and negative response to the medications (Agarwal, Sharma, Kumar, & Lowe, 1998; Johnston, Ahmad, Smith, & Rose, 1998; M. Y. Smith, Rapkin, Morrison, & Kammerman, 1997) have been associated with adherence. Self-efficacy has been investigated as well, with varying results. Both positive relationships (Granlund, Brulin, Johansson, & Sojka, 1998; Hellman, 1997; Skelly, Marshall, Haughey, Davis, & Dunford, 1995;

Taylor & May, 1996) and the absence of relationships (Barlow, 1998; Demyttenaere et al., 1998) have been reported.

## Symptoms

Side effects have contributed to stopping treatment (Ash, Chen, & Dolkhani, 1998; Berman, Epstein, & Lydick, 1997; Silva et al., 1996), and positive benefits have been associated with good adherence (Carr, Smith, Pryor, & Partridge, 1996; Engleman et al., 1996).

## Social Support

Support and communication also appear to play a role in adherence. Direct involvement in the regimen (Anderson et al., 1997) has been important in pediatrics and in tuberculosis care. General family support has been important in some studies (Brown et al., 1998; Courneya & McAuley, 1995; Garay-Sevilla et al., 1995) though not in all (Moran, Christensen, & Lawton, 1998). The nature of the patient-provider interaction also seems to be important (Apter et al., 1998; Cecil, 1998; Cecil & Killeen, 1997; Harris, Luft, Rudy, & Tierney, 1995).

## Personal Characteristics

In addition, personal characteristics may be important, although the data are less strong. Stress (Stetson, Rahn, Dubbert, Wilner, & Mercury, 1997), depression (Carney et al., 1995; N. Singh et al., 1996; Spiers & Kutzik, 1995; Williams & Lord, 1995), and conscientiousness (Christensen & Smith, 1995; Wiebe & Christensen, 1997) have been linked to adherence.

## Summary

Multiple factors have an impact on adherence. The variations in populations, regimen, and measures make the identification of any robust predictor difficult. Indeed, a further complication is that recent work has found that different predictors of adherence are identified in the same population at the same time when different adherence measures are used (Dunbar-Jacob, Sereika, Rohay, & Burke, 1998).

# COGNITIVE FUNCTION

Adherence to medical regimens is a cognitively demanding task, yet most discussions of adherence completely overlook the potentially important role played by cognitive processes. To fully understand instructions for taking medications, patients must pay attention to the health professional, encode or learn the treatment plan so that it can be recalled accurately from long-term memory at a later time, and integrate this new regimen into their already scheduled daily activities. Yet understanding what *ought* to be done is not enough. Patients must actually follow the regimen prospectively and remember that, at some time in the near future, a specific dose must be taken—often under certain conditions (e.g., with milk or on an empty stomach). They also must be able to monitor their own adherence behavior over the course of a day by updating "working memory" efficiently and thereby remembering, for example, that they already took their big blue pill in the morning, but did not take the little clear pill.

Given these types of cognitive demands, one would expect to find that patients who have difficulty paying attention, comprehending verbal instructions, or remembering also ought to be less adherent than their cognitively intact peers. As a corollary, one also would predict that cognitively impaired patients who are provided with external environmental supports (or "cognitive prostheses") that facilitate comprehension or improve memory ought to manifest a corresponding improvement in adherence behaviors.

Two recent studies have explicitly tested the hypothesis that medication-taking behaviors in medically ill patients are influenced by their cognitive abilities. In the first of these, Morrell and his associates (1997) evaluated 48 adults, 36 to 87 years of age, who were diagnosed with hypertension. Bar-code scanners were used to track medication-taking behaviors over a 2-month period, and cognitive function was assessed with a test of working memory and with a vocabulary knowledge test. Contrary to expectation, there was no relationship between patients' nonadherence and performance on either cognitive test. Although it is tempting to speculate that these null results reflect limited statistical power, it may be more reasonable to conclude that the hypothesis was never adequately tested because of the use of limited and insensitive cognitive assessment measures.

A second study, conducted with 121 patients with rheumatoid arthritis, assessed cognitive functioning with a more extensive battery and measured adherence with microelectronic monitoring techniques system (MEMS) (Park et al., 1999). Subjects completed questionnaires on health and physical functioning, beliefs about their illness and medications, and lifestyle (including "busyness") and also were evaluated with cognitive tests assessing working memory, long-term memory, speed of information processing, text comprehension, reasoning, and vocabulary. Most of these measures had been developed in the cognitive psychology laboratory to evaluate specific cognitive processes; none had been designed to identify people with clinically significant cognitive impairments.

Although the investigators found (as expected) a significant age-related decline in cognitive performance, they did not find a corresponding age-related decline in adherence behaviors. Rather, older patients (55 to 84 years of age) were more likely to be perfectly adherent, compared to patients 34 to 54 years of age (47% vs. 28%, respectively). Further, the researchers found no evidence that older patients or those with poorer cognitive test scores were more likely to rely on external prostheses (e.g., pillbox organizers, use of reminder notes, etc). That is, contrary to their hypothesis, Park et al. (1999) did not find a striking relationship between adherence behavior and cognitive abilities—measured either directly, with cognitive tests, or inferred from patients' use of environmental supports.

One possible reason for these negative findings is that age may be serving as a suppressor variable that serves, statistically, to mask the relationship between cognitive function and adherence. Although older adults ordinarily show a decline in cognitive function, it is also true that older adults are more vigilant about health issues than are younger adults (Leventhal & Crouch, 1997; Leventhal, Leventhal, Schaefer, & Easterling, 1993) and that this vigilance may lead to better adherence. To control statistically for age-associated variance in cognitive function, Park and her associates (1999) used structural equation modeling techniques and found a direct relationship between cognitive function and nonadherence. Despite this empirical support for their hypothesis that lower cognitive function may contribute somewhat to poorer adherence, the extensive statistical legerdemain needed to demonstrate such a relationship suggests either that these associations are clinically inconsequential, that the assessment of cognitive function is inadequate, or that the measures of adherence are weak (Cuffel, Alford, Fischer, & Owen, 1996; Incalzi, Gemma, Marra, Capparella, Fuso, & Carbonin, 1997; Kemp & David, 1996; McKee, Hull, & Smith, 1997; Rost, Roter, Quill, Bertakis, & Collaborative Study Group, 1990).

The potential role of cognitive function in adherence is enticing. Yet studies to date are fraught with methodological flaws. Clearly, investigation of this potential predictor, which lends itself to compensatory strategies, is recommended, using methodologically and theoretically sound approaches.

## PREDICTORS OF ADHERENCE IN CHILDREN AND YOUTH

Research on the predictors of adherence, from a developmental perspective, has focused primarily on the adult and older adult, with a limited examination of the pediatric and adolescent populations. Where the younger populations have been examined, developmental predictors have rarely been addressed. Such issues of developmental level, cognitive ability, ability to conduct self-management regimens, peer and cultural contextual influences, and other potentially relevant factors have been discussed but rarely examined.

Psychosocial factors, such as attention, motivation, and self-esteem, that have been associated with poor adherence have been enumerated in detail in earlier reviews of adherence literature (Rapoff, 1998). Disintegrated family structure and functioning also have been associated with poor adherence in children and adolescents with chronic disorders (Hanson, DeGuire, Schinkel, & Kolterman, 1995; Pollock, Kovacs, & Charron-Prochownik, 1995; Schreiber, Effgen, & Palisano, 1995; Wamboldt et al., 1995).

Although the linkage is not persuasive, some research has examined knowledge, attitudes, and health beliefs with poor patient adherence (Anderson et al., 1997; Bastiaens, 1995; Bender et al., 1998; Holmbeck et al., 1998; Kyngas, Hentinen, & Barlow, 1998; Moore-Caldwell et al., 1997). Parental monitoring also has been identified as a positive factor influencing adherence (Alperstein, Morgan, Mills, & Daniels, 1998; Higa, Chan, Bass, & Alfaro, 1997; King et al., 1997).

Disease factors play a role in adherence with therapeutic regimens and interventions in pediatric and adolescent populations, as well as complexity in treatment regimens (Urban et al., 1997; Watson, Farley, Lovelace, & Vink, 1998), side effects of treatments (Polaneczky & Liblanc, 1998), and taste of medications and administration route (Gross, Burr, Storm, Czarniecki, & D'Orlando, 1998; Higa et al., 1997).

The limited investigations of predictors of adherence from a developmental perspective in pediatrics suggest the need for further study. The role of the family as well as the developmental capabilities of the child are of major importance in this group.

## INTERVENTION STRATEGIES TO PROMOTE IMPROVED ADHERENCE

Although there is a voluminous literature on adherence to treatment, very little research has examined strategies to promote adherence. When one examines the proportion of those studies that have been randomized, controlled studies, the number decreases even further. There are fewer still that have measured both adherence and its impact on clinical outcomes or have followed the study subjects to determine the duration of intervention effects. This section reviews the literature on adherence interventions, focusing on those that have used a randomized, controlled design.

A recent metanalysis of 153 studies published between 1977 and 1994 that synthesizes the literature examining the effectiveness of interventions to improve adherence is of significance (Roter et al., 1998). This metanalysis included 116 randomized trials addressing both acute and chronic disorders. Regardless of the adherence measure used, the interventions yielded mean effect sizes ranging from small to large that were highly significant. An examination of the focus of the intervention (educational, behavioral, affective, or some combination) showed that a combined focus resulted in larger effects than did the single-focus interventions. These researchers pointed out that intervention studies examining adherence should include additional outcomes, such as quality of life, patient satisfaction, understanding, and functional status in order to have a more comprehensive picture of adherence.

This review of current research uses the classification scheme for intervention strategies described by Roter et al. (1998). Educational interventions include written and/or verbal instructions delivered individually, in a group, or by telephone, as well as the use of audiovisual material. Behavioral strategies include the use of incentives, tailoring, reminders, modeling, contracting, and skill building. Affective approaches used social supports, counseling, and home visits as a means to appeal to feelings and emotions. Combined strategies included any combination of the three broad intervention classifications. The studies that are included in this review focus on medication, diet, and exercise adherence, as well as appointment keeping.

Studies examining the effect of an educational intervention to enhance medication adherence demonstrated variable results. Research using educational interventions with patients with asthma demonstrated a positive effect on medication adherence (Holzheimer, Mohay, & Masters, 1998), partial adherence (van der Palen, Klein, & Rovers, 1997), and no differences between groups (M. O. Turner, Taylor, Bennett, & Fitzgerald, 1998). Powell and Edgren (1995), finding no differences in medication adherence ratio between the control and any of the treatment groups, concluded that the mailing of a videotape did not improve adherence.

Direct observation was found to have less effect (Zwarenstein, Schoeman, Vundule, Lombard, & Tatley, 1998) and a greater effect (B. L. Davidson, 1998) than self-management in patients with tuberculosis. Self-management improved adherence to asthma medications (Berg, Dunbar-Jacob, & Sereika, 1997), whereas supervised therapy and dispensing zidovudine improved adherence in HIV-infected patients (Wall et al., 1995). Counseling had an enhancing effect on medication adherence (Cheng et al., 1998; Goodyer, Miskelly, & Milligan, 1995), as well as a limited effect on adherence (Williford & Johnson, 1995). Integrating a computer-controlled telephone system with usual care increased adherence to antihypertensive medication (Friedman, Furberg, & Demets, 1996).

Combined approaches sustained improved adherence to medication regimen (Kemp, Hayward, Applewhaite, Everitt, & David, 1996) and showed variable rates of adherence over time (Berkovitch et al., 1998). Use of multiple strategies improved medication adherence (Azrin & Teichner, 1998; Katon et al., 1995; Knobel et al., 1998; Rich, Gray, Beckham, Wittenberg, & Luther, 1996), and improved overall functioning (Clarkin,

Carpenter, Hull, Wilner, & Glick, 1998), but also had no effect on adherence (Wadibia, Lucas, Stading, Hilleman, & Mohiuddin, 1995).

Researchers addressing exercise adherence found that educational strategies increased adherence to physical exercise (Jakicic, Wing, Butler, & Robertson, 1995; Schneiders, Zusman, & Singer, 1998) and improved joint protection and energy conservation in patients with rheumatoid arthritis (Brus, van de Laar, Taal, Rasker, & Wiegman, 1998). Patients assigned to a fitness center had a greater exercise adherence rate than those in a home training program (Bentsen et al. 1997). Sustained effects on exercise participation in 49 obese women were demonstrated with a home exercise program instead of group intervention (Perri et al., 1997). Patients with low back pain assigned to an exercise and motivation program were more likely to attend exercise appointments at the 4-month follow-up than were controls who received only the exercise program. However, there were no sustaining effects at 12 months (Friedrich, Gittler, Halberstadt, Cermak, & Heiller, 1998).

Researchers studying overweight subjects in a behavioral weight loss program found that neither the use of a personal trainer nor a lottery incentive improved adherence over the control subjects (Jeffery, Wing, Thorson, & Burton, 1998; Wing, Jeffery, Pronk, & Hellerstedt, 1996). Subjects with musculoskeletal pain who received the addition of a cognitive-behavioral technique to enhance exercise adherence had greater adherence and exercised more; however, there was no reduction in pain (Linton, Hellsing, & Bergstroem, 1996).

Behavioral interventions have been tested for their effects on dietary adherence. Toobert and colleagues (Toobert, Glasgow, Nettekoven, & Brown, 1998) found that the PrimeTime comprehensive lifestyle management program for postmenopausal women with coronary heart disease (CHD) yielded significant changes in both short-term (4 months) and long-term (12 months) adherence to diet, as well as to exercise and stress management. Other researchers, studying healthy premenopausal women to determine if a dietary and behavioral intervention can prevent elevations in risk factors for CHD as women reach menopause, found that short-term results (6 months) showed significant increases in exercise and significant reductions in CHD risk factors (Simkin-Silverman et al., 1995).

Telephone counseling was determined to enhance a dietary intervention designed to increase fruits and vegetables and lower fat in the diet in a sample of breast cancer survivors (Pierce et al., 1997). Using a sample of 560 men and women with cardiac risk factors, McCarron et al. (1997) examined the effects of the Campbell's Center for Nutrition and Wellness (CCNW) plan compared to the American Heart Association Step I and Step II diet. While patient outcomes improved on both plans, subjects in the CCNW plan had significantly better dietary adherence and clinical outcomes. Comparing both a home-based (HB) and a clinic-based (CB) program with a control group to prevent weight gain in sedentary men aged 25–40, Leermarkers, Jakicic, Viteri, and Wing (1998) found that both the HB and the CB programs achieved similar outcomes.

Testing interventions to enable appointment keeping was a health concern addressed by many researchers. Telephone call and mail reminders had variable degrees of success. For example, significant positive effects were found with adolescents (O'Brien & Lazebnik, 1998), adults at risk for sexually transmitted diseases (Martin, 1998), substance abusers (Gariti et al., 1995), and children seen in an emergency room (Komoroski, Graham, & Kirby, 1996). Researchers found that mailed postcards (Ahluwalia, McNagny, & Kanvru, 1996) and mail and telephone reminders (Keder, Rulin, & Gruss, 1998) made no difference in adherence to appointments.

Interventions also have addressed compensatory strategies for cognitive dysfunction, particularly the memory disorders that may affect older adults. Morrow and his colleagues demonstrated that comprehension and recall of medication information was facilitated significantly when drug-taking instructions were explicit (Morrow, Leirer, & Altieri, 1995) and highly organized (Morrow, Leirer, Andrassy, Hier, & Menard, 1998), when pictorial icons were used to supplement written medication instructions (Morrow, Hier, Menard, & Leirer, 1998), and when these instructions were consistent with elders' internal schemas (i.e., mental representations of how they ordinarily take medications and handle problems like missed doses) (Morrow, Leirer, Altieri, & Tanke, 1991). Individual differences in cognitive ability played a most important role, as demonstrated by data showing that the facilitative effect of schema-compatible instructions on recall was enhanced by subjects' verbal ability (i.e., vocabulary scores) (Morrow, Leirer, Andrassy, Tanke, & Stine-Morrow, 1996). Not all prostheses are beneficial, however. Morrell and associates (1997) reported that older adults' comprehension of prescription information may be hampered, rather than facilitated, by certain types of pictorial stimuli, and they noted that this was most likely to occur when the use of pictograms increased (rather than decreased) cognitive processing by requiring the patient to draw inferences (e.g., interpreting a milk carton on a label as indicating that the pills should be taken with milk).

External devices certainly help older adults comprehend and recall medication information. Do they actually improve adherence behaviors? Research studies have demonstrated that they may—but only under certain conditions. Measuring medication-taking behavior directly by having subjects record each drug dosing electronically with the Videx Time Wand bar-code reader, Park, Morrell, Frieske, and Kincaid (1992) found that old-old adults (i.e., over the age of 70) showed better adherence when they were given two types of external organizers (*both* a 1-week medication organizer pillbox and an hour-by-hour chart of their medication regimen). In contrast, those given only one type of organizer showed no improvement in their medication-taking behavior when compared to subjects given none.

Focusing on memory, rather than comprehension, Leirer and associates (Leirer, Morrow, Tanke, & Pariante, 1991) examined the effects of voice mail reminders on adherence behaviors in a group of pseudopatients. Those who received personalized voice messages every time they were scheduled to take a pill showed significantly less nonadherence over a 14-day period (2.1%), as measured with portable bar code readers, compared to control subjects who received no reminders (14.2%).

### Summary

Educational, behavioral, cognitive, affective interventions to enhance adherence have been studied with persons with various chronic disorders. These studies have produced mixed results. Further work is needed, using carefully designed and theoretically based interventions. Work also is needed to determine the sustaining effects of adherence-promoting strategies. Researchers should investigate the use of maintenance programs and the use of boosters to sustain adherence.

## MEASUREMENT OF ADHERENCE

The estimation of the magnitude of adherence, the identification of impact and of predictors, as well as the evaluation of interventions, are all dependent on adequate measurement of adherence. Historically, the primary measure in both children and adults across regimen has been self-report. This has taken various forms, including interviews, structured questionnaires (e.g., Connor et al., 1992; Morisky, Green, & Levine, 1986; Paffenbarger, Wing, & Hyde, 1978; Shea, Misra, Ehrlich, Field, & Francis, 1992; Willet, Sampson, & Stampfer, 1985), and daily diaries (Berg et al., 1998; Buzzard et al., 1996; Van Horn et al., 1997). Adherence is generally overestimated by these strategies (Sereika et al., 1998; Wagner, Schnoll, & Gipson, 1998). The tendency is for self-report to overestimate adherence (Bender et al., 1998; Burney, Krishnan, Ruffin, Zhang, & Brenner, 1996; Straka et al., 1997).

Pharmacy records offer another source of adherence data. These records have been shown to approximate electronic assessment, with a tendency to overestimate adherence (Frick et al., 1998). However, they have been considered adequate (Gregoire, Guilbert, Archambault, & Contandriopoulos, 1997) if an adequate exposure time window is used (Lau, de Boer, Beuning, & Porsius, 1997). Pill counts also have underestimated adherence (Mason et al., 1995), and data suggest that canister weights may underestimate overuse (Rand et al., 1995).

A variety of biochemical measures of adherence have been used. Included in these are markers (Del Boca, Kranzler, Brown, & Korner, 1996; Shine & McDonald, 1997; Switzer et al., 1997; Thilothammal, Krishnamurthy, Banu, & Gandhimathy, 1995; Tynan et al., 1995) for both dietary and pharmacological treatments. Blood levels (Elizaga & Friedland, 1997; Gomes, Filho, & Noe, 1998), saliva levels (Hugen et al., 1998), drug metabolites (Lennard, Welch, & Lilleyman, 1995), and hair samples (Tracqui, Kintz, & Mangin, 1995; Williams, Patsalos, & Wilson, 1997) have been used to assess drug adherence with varying degrees of utility. These methods do not offer a sensitive measurer of daily variations in adherence nor of overall levels of adherence.

Perhaps the most accepted measure of adherence is the use of electronic monitoring. Such methods are available for medication (Detry, Block, DeBacker, & Degaute, 1995; Fallab-Stubi et al., 1998; J. Y. Lee, Kusek, et al., 1996), inhaled medication (Bender et al., 1998; Gonda et al., 1998), peak flow monitoring (Cote et al., 1998), exercise (Matthews & Freedson, 1995), and patch contact (Fielder et al., 1995), with palm-top diaries for diary assessment (Shiffman & Stone, 1998). These monitors use microprocessor technology to record and store timed adherence events. Data can be downloaded to a desktop computer for review and analysis.

## ANALYSES OF ADHERENCE DATA

For the investigator interested in studying adherence, attention should be given to analysis issues. Adherence data present a unique challenge. Nonadherence to a regimen can lead to the underreporting of both therapeutic and adverse effects and can seriously undermine even the best-designed study (Feinstein, 1974; Goldsmith, 1979). Since such protocol deviations may affect the evaluation of treatment efficacy (i.e., whether a treatment biologically reduces or increases the occurrence of a desired outcome), the monitoring of patient adherence has become increasingly commonplace in experimental studies, and adherence information has become essential to the interpretation of findings (Freedman, 1990). Research efforts have been made to limit the impact of adherence in the design phase when estimating sample size (Halperin, Rogot, Gurian, & Ederer, 1968; Lachin, 1981; Lachin & Foulkes, 1986; Palta & McHugh, 1980; Schork & Remington, 1967) and selecting subjects (Lang, 1990; Probstfield, 1991). Because perfect adherence is nearly impossible, statisticians and researchers alike, especially in the clinical trials community, have considered patient adherence in a dual role in data analysis, treated as both the *outcome* of interest (Dunbar-Jacob et al., 1995; L. M. Friedman et al., 1996; Pocock, 1983) and as an important *explanatory variable* (Efron & Feldman, 1991; Oakes et al., 1993).

## Use of Adherence Information in the Design Stage

The presence of treatment nonadherence (i.e., partial adherers, drop-ins, or dropouts) may result in a loss of precision and power when estimation and hypothesis testing of treatment efficacy are of interest (Feinstein, 1974). Several methods have been proposed to limit the impact of nonadherence on assessing treatment efficacy, such as the inflation of sample size when designing a study and prerandomization run-ins when selecting subjects for participation. To compensate for the potential loss in power or precision due to nonadherence, Lachin (1981) presents a simple multiplier that inflates sample sizes to account for dropouts that can be generalized to consider drop-ins as well (L. M. Friedman et al., 1996). More elaborate model-based approaches also have been proposed that take into consideration not only the impact of nonadherence on the efficacy estimates but also the time to maximum treatment effectiveness (Halperin et al., 1968; Lachin, 1981; Lakatos, 1986; Newcombe, 1988; Palta & McHugh, 1980; Schork & Remington, 1967; Wu, Fisher, & DeMets, 1980).

The use of run-ins prior to randomization has been suggested as a means of enhancing treatment adherence during the conduct of treatment efficacy studies (Lang, 1990; Probstfield, 1991). The belief is that the adherence behavior exhibited during a prerandomization run-in is a reasonable proxy for the behavior witnessed during postrandomization (Lang, 1990). Subjects are then selected for participation on the basis of their run-in adherence, with those demonstrating poor adherence to selected components of the treatment protocol being screened from later participation (Probstfield, 1991). Lang and Probstfield caution that careful consideration be given for the inclusion of an adherence run-in as the net benefit in enhanced treatment, where adherence may be minimal due to limitations and problems related to recruitment, utility, cost, and generalizability. Davis et al. (Davis, Applegate, Gordon, Curtis, & McCormick, 1995) empirically evaluated the effectiveness of a prerandomization placebo run-in and found that the exclusion of subjects with poor run-in adherence had little impact on adherence and outcome assessments but would lead to recruitment difficulties and possible sampling bias. Furthermore, there may be misclassification of patients on the basis of information collected during the run-in (Brittain & Wittes, 1990; Davis, 1998), further limiting the desired gain in statistical power.

### The Analysis of Adherence as an Outcome

Adherence has often been viewed as the response of interest, as when evaluating the feasibility of protocol specifications in treatment effectiveness studies (L. M. Friedman et al., 1996; Pocock, 1983) and when assessing the impact of adherence-enhancing interventions (Dunbar-Jacob et al., 1995). To achieve these ends, research endeavors have focused on describing and quantifying adherence. Unfortunately, the analysis of adherence often has been greatly limited by the method of adherence measurement and frequency of assessment.

Early efforts toward quantifying adherence involved reporting dropout rates, comparison of dropout rates across groups, and analysis of time until dropout (E. O. Smith et al., 1980). More recent endeavors have tried to account more fully for a subject's adherence history over the full study period and have utilized various measures of adherence when modeling. E. O. Smith and colleagues modeled the transitions from active to inactive study participation based on clinic visits, using a two-compartment regression model, which allows for the simultaneous identification of subject factors related to transitions. Lim (1992) utilized a random-effects model (Laird & Ware, 1982) to obtain estimates of adherence based on serum drug levels of zidovudine in AIDS patients by incorporating accessory information on the properties of serum assays for and pharmacokinetic behavior of zidovudine when modeling. Kim and Lagakos (1994, 1996) proposed two analytic strategies for estimating nonadherence to AZT, based on the longitudinal data of laboratory markers, using a modified change-point approach to estimate the time of drug initiation (Kim & Lagakos, 1994). Kim and Lagakos (1996) later proposed using these estimated initiation times to then estimate the times to nonadherence.

With the advent of electronic monitoring technology (Cramer, Mattson, Prevey, Scheyer, & Ouellette, 1989; Kruse & Weber, 1990; Urquhart, 1990), the measurement of patient adherence to oral and inhaled medications has become even more precise, generating a wealth of information that yields an indirect objective assessment of adherence in real time. Recent efforts have been made to analyze adherence information by electronic event monitoring (Girard, Blaschke, Kastrissios, & Sheiner, 1998; Rohay, Dunbar-Jacob, Sereika, Kwoh, & Burke, 1996; Rohay, Marsh, Sereika, Mazumdar, & Dunbar-Jacob, 1994; D. Smith & Diggle, 1998; Vrijens & Goetghebeur, 1997). Several studies have investigated the impact of the aggregation of adherence data and method of summarization (Rohay et al., 1994, 1996; Vrijens & Goetghebeur, 1997). Their results indicated that summary measures that account for the relative timing of doses tend to be more informative than measures that consider only the number of daily doses. Nevertheless, Rohay et al. (1996) and Vrijens and Goetghebeur (1997) concluded that the summarization of data may lead to a substantial loss of information on adherence patterns over time and a subsequent loss of power when investigating time effects for adherence.

To capture information regarding temporal adherence patterns, researchers have begun to consider longitudinal data analytic methods (Girard et al., 1998; D. Smith & Diggle, 1998; Vrijens & Goetghebeur, 1997). Vrijens and Goetghebeur (1997) fitted models to binary adherence data of a once-daily regimen of antihypertensive medication to test for differences in adherence between subjects randomized to home blood pressure monitoring compared to no monitoring. Using a conditional model, Vrijens and Goetghebeur showed that current adherence behavior was dependent on past adherence behavior and treatment assignment. Vrijens and Goetghebeur also used marginal modeling with generalized estimating equations (Liang & Zeger, 1986) to better depict the effect of randomized assignment. A limitation to this approach is that it cannot handle longtime series of repeated measurements. To address this limitation, D. Smith and Diggle (1998) modeled binary adherence data showing that a subject's likelihood to adhere at any given time is governed by an underlying latent, stationary, and continuous process and time-dependent covariates.

## Impact of Nonadherence on Treatment Efficacy

Nonadherence also has been considered as an explanatory variable when determining treatment efficacy (Efron & Feldman, 1991; L. M. Friedman et al., 1996; Oakes et al., 1993). Traditionally, in clinical efficacy studies, outcome variables are analyzed using an "intent-to-treat" approach, where all subjects are included in data analysis as randomized regardless of their adherence to the assigned treatment (Fisher et al., 1990). There has been considerable debate between clinicians and statisticians, as well as among members of the statistical community, over this policy of inclusion versus an approach in which subjects are analyzed on the basis of treatment actually received (Lewis & Machin, 1993). Feinstein (1985) and Sheiner and Rubin (1995) have noted that the intention-to-treat approach provides valid inference on use-effectiveness—the effect of assignment to treatment on an outcome—in a study setting but fails to provide valid inference of use-effectiveness in a practice setting or of method-effectiveness, the effect of the actual treatment received. However, concerns related to potential for selection bias have supported the use of the intention-to-treat approach as the primary method of analysis for treatment efficacy data (Y. J. Lee, Ellenberg, Hirtz, & Nelson, 1991; Peduzzi, Wittes, & Detre, 1993). Recent work has sought to refine efficacy estimation procedures in the presence of treatment nonadherence and to limit biases related to nonadherence through the complex modeling of adherence (Angrist, Imbens, & Rubin, 1996; Balke & Pearl, 1997; Cuzick, Edwards, & Seganan, 1997; Efron & Feldman, 1991; Goetghebeur & Lapp, 1997; Goetghebeur & Molenberghs, 1996; Goetghebeur, Molenberghs, & Katz, 1998; Goetghebeur & Shapiro, 1996; Imbens & Rubin, 1997; Little & Yau, 1998; Mark & Robins, 1993; Oakes et al., 1993; Robbins, 1998; Robins & Tsiatis, 1991; Rubin, 1998; Sommer & Zeger, 1991; Wang, Husan, & Chow, 1996; White & Goetghebeur, 1998). This extensive body of work supports the use of supplementary comparative analyses for treatment efficacy, which incorporate information on adherence to assignment treatment, especially when treatment adherence is comprehensively, consistently, and reliably measured (Pocock & Abdalla, 1998).

## SUMMARY

Adherence to treatment among persons with chronic disorders constitutes a significant problem. Approximately half of patients have difficulty following their regimen, leading to costly and clinically adverse outcomes. Multiple factors have been associated with poor adherence but none of sufficiently robust an effect to lead to the reliable identification of poor adherers. Although an array of strategies has been evaluated for their ability to improve adherence, including educational, behavioral, cognitive, and affective interventions, very few randomized, controlled studies have been carried out. Thus, the data supporting interventions are weak. Further, in the area of pediatrics, developmental issues have not been adequately addressed. Problems in the field still exist as a function of the multiple methods of assessment, with inconsistent findings. Clearly, considerable research efforts are necessary to better understand and improve adherence. Progress in analysis strategies and in measurement methodology will support these needed advances in the field.

## ACKNOWLEDGMENTS

This chapter is supported in part by the National Institute of Nursing Research (5 P30 NR03924). We acknowledge the assistance of Sherri Ciocoi and Stephanine Duplaga with literature searches and manuscript preparation.

## REFERENCES

Abel, S., Sobesky, G., Cabie, A., Conlan-Nayaud, G., & Durocher, A. (1998). Role of compliance in the efficacy of highly active antiretroviral therapy (HAART) among a Caribbean cohort of unselected patients. *International Conference on AIDS, 12,* 599.

Achusim, L. E., Caselnova, D. A., & Cosgrove, R. (1998). Consequences of unclaimed prescriptions in a university health system. *ASHP Midyear Clinical Meeting, 33*(Dec.), P–374D.

Acurcio, F. A., & Guimares, M. D. (1998). Utilization of prescribed drugs by HIV infected individuals: A qualitative approach. *International Conference on AIDS, 12,* 835.

Adarmes, C. J., & Sunahara, J. F. (1997). Hypertensive urgencies and emergencies in ambulatory care clinics. *ASHP Midyear Clinical Meeting, 32*(Dec.), P–93E.

Agarwal, M. R., Sharma, V. K., Kishar, Kumar, K. V., & Lowe, D. (1998). Noncompliance with treatment in patients suffering from schizophrenia: A study to evaluate possible contributing factors. *International Journal of Social Psychiatry, 44*(2), 92–106.

Agi, R. O., Egbunike, I. G., Osemene, N. I., Plattenburg, J. P., Plattenburg, P., & Jackson, D. M. (1996). Evaluation and impact of unclaimed prescriptions in a county hospital district institution. *ASHP Midyear Clinical Meeting, 31*(Dec.), P–447E.

Agostoni, C., Riva, E., Galli, C., Marangoni, F., Luotti, D., & Giovannini, M. (1998). Plasma arachidonic acid and serum thromboxane B2 concentrations in phenylketonuric children are correlated with dietary compliance. *Zeitschrift für Ernahrungswissenschaft, 37*(S1), 122–124.

Ahluwalia, J. S., McNagny, S. E., & Kanuru, N. K. (1996). A randomized trial to improve follow-up care in severe uncontrolled hypertensives at an inner-city walk-in clinic. *Journal of Health Care for the Poor and Underserved, 7*(4), 377–389.

Ailinger, R. L., & Dear, M. R. (1998). Adherence to tuberculosis preventive therapy among Latino immigrants. *Public Health Nursing, 15*(1), 19–24.

Alperstein, G., Morgan, K. R., Mills, K., & Daniels, L. (1998). Compliance with antituberculosis preventive therapy among 6-year-old children. *Australian and New Zealand Journal of Public Health, 22*(2), 210–213.

Amici, G., Viglino, G., Virga, G., Gandolfo, C., Da Rin, G., Bocci, C., & Cavalli, P. L. (1996). Compliance study in peritoneal dialysis using PD Adequest software. *Peritoneal Dialysis International, 16S1,* S176–S178.

Anderson, B., Ho, J., Brackett, J., Finkelstein, D., & Laffel, L. (1997). Parental involvement in diabetes management tasks: Relationships to blood glucose monitoring adherence and metabolic control in young adolescents with insulin-dependent diabetes mellitus. *Journal of Pediatrics, 130*(2), 257–265.

Andrade, S. E., Walker, A. M., Gottlief, L. K., Hollenberg, N. K., Testa, M. A., Saperia, E. M., & Platt, R. (1995). Discontinuation of antihyperlipidemic drugs: Do rates reported in clinical trials reflect rates in primary care settings? *New England Journal of Medicine, 332,* 1125–1131.

Angrist, J. D., Imbens, G. W., & Rubin, D. B. (1996). Identification of causal effects using instrumental variables (with discussion). *Journal of the American Statistical Association, 91,* 444–472.

Apter, A. J., Reisine, S. T., Affleck, G., Barrows, E., & ZuWallack, R. L. (1998). Adherence with twice-daily dosing of inhaled steroids. Socioeconomic and health-belief differences. *American Journal of Respiratory and Critical Care Medicine, 157*(Pt 1), 1810–1817.

Arabe, J., Rubini, N. P., Rodriques, A. C., Leal, D. W., Freitas, E. H., Sion, F. S., & Morais-de-sa, C. A. (1998). Factors which influence adherence to the use of protease inhibitors. *International Conference on AIDS, 12,* 602–603.

Arbyn, M., Quataert, P., Van Hal, G., & Van Oyen, H. (1997). Cervical cancer screening in the Flemish region (Belgium): Measurement of the attendance rate by telephone interview. *European Journal of Cancer Prevention, 6*(4), 389–398.

Ash, A. L., Chen, S. W., & Dolkhani, N. (1998). Factors influencing noncompliance or lack of initiation of hormone replacement therapy in appropriately indicated post-menopausal women. *ASHP Midyear Clinical Meeting, 33*(Dec.), P–246D.

Atwood, J. R., Giordano, L, Vargas, P., Blackwell, G. G., Earnest, D. L., Meyskens, F., & Alberts, D. (1996). Adherence enhancers in pill-related clinical trials: A health behavior in cancer prevention model-based approach. *Patient Education and Counseling, 28*(1), 15–23.

Aversa, S. L., & Kimberlin, C. (1996). Psychosocial aspects of antiretroviral medication use among HIV patients. *Patient Education and Counseling, 29*(2), 207–219.

Ayuso-Gutierrez, J. L., & del Rio Vega, J. M. (1997). Factors influencing relapse in the long-term course of schizophrenia. *Schizophrenia Research, 28*(2–3), 199–206.

Azrin, N. H., & Teichner, G. (1998). Evaluation of an instructional program for improving medication compliance for chronically mentally ill outpatients. *Behaviour Research and Therapy, 36*(9), 849–861.

Baier, M., Murray, R., North, C., Lato, M., & Eskew, C. (1996). Comparison of completers and noncompleters in a transitional residential program for homeless mentally ill. *Issues in Mental Health Nursing, 17*(4), 337–352.

Balestra, P., Ferri, F., Galgani, S., Narciso, P., Pellicelli, A., Tozzi, V., Zaccarelli, M., & Visco, G. (1996). Clinical, psychological and behavioral characteristics of HIV patients reporting low compliance to treatments. *International Conference on AIDS, 11*(1), 290.

Balke, A., & Pearl, J. (1997). Bounds on treatment effects from studies with imperfect compliance. *Journal of the American Statistical Association, 92*, 1171–1176.

Bangsberg, D. R., Zolopa, A. R., Charlebois, E., Tulsky, J., Hecht, F. M., Robertson, M., Chesney, M., Holodniy, M., Merigan, T. C., & Moss, A. R. (1998). HIV-infected homeless and marginally housed (H/M) patients adhere to and receive early virologic benefit from protease inhibitors (PI). *5th Conference on Retroviral Opportunistic Infections* (p. 107).

Barlow, J. H. (1998). Understanding exercise in the context of chronic disease: An exploratory investigation of self-efficacy. *Perceptual and Motor Skills, 87*(2), 439–446.

Barnowski, T. L., Blessinger, S. C., Britton, K. J., Flanagan, K. E., Mieling, P. A., Ptacek, M. N., & Moyers, P. A. (1998). The relationship of compliance and grip strength return post-carpal tunnel release surgery. *Work: A Journal of Prevention, Assessment and Rehabilitation, 10*(2), 181–191.

Bastiaens, L. (1995). Compliance with pharmocotherapy in adolescents: Effects of patients' and parents' knowledge and attitudes toward treatment. *Journal of Child and Adolescent Psychopharmacology, 5*(1), 39–48.

Battegay, M., Bassetti, S., Rickenbach, M., Flepp, M., Furrer, H. J., Telenti, A., Vernazza, P., Bernasconi, E., & Sudre, P. (1998). Why is highly active anti-retroviral therapy (HAART) not prescribed or why is it discontinued: A prospective analysis in the Swiss HIV Cohort Study (SHCS). *International Conference on AIDS, 12*, 588.

Bender, B., Milgrom, H., Rand, C., & Ackerson, L. (1998). Psychological factors associated with medication nonadherence in asthmatic children. *Journal of Asthma, 35*(4), 347–353.

Bentsen, H., Lindgarde, F., & Manthorpe, R. (1997). The effect of dynamic strength back exercise and/or a home training program in 57-year-old women with chronic back pain. *Spine, 22*(13), 1494–1500.

Berg, J., Dunbar-Jacob, J., & Rohay, J. M. (1998). Compliance with inhaled medications: The relationship between diary and electronic monitor. *Annals of Behavior Medicine, 20*(1), 36–38.

Berg, J., Dunbar-Jacob, J., & Sereika, S. (1997). An evaluation of a self-management program for adults with asthma. *Clinical Nursing Research, 6*(3), 225–238.

Bergeron, K., Gormley, J., Sousa, H., Tashima, K., Flanigan, T. P., & Merriman, N. A. (1998). Adherence to HAART in clinical trials vs. clinical care setting. *International Conference on AIDS, 12*, 1065.

Berkovitch, M., Papadouris, D., Shaw, D., Onuaha, N., Dias, C., & Olivieri, N. F. (1998). *British Journal of Clinical Pharmacology, 45*(6), 605–607.

Bernardini, J., & Piraino, B. (1998). Compliance in CAPD and CCPD patients as measured by supply inventories during home visits. *American Journal of Kidney Diseases, 31*(1), 101–107.

Besch, C. L., Morse, E., Simon, P., Hodges, J., & Franchino, B. (1997, January). *Preliminary results of compliance study with CPCRA 007 combination nucleoside study.* Paper presented at the 4th Conference on Retroviral Opportunistic Infections (p. 111).

Bocchetta, A., Ardau, R., Burrai, C., Chillotti, C., Quesada, G., & DelZomp, M. (1998). Suicidal behavior on and off lithium prophylaxis in a group of patients with prior suicide attempts. *Journal of Clinical Psychopharmacology, 18*(5), 384–389.

Bosley, C. M., Fosbury, J. A., & Cochrane, G. M. (1995). The psychological factors associated with poor compliance with treatment in asthma. *European Respiratory Journal, 8*(6), 899–904.

Brill, K. (1997). Minimizing the problem of poor compliance in adolescents: Clinical experience with a modern low-dose gestodene-containing oral contraceptive. In G. Creatsas, G. Mastorakos et al. (Eds.), *Adolescent gynecology and endocrinology: Basic and clinical aspects* (Vol. 816, pp. 457–465). New York: New York Academy of Sciences.

Brittain, E., & Wittes, J. (1990). The run-in period in clinical trials: The effect of misclassification on efficiency. *Controlled Clinical Trials, 11*, 327–338.

Brown, M. A., Inouye, J., Powell-Cope, G. M., Holzemer, W. L., Nokes, K. M., Corless, I. B., & Turner, J. G. (1998). Social support and adherence in HIV+ persons. *International Conference on AIDS, 12*, 590.

Brus, H. L., van de Laar, M. A., Taal, E., Rasker, J. J., & Wiegman, O. (1998). Effects of patient education on compliance with basic treatment regimens and health in recent onset active rheumatoid arthritis. *Annals of the Rheumatic Diseases, 57*(3), 146–151.

Buck, D., Jacoby, A., Baker, G. A., & Chadwick, D. W. (1997). Factors influencing compliance with antiepileptic drug regimes. *Seizure, 6*(2), 87–93.

Burkhart, P., & Dunbar-Jacob, J. (in press). Adherence research in the pediatric and adolescent populations: A decade in review. In L. Hayman, R. Turner, & M. Mahon (Eds.), *Health and behavior in childhood and adolescence: Cross-disciplinary perspectives.* Hillsdale, NJ: Lawrence Erlbaum.

Burman, R. S., Epstein, R. S., & Lydick, E. (1997). Risk factors associated with women's compliance with estrogen replacement therapy. *Journal of Women's Health, 6*(2), 219–226.

Burney, K. D., Krishnan, K., Ruffin, M. T., Zhang, D., & Brenner, D. E. (1996). Adherence to single daily dose of aspirin in a chemoprevention trial. An evaluation of self-report and microelectronic monitoring. *Archives of Family Medicine, 5*(5), 297–300.

Buzzard, I. M., Faucett, C. L., Jeffrey, R. W., McBane, L., McGovern, P., Baxter, J. S., Shapiro, A. C., Blackburn, G. L., Chlebowski, R. T., Elashoff, R. M., & Wynder, E. L. (1996). Monitoring dietary change in a low-fat diet intervention study: Advantages of using 24-hour dietary recalls vs food records. *Journal of the American Dietetic Association, 96*(6), 574–579.

Carney, R. M., Freedland, K. E., Eisen, S. A., Rich, M. W., & Jaffe, A. S. (1995). Major depression and medication adherence in elderly patients with coronary artery disease. *Health Psychology, 14*(1), 88–90.

Carney, R. M., Freedland, K. E., Eisen, S. A., Rich, M. W., Sakala, J. A., & Jaffe, A. S. (1998). Adherence to a prophylactic medication regimen in patients with symptomatic versus asymptomatic ischemic heart disease. *Behavioral Medicine, 24*(1), 35–39.

Carr, L., Smith, R. E., Pryor, J. A., & Patridge, C. (1996). Cystic fibrosis patients' views and beliefs about chest clearance and exercise: A pilot study. *Physiotherapy, 82*(11), 621–627.

Caserta, M. S., & Gillett, P. A. (1998). Older women's feelings about exercise and their adherence to an aerobic regimen over time. *Gerontologist, 38*(5), 602–609.

Catz, S., & McClure, J. B. (1998). HIV outpatient adherence: Relation of disease status to appointment-keeping. *International Conference on AIDS, 12,* 864.

Cecil, D. W. (1998). Relational control patterns in physician-patient clinical encounters: Continuing the conversation. *Health Communication, 10*(2), 15–25, 149.

Cecil, D. W., & Killeen, I. (1997). Control, compliance, and satisfaction in the family practice encounter. *Family Medicine, 29*(9), 653–657.

Chang, S., Chan, G. M., Chan, J. C., Raymond, K., & Critchley, J. A., (1998). Compliance with prescriptions of nine or more medications daily. *ASHP Midyear Clinical Meeting, 33*(Dec.), INTL-9.

Cheng, J. W., Rozenfeld, V., Pflomm, J. M., Singh, K. K., & Bazil, M. K. (1998). Impact of providing pharmaceutical care in a cardiology clinic on patients' medication knowledge and adherence. *ASHP Midyear Clinical Meeting, 33*(Dec.), FGF-1.

Chizzola, P. R., Mansur, A. J., da Luz, P. L., & Bellotti, G. (1996). Compliance with pharmacological treatment in outpatients from a Brazilian cardiology referral center. *Revista Paulista de Medicina 114*(5), 1259–1264.

Christensen, A. J., & Smith, T. W. (1995). Personality and patient adherence: Correlates of the five-factor model in renal analysis. *Journal of Behavioral Medicine 18*(3), 305–313.

Clarkin, J. F., Carpenter, D., Hull, J., Wilner, P., & Glick, I. (1998). Effects of psychoeducational intervention for married persons with bipolar disorder and their spouses. *Psychiatric Services, 49*(4), 531–533.

Cline, J. C., Foster, A. C., Lee, T. J., & Pait, L.D. (1998). Unclaimed prescriptions in an outpatient pharmacy within an academic medical center. *ASHP Midyear Clinical Meeting, 33,* P–376E.

Conner, S. L. Gustafson, J. R., Sexton, G., Becker, N., Artaud-Wild, S., & Conner, W. E. (1992). The Diet Habit Survey: A new method of dietary assessment that relates to plasma cholesterol changes. *Journal of the American Dietetic Association, 92*, 41–47.

Conte, G., Ferrari, R., Guarneri, L., Calzeroni, A., & Sacchetti, E. (1996). Reducing the "revolving door" phenomenon. *American Journal of Psychiatry, 153*(11), 1512.

Conway, S. P., Pond, M. N., Hamnett, T., & Watson, A. (1996). Compliance with treatment in adult patients with cystic fibrosis. *Thorax, 51*(1), 29–33.

Corden, Z. M., Bosley, C. M., Rees, P. J., & Cochrane, G. M. (1997). Home nebulizer therapy for patients with COPD: Patient compliance with treatment and its relation to quality of life. *Chest ,112*(5), 1278–1282.

Cosler , L. E., Markson, L. E., Fanning, T. R., & Turner, B. J. (1996). Compliance with tuberculosis treatment in a symptomatic HIV cohort, *AHSR and FHSR Annual Meeting Abstract Book, 13*, 48–49.

Cote, J., Cartier, A., Malo, J., Rouleau, M., & Boulet, L. (1998). Compliance with peak expiratory flow monitoring in home management of asthma. *Chest: The Cardiopulmonary Journal, 113*(4), 968–972.

Courneya, K. S., & McAuley, E. (1995). Cognitive mediators of the social influence exercise adherence relationship: A test of the theory of planned behavior. *Journal of Behavioral Medicine, 18*(5), 499–515.

Cox, K. L., Puddey, I. B., Burke, V., Beilin, L. J., Morton, A. R., & Bettridge, H. F. (1996). Determinants of change in blood pressure during S.W.E.A.T.: The sedentary women exercise adherence trial. *Clinical and Experimental Pharmacology and Physiology, 23*(6–7), 567–569.

Cramer, J. A., Scheyer, R. D., & Mattson, R. H. (1990). Compliance declines between clinic visits. *Archives of Internal Medicine, 150*(7), 1509–1510.

Cramer, J., Vachon, L., Desforges, C., & Sussman, N. M. (1995). Dose frequency and dose interval compliance with multiple antiepileptic medications during a controlled clinical trial. *Epilepsia, 36*(11), 1111–1117.

Cramer, J. A., Mattson, R. H., Prevey, M. L., Scheyer, R. D., & Ouellette, V. L. (1989). How often is medication taken as prescribed? A novel assessment technique. *Journal of the American Medical Association, 261*, 3273–3277.

Cuffel, B. J., Alford, J., Fischer, E. P., & Owen, R. R. (1996). Awareness of illness in schizophrenia and outpatient treatment adherence. *Journal of Nervous and Mental Disease, 184*, 653–659.

Cuzick, J., Edwards, R., & Seganan, N. (1997). Adjusting for non-compliance and contamination in randomized clinical trials. *Statistics in Medicine, 16*, 1017–1029.

Daley, D. C., Salloum, I. M., Zuckoff, A., Kirisci, L., & Thase, M. E. (1998). Increasing treatment adherence among outpatients with depression and cocaine dependence. Results of a pilot study. *American Journal of Psychiatry, 155*(11), 1611–1613.

Davidson, B. L. (1998). A controlled comparison of directly observed therapy vs self-administered therapy for active tuberculosis in the urban United States. *Chest, 114*(5), 1239–1243.

Davidson, M. H., Kong, J. C., Drennan, K. B., Story, K., & Anderson, G. H. (1996). Efficacy of the National Cholesterol Education Program Step I diet: A randomized trial incorporating quick-service foods. *Archives of Internal Medicine, 156*(3), 305–312.

Davis, C. E. (1998). Prerandomization compliance screening. In S. A. Shumaker &

E. B. Schron (Eds.), *The handbook of health behavior change* (2nd ed., pp. 485–490). New York: Springer Publishing Co.

Davis, C. E., Applegate, W. B., Gordon, D. J., Curtis, R. C., & McCormick, M. (1995). An empirical evaluation of the placebo run-in. *Controlled Clinical Trials, 16*(1), 41–50.

De Geest, S., Abraham, I., Moons, P., Vandeputte, M., Van Cleemput, J., Evers, G., Daenen, W., & Vanhaecke, J. (1998). Late acute rejection and subclinical non-compliance with cyclosporine thearpy in heart transplant recipients. *Journal of Heart and Lung Transplantation, 17*(9), 854–863.

De Klerk, E., & van der Linden, S. J. (1996). Compliance monitoring of NSAID drug therapy in ankylosing spondylitis, experiences with and electronic monitoring device. *British Journal of Rheumatology, 35*(1), 60–65.

Del Boca, F. K., Kranzler, H. R., Brown, J., & Korner, P. F. (1996). Assessment of medication compliance in alcololics through UV light detection of a riboflavin tracer. *Alcoholism, Clinical and Experimental Research, 20*(8), 1412–1417.

Demyttenaere, K., Van Ganse, E., Gregoire, J., Gaens, E., Mesters, P., & Belgian Compliance Study Group. (1998). Compliance in depressed patients treated with fluoxetine or amitriptyline. *International Clinical Psychopharmacology, 13*(1), 11–17.

DeProspero, T., & Riffle, W. A. (1997). Improving patients' drug compliance. *Psychiatric Services, 48*(11), 1468.

Detry, J. M., Block, P., DeBacker, G., & Degaute, J. P. (1995). Patient compliance and therapeutic coverage: Comparison of amlodipine and slow release nifedipine in the treatment of hypertension. The Belgian Collaborative Study Group. *European Journal of Clinical Pharmacology, 47*(6), 477–481.

Dew, M. A., Roth, L. H., Thompson, M. E., Kormos, R. L., & Griffith, B. P. (1996). Medical compliance and its predictors in the first year after heart transplantation. *Journal of Heart and Lung Transplantation, 15*(6), 631–645.

Dooley, R., Kunik, M. E., & Molinari, V. (1998). Reminder call on appointment compliance in geropsychiatric outpatients. *Clinical Gerontologist, 19*(2), 82–88.

Douglas, S., Blixen, C., & Bartucci, R. (1996). Relationship between pretransplant noncompliance and posttransplant outcomes in renal transplant recipients. *Journal of Transplant Coordination, 6*(2), 53–58.

Dunbar-Jacob, J., Sereika, S., Burke, L. E., Starz, T., Rohay, J. M., & Kwoh, C. K. (1995). Can poor adherence be improved? *Annals of Behavioral Medicine, 17S,* 50–61.

Dunbar-Jacob, J., Sereika, S., Rohay, J., & Burke, L. E. (1998). Electronic methods in assessing adherence to medical regimens. In D. S. Krantz & A. Baum (Eds.), *Technology and methods in behavioral medicine* (pp. 95–113). Mahwah, NJ: Lawrence Erlbaum.

Duncan, J. C., & Rogers, R. (1998). Medication compliance in patients with chronic schizophrenia: Implications for the community management of mentally disordered offenders. *Journal of Forensic Sciences, 43*(6), 1133–1137.

Dyer, P. H., Lloyd, C. E., Lancashire, R. J., Bain, S. C., & Barnett, A. H. (1998). Factors associated with clinic non-attendance in adults with type 1 diabetes mellitus. *Diabetic Medicine, 15*(4), 339–343.

Ecclestone, N. A., Myers, A. M., & Paterson, D. H. (1998). Tracking older participants of twelve physical activity classes over a three-year period. *Journal of Aging and Physical Activity, 6*(1), 70–82.

Efron, B., & Feldman, D. (1991). Compliance as an explanatory variable in clinical trials (with discussion). *Journal of the American Statistical Association, 86,* 9–26.

Ecclestone, M. A., Myers, A. M., & Paterson, D. H. (1998). Tracking older participants of twelve physical activity classes over a three-year period. *Journal of Aging and Physical Activity, 6*(1), 70–82.

Elizaga, J., & Friedland, J. S. (1997). Monitoring compliance with antituberculosis treatment by detection of isoniazid in urine. *Lancet, 350,* 1225–1226.

Engleman, H. M., Asgari-Jirhandeh, N., McLeod, A. L., Ramsay, C. F., Deary, I. J., & Douglas, N. J. (1996). Self-reported use of CPAP and benfits of CPAP therapy: A patient survey . . . continuous positive airway pressure. *Chest: The Cardiopulmonary Journal, 109*(6), 1470–1476.

Erickson, S. R., Slaughter, R., & Halapy, H. (1997). Pharmacists' ability to influence outcomes of hypertension therapy. *Pharmacotherapy, 17*(1), 140–147.

Erlen, J. A., & Mellors, M. P. (1999). Adherence to combination therapy in persons living with HIV: Balancing the hardships and the blessings. *Journal of the Association of Nurses in AIDS Care, 10*(4), 75–84.

Esch, L. D. Shelton, M. J., Esch, A. E., Morse, G. D., & Hewitt, R. G. (1998). Medication adherenec enhancement after viral genotyping in HIV+ patients failing highly active antiretroviral therapy (HAART). *International Conference on AIDS, 12,* 592–593, (abstract no. 32357).

Fallab-Stubi, C. L., Zellweger, J. P., Sauty, A., Uldry, C., Iorillo, D., & Burnier, M. (1998). Electronic monitoring of adherence to treatment in the preventive chemotherapy of tuberculosis. *International Journal of Tuberculosis and Lung Disease, 2*(7), 525–530.

Favre, S., Huguelet, M. A., Vogel, S., & Gonzalez, M. A. (1997). Neuroleptic compliance in a cohort of first episode schizophrenics: A naturalistic study. *European Journal of Psychiatry, 11*(1), 35–42.

Feinstein, A. (1974). Clinical biostatistics: 30. Biostatistical problems in "compliance bias." *Clinical Pharmacology and Therapies, 16,* 846–857.

Feinstein, A. R. (1985). *The architecture of clinical research.* Philadelphia: W. B. Saunders.

Fielder, A. R., Irwin, M., Auld, R., Cocker, K. D., Jones, H. S., & Moseley, M. J. (1995). Compliance in amblyopia therapy: Objective monitoring of occlusion. *British Journal of Ophthalmology, 79*(6), 585–589.

Fisher, L. D., Dixon, D. O., Herson, J., Frankowski, R. K., Hearron, M. S., & Peace, K. E. (1990). Intention-to-treat in clinical trials. In K. E. Peace (Ed.), *Statistical issues in drug research and development* (pp. 331–350). New York: Marcel Dekker.

Flack, J. M., Novikov, S. V., & Ferrario, C. M. (1996). Benefits of adherence to antihypertensive drug therapy. *European Heart Journal, 17*(Suppl A), 166–220.

Fleury, B., Rakotonanshary, D., Hausser-Hauw, C., Lebeau, B., & Guilleminault, C. (1996). Objective patient compliance in long-term use of nCPAP. *European Respiratory Journal, 9*(11), 2356–2359.

Flexner, C., Noe, D., Benson, C., Currier, J., Andrade, A., & Shaver, A. (1998). Adherence patterns in patients with symptomatic Mycobacterium avium complex (MAC) infection taking a twice-daily clarithromycon regimen. *International Conference on AIDS, 12,* 585.

Frank, M. (1996). Factors associated with non-compliance with a medical follow-up regimen after discharge from a pediatric diabetes clinic. *Canadian Journal of Diabetes Care, 20*(3), 13–20.

Franklin, T. L., Kolasa, K. M., Griffin, K., Mayo, C., & Badenhop, D. T. (1995). Adherence to very-low-fat diet by a group of cardiac rehabilitation patients in the rural southeastern United States. *Archives of Family Medicine, 4*(6), 551–554.

Freedman, L. S. (1990). The effect of partial noncompliance on the power of a clinical trial. *Controlled Clinical Trials, 11,* 157–168.

Frick, P. A., Gal, P., Lane, T. W., & Swell, P. C. (1998). Antiretroviral medication compliance in patients with AIDS. *AIDS Patient Care and STDs, 12*(6), 463–470.

Friedman, L. M., Furberg, C. D., & Demets, D. L. (1996). *Fundamentals of clinical trials* (3rd ed.). St. Louis: Mosby-Year Book.

Friedman, R. H., Kazis, L. E., Jette, A., Smith, M. B., Stollerman, J., Torgerson, J., & Carey, K. (1996). A telecommunication system for monitoring and counseling patients with hypertensions. Impact on medication adherence and blood pressure. *American Journal of Hypertension, 9*(4, pt. 1), 285–292.

Friedrich, M., Gittler, G., Halberstadi, Y., Cermak, T., & Heiller, I. (1998). Combined exercise and motivation program: Effect on the compliance and level of disability of patients with chronic low back pain: A randomized controlled trial. *Archives of Physical Medicine and Rehabilitation, 79*(5), 475–487.

Gallant, J. E., & Block, D. S. (1998). Adherence to antiretroviral regimes in HIV-infected patents: Results of a survey among physcians and patents. *Journal of the International Association of Physicians in AIDS Care, 4*(5), 32–35.

Gallo, A. M., & Knafl, K. A. (1998). Parents' reports of "tricks of the trade" for managing childhood chronic illness. *Journal of the Society of Pediatric Nurses, 3*(3), 93–100.

Garay-Sevila, M. E., Nava, L. E., Malacara, J. M., Huerta, R., Diaz de Leon, J., Mena, A., & Fajardo, M. E. (1995). Adherence to treatment and social support in patents with non-insulin dependent diabetes mellitus. *Journal of Diabetes and Its Complications, 9*(2), 81–86.

Gariti, P., Alterman, A. I., Holub-Beyer, E., Volpicelli, J. R., Prentice, N., & O'Brien, C. P. (1995). Effects of an appointment reminder call on patient show rates. *Journal of Substance Abuse Treatment, 12*(3), 207–212.

Gearhart, G. G., Stowers, A. D., & Hope, J. C. (1997). Impact of multidisciplinary patinet education on blood pressure control. *ASHP Midyear Clinical Meeting, 32,* 215E.

Geil, P. B., Anderson, J. W., & Gustafson, N. J. (1995). Women and men with hypercholesterolemia respond similarly to an American Heart Association step 1 diet. *Journal of the American Dietetic Association, 95*(4), 436–441.

Gibson, N. A., Ferguson, A. E., Aitchison, T. C., & Paton, J. Y. (1995). Compliance with inhaled asthma medication in preschool children. *Thorax, 50*(12), 1274–1279.

Gifford, A. L., Shively, M. J., Bormann, J. E., Timberlake, D., & Bozzettte, S. A. (1998). Self-reported adherence to combination antiretroviral medication (ARV) regimens in a community-based sample of HIV-infected adults. *International Conference on AIDS, 12,* 88 (abstract no. 32338).

Gir, E., Pratt, R., Bunch, E. H., & Holzemer, W. L. (1998). Adherence to antiretroviral therapy: A four country comparison. *International Conference on AIDS, 12,* 1023 (abstract no. 60129).

Girard, P., Blaschke, T. F., Kastrissios, H., & Sheiner, L. B. (1998). A Markov mixed effect regression model for drug compliance. *Statistics in Medicine, 17,* 2313–2333.

Glasgow, R. E., Hampson, S. E., Strycker, L. A., & Ruggerio, L. (1997). Personal-model beliefs and social environmental barriers related to diabetes self-management. *Diabetes Care, 20*(4), 556–561.

Goetchebeur, E., & Lapp, K. (1997). The effect of treatment compliance in a placebo-controlled trial: Regression with unpaired data. *Applied Statistics, 46*(3), 351–364.

Goetghebeur, E., & Molenberghs, G. (1996). Causal inference in a placebo-controlled clinicial trial with binary outcome and ordered compliance. *Journal of the American Statistical Association, 91,* 928–934.

Goetghebeur, E., Molenberghs, G., & Katz, J. (1998). Estimating the causal effect of compliance on binary outcome in randomized controlled trials. *Statistics in Medicine, 17,* 341–355.

Goetghebeur, E., & Shapiro, S. H. (1996). Analysing non-compliance in clinical trials: Ethical imperative or mission impossible? *Statistics in Medicine, 15,* 2813–2826.

Goldsmith, C. H. (1979). The effect of compliance distributions on therapeutic trials. In R. B. Hayes, D. W. Taylor, & D. L. Sackett (Eds.), *Compliance in health care* (pp. 297–308). Baltimore: Johns Hopkins University Press.

Gomes, M., Filho, H., & Noe, R. A. (1998). Anti-epileptic drug intake adherence. *Arquivos de Neuro-Psiquiatria, 56*(4), 708–713.

Gonda, I., Schuster, J. A., Rubsamen, R. M., Lloyd, P., Cipolla, D., & Farr, S. J. (1998). Inhalation delivery systems with compliance and disease management capabilities. *Journal of Controlled Release, 53*(1–3), 269–274.

Goodyer, L. I., Miskelly, F., & Milligan, P. (1995). Does encouraging good compliance improve patients' clinical condition in heart failure? *British Journal of Clinical Practice, 49*(4), 173–176.

Gowers, S. G., Jones, J. C., Kiana, S., & North, C. D. (1995). Family functioning: A correlate of diabetic control? *Journal of Child Psychology and Psychiatry and Allied Disciplines, 36*(6), 993–1001.

Grady, K. L., Jalowiec, A., & White-Williams, C. (1998). Patient compliance at one year and two years after heart transplantation. *Journal of Heart and Lung Transplantation, 17*(4), 383–394.

Granlund, B., Brulin, C., Johansson, H., & Sojka, P. (1998). Can motivational factors predict adherence to an exercise program for subjects with low back pain? *Scandinavian Journal of Behaviour Therapy, 27*(2), 81–96.

Gregoire, J. P., Guilbert, R., Archambault, A., & Contandriopoulos, A. P. (1997). Measurement of noncompliance to antihypertensive medication using pill counts and pharmacy records. *Journal of Social and Administrative Pharmacy, 14*(4), 198–207.

Gross, E., Burr, C. K., Storm, D., Czarniecki, L., & D'Orlando, D. (1998). Monitoring treatment adherence in pediatric HIV: Identifying the issues from providers and familiies. *International Conference on AIDS. 12,* 609 (abstract no. 32438).

Habib, A., Sanchez, M., Pervez, R., & Devanand, D. P. (1998). Compliance with disposition to primary care physicians and psychiatrist in elderly homebound mentally ill patients. *American Journal of Geriatric Psychiatry, 6*(4), 290–295.

Hales, G., Mitchell, J., Smith, D. E., & Kippex, S. (1998). Validity of patient questioning versus pill count as an assessment of compliance. *International Conference on AIDS, 12,* 596.

Hallert, C., Granno, C., Grant, C., Hulten, S., Midhagen, G., Strom, M., Svensson, H., Valdimarsson, T., & Wickstrom, T. (1998). Quality of life of adult coeliac patients treated for 10 years. *Scandinavian Journal of Gastroenterology, 33*(9), 933–938.

Halperin, M., Rogot, E., Gurian, J., & Ederer, F. (1968). Sample sizes for medical trials with special reference to long-term therapy. *Journal of Chronic Disease, 21,* 13–24.

Hanson, C. L., De Guire, M. J., Schinkel, A. M., & Kolterman, O. G. (1995). Empirical validation for a family-centered model of care. *Diabetes Care, 18*(10), 1347–1356.

Harel, Z., Biro, F. M., Kollar, L. M., & Rauh, J. L. (1996). Adolescents' reasons for and experience after discontinuation of the long-acting contraceptives Depo-Provera and Norplant. *Journal of Adolescent Health, 19*(2), 118–123.

Harris, L. E., Luft, F. C., Rudy, D. W., & Tierney, W. M. (1995). Correlates of health care satisfaction in inner-city patients with hypertension and chronic renal insufficiency. *Social Science and Medicine, 41*(12), 1639–1645.

Hecht, F. M., Colfax, G., Swanson, M., & Chesney, M. A. (1998, February). *Adherence and effectiveness of protease inhibitors in clinical practice.* Paper presented at the 5th Conference on Retroviral Opportunistic Infections (p. 107).

Hedge, B., & Petrak, J. A. (1998). Take as prescribed: A study of adherence behaviors in people taking anti-retroviral medications. *International Conference on AIDS, 12,* 590–591.

Heinasmaki, T., Shi, Q., Creagh, T., Mathur-Wagh, H., Marshak, A., Kanmaz, T., & Mildvan, D. (1998). Adherence and antiretroviral responses to highly active antiretroviral therapy (HAART) in patients infected with human immunodeficiency virus (HIV): Comparison between an outpatient clinic and clinical trials unit. *International Conference on AIDS, 12,* 597–598.

Hellman, E. A. (1997). Use of the stages of change in exercise adherence model among older adults with a cardiac diagnosis. *Journal of Cardiopulmonary Rehabilitation, 17*(3), 145–155.

Higa, S. K., Chan, D. S., Bass, J. W., & Alfaro, P. J. (1997). Oral antibiotic suspension: Do adult taste tests predict compliance in infants and young children? *Journal of Pediatric Pharmacy Practice, 2*(5), 265–270.

Hilbrands, L. B., Hoitsma, A. J., & Koene, R. A. (1995). Medication compliance after renal transplantation. *Transplantation, 60*(9), 914–920.

Holmbeck, G. N., Belvedere, M. C., Christensen, M., Czerwinski, A. M., Hommeyer, J. S., Johnson, S. Z., & Kung, E. (1998). Assessment of adherence with multiple informants in preadolescents with spina bifida. Initial development of a multidimensional, multitask parent-report questionnaire. *Journal of Personality Assessment, 70*(3), 427–440.

Holzheimer, L., Mohay, H., & Masters, I. B. (1998). Educating young children about asthma: Comparing the effectiveness of a developmentally appropriate asthma education video tape and picture book. *Child: Care, Health and Development, 24*(1), 85–99.

Hugen, P. W., Burger, D. M., Hoetelmans, R. M., Meenhorst, P. L., Mulder, J. W., & Koopmans, P. P. (1998). Saliva as a possible specimen for monitoring compliance and plasma levels in patients treated with indinavir (IDV). *International Conference on AIDS, 12,* 586–587.

Hylan, T. R., Dunn, R. L., Tepner, R. G., & Meurgey, F. (1998). Gaps in antidepressant prescribing in primary care in the United Kingdom. *International Clinical Psychopharmacology, 13*(6), 235–243.

Ibach, M. B. (1995). Predictors of compliance after hospitalization. *Journal of the Louisiana State Medical Society, 147*(7), 321–324.

Ifudu, O., Chan, P. E., Mayers, J. D., Choen, L. S., Brezsnyak, W. F., Herman, A. I., Avram, M. M., & Friedman, E. A. (1996). Anemia severity and missed dialysis treatments in erythropoietin-treated hemodialysis patients. *ASAIO Journal, 42*(3), 146–149.

Imbens, G. W., & Rubin, D. B. (1997). Bayesian inference for causal effects in randomized experiments with noncompliance. *Annals of Statistics, 25*(1), 305–327.

Incalzi, R. A., Gemma, A., Marra, C., Capparella, O., Fuso, L., & Carbonin, P. (1997). Verbal memory impairment in COD: Its mechanisms and relevance. *Chest, 112,* 1506–1513.

Jakicic, J. M., Wing, R. R., Butler, B. A., & Robertson, R. J. (1995). Prescribing exercise in mutlple short bouts versus one continuous bout: Effect on adherence, cardiorespiratory fitness, and weight loss in overweight women. *International Journal of Obesity and Related Metabolic Disorders, 19*(12), 893–901.

Jeffrey, R. W., Wing, R. R., Thorson, C., & Burton, L. R. (1998). Use of personal trainers and financial incentives to increase exercise in a behavioral weight-loss program. *Journal of Consulting and Clinical Psychology, 66*(5), 777–783.

Jeng, C., & Braun, L. T. (1997). The influence of self-efficacy on exercise intensity, compliance rate and cardiac rehabilitation outcomes among coronary artery disease patients. *Progress in Cardiovascular Nursing, 12*(1), 13–24.

Johnston, B. E., Ahmad, K., Smith C., & Rose, D. N. (1998). Adherence to highly active antiretroviral therapy among HIV-infected patients of the inner city. *International Conference on AIDS, 12,* 599 (abstract no. 32389).

Jones, J. K., Gorkin, L., Lian, J. F., Staffa, J. A., & Fletcher, A. P. (1995). Discontinuation of and changes in treatment after start of new courses of antihypertensive drugs: A study of a United Kingdom population. *British Medical Journal, 311,* 293–295.

Kastrissios, H., Suarez, J., Katzenstein, D., Girard, P., Sheiner, L. B., & Blaschke, T. F. (1998). Characterizing patterns of drug-taking behavior with a multiple drug regimen in an AIDS clinical trial. *AIDS, 12*(17), 2295–2303.

Katon, W., Von Korff, M., Lin, E., Walker, E., Simon, G. E., Bush, T., Robinson, P., & Russo, J. (1995). Collaborative management to achieve treatment guidelines. Impact on depression in primary care. *Journal of the American Medical Association, 273*(13), 1026–1031.

Katz, D. L., Brunner, R. L., St. Jeor, S. T., Scott, B., Jekel, J. F., & Brownell, K. D. (1998). Dietary fat consumption in a cohort of American adults, 1985–1991: Covariates, secular trends, and compliance with guidelines. *American Journal of Health Promotion, 12*(6), 382–390.

Katz, R. C., Ashmore, J., Barboa, E., Trueblood, K., McLaughlin, V., & Mathews, L.

(1998). Knowledge of disease and dietary compliance in patients with end-stage renal disease. *Psychological Reports, 82*(1), 331–336.

Keder, L. M., Rulin, M. C., & Gruss, J. (1998). Compliance with depot medroxyprogesterone acetate: A randomized, controlled trial of intensive reminders. *American Journal of Obstetrics and Gynecology, 179*(3, pt. 1), 583–585.

Kemp, R., & David, A. (1996). Psychological predictors of insight and compliance in psychotic patients. *British Journal of Psychiatry, 169,* 444–450.

Kemp, R., Hayward, P., Applewhaite, G., Everitt, B., & David, A. (1996). Compliance therapy in psychotic patients: Randomized controlled trial. *British Medical Journal, 312,* 345–349.

Khalil, S. A., & Elzubier, A. G. (1997). Drug compliance among hypertensive patients in Tabuk, Saudi Arabia. *Journal of Hypertension, 15*(5), 561–565.

Kim, H. M., & Lagakos, S. (1994). Assessing drug compliance using longitudinal marker data, with application to AIDS. *Statistics in Medicine, 12,* 1185–1195.

Kim, H. M., & Lagakos, S. (1996). Non-parametric inference of a failure time distribution when the failure times are estimated. *Statistics in Medicine, 15,* 2475–2490.

King, C. A., Hovey, J. D., Brand, E., Wilson, R., & Ghaziuddin, N. (1997). Suicidal adolescents after hospitalization: Parent and family impacts on treatment follow-through. *Journal of the American Academy of Child and Adolescent Psychiatry, 36*(1), 85–93.

Kissinger, P., Cohen, D., Brandon, W., Rice, J., Morse, A., & Clark, R. (1995). Compliance with public sector HIV medical care. *Journal of the National Medical Association, 87*(1), 19–24.

Knobel, H., Carmona, A., Grau, S., Saballs, P., Gimeno, J. L., & Lopez Colomes, J. L. (1998). Strategies to optimise adherence to highly active antiretroviral treatment. *International Conference on AIDS, 12,* 585.

Knopp, R. H., Retzlaff, B. M., Walden, C. E., Dowdy, A. A., Tsunehara, C. H., Austin, M. A., & Nguyen, T. (1997). A double-blind, randomized, controlled trial of the effects of two eggs per day in moderately hypercholesterolemic and combined hyperlipidemic subjects taught the NCEP step I diet. *Journal of the American College of Nutrition, 16*(6), 551–561.

Komoroski, E. M., Graham, C. J., & Kirby, R. S. (1996). A comparison of interventions to improve clinic follow-up compliance after a pediatric emergency department visit. *Pediatric Emergency Care, 12*(2), 87–90.

Kruse, W., & Weber, E. (1990). Dynamics of drug regimen compliance: Its assessment by microprocessor-based monitoring. *European Journal of Clinical Pharmacology, 38,* 561–565.

Kyngas, H., Hentinen, M., & Barlow, J. H. (1998). Adolescents' perceptions of physicians, nurses, parents and friends: Help or hindrance in compliance with diabetes self-care? *Journal of Advanced Nursing, 27*(4), 760–769.

Kyngas, H., Hentinen, M., Koivukangas, P., & Ohinmaa, A. (1996). Young diabetics' compliance in the framework of the mimic model. *Journal of Advanced Nursing, 24*(5), 997–1005.

La Greca, A., Auslander, W., Greco, P., Spetter, D., Fisher, E., & Santiago, J. (1995). I get by with a little help from my family and friends: Adolescents' support for diabetes care. *Journal of Pediatric Psychology, 20*(4), 449–476.

Lachin, J. M. (1981). Introduction to sample size determination and power analysis for clinical trials. *Controlled Clinical Trials, 2,* 93–113.

Lachin, J. M., & Foulkes, M. A. (1986). Evaluation of sample size and power for anlyses of survival with allowance for nonuniform patient entry, losses to follow-up, noncompliance, and stratification. *Biometrics, 42,* 507–519.

Laird, N. M., & Ware, J. H (1982). Random effects models for longitudinal data. *Biometrics, 38,* 963–974.

Lakatos, E. (1986). Sample size determination in clinical trials with time-dependent rates of losses and non-compliance. *Controlled Clinical Trials, 7,* 189–199.

Lang, J. M. (1990). The use of a run-in to enhance compliance. *Statistics in Medicine, 9,* 87–95.

Lau, H. S., de Boer, A., Beuning, K. S., & Porsius, A. (1997). Validation of pharmacy records in drug exposure assessment. *Journal of Clinical Epidemiology, 50*(5), 619–625.

Laumann, J. M., & Bjornson, D. C. (1997). Treatment of Medicaid patient with asthma: Comparison with treatment guidelines using disease-based drug utilization review methodology. *ASHP Midyear Clinical Meeting, 32*(Dec), P–52E.

Lee, C. R., Nicholson, P. W., Ledermann, J. A., & Rustin, G. J. (1996). Patient compliance with prolonged oral altretamine treatment in relapsed ovarian cancer. *European Journal of Gynaecological Oncology, 17*(2), 99–103.

Lee, J. Y., Jensen, B. E., Oberman, A., Fletcher, G. F., Fletcher, B. J., & Raczynski, J. M. (1996). Adherence in the training levels comparison trial. *Medicine and Science in Sports and Exercise, 28*(1), 47–52.

Lee, J. Y., Kusek, J. W., Greene, P. G., Bernhard, S., Norris, K., Smith, D., Wilkening, B., & Wright, J. T. Jr. (1996). Assessing medication adherence by pill count and electronic monitoring in the African American Study of Kidney Disease and Hypertension. *American Journal of Hypertension, 9*(8), 719–725.

Lee, Y. J., Ellenberg, J. H., Hirtz, D. G., & Nelson, K. B. (1991). Analysis of clinicial trials by treatment actually received: Is it really an option? *Statistics in Medicine, 10,* 1595–1605.

Leermarkers, E. A., Jakicic, J. M., Viteri, J., & Wing, R. R. (1998). Clinic-based vs. home-based interventions for preventing weight gain in men. *Obesity Research, 6*(5), 346–352.

Leggat, J. E. Jr., Orzol, S. M., Hulbert-Shearon, T. E., Golper, T. A., Jones, C. A., Held, P. J., & Port, F. K. (1998). Noncompliance in hemodialysis: Predictors and survival analysis. *American Journal of Kidney Disease, 32*(1), 139–145.

Leirer, V. O., Morrow, D. G., Tanke, E. D., & Pariante, G. M. (1991). Elders' nonadherence: Its assessment and medication reminding by voice mail. *Gerontologist, 31,* 514–520.

Lennard, L., Welch, J., & Lilleyman, J. S. (1995). Intracellular metabolites of mercaptopurine in children with lymphoblastic leukaemia: A possible indicator of noncompliance? *British Journal of Cancer, 72*(4), 1004–1006.

Leventhal, E. A., & Crouch, M. (1997). Are there differences in perceptions of illness across the lifespan? In K. J. Petrie & J. A. Weinman (Eds.), *Perceptions of health and illness: Current research and applications* (pp. 77–102). Amsterdam: Harwood Academic.

Leventhal, E. A., Leventhal, H., Schaefer, P., & Easterling, D. (1993). Conservation of energy, uncertainty reduction and swift utilization of medical care among the elderly. *Journal of Gerontology, 48,* 78–86.

Lewis, A. (1997). Non-compliance: A $100 billion problem. *Remington Report, 5*(4), 14–15.

Lewis, J. A., & Machin, D. (1993). Intention-to-treat: Who should use ITT? *British Journal of Cancer, 68,* 647–650.

Liang, K.-Y., & Zeger, S. L. (1986). Longitudinal data analysis using generalized linear models. *Biometrika, 73,* 13–22.

Lim, L. L.-Y. (1992). Estimating compliance to study medication from serum drug levels: Application to an AIDS clinical trial of zidovudine. *Biometrics, 48,* 619–630.

Lin, E. H., Von Korff, M., Katon, W., & Bush, T. (1995). The role of the primary care physician in patients' adherence to antidepressant therapy. *Medical Care, 33*(1), 67–74.

Linton, S. J., Hellsing, A. L., & Bergstroem, G. (1996). Exercise for workers with musculoskeletal pain: Does enhancing compliance decrease pain? *Journal of Occupational Rehabilitation, 6*(3), 177–190.

Lipid Research Clinics Program. (1984a). The Lipid Research Clinics Coronary Primary Prevention Program Trial results: 1. Reduction in incidence of coronary heart disease. *Journal of the American Medical Association, 251*(3), 351–364.

Lipid Research Clinics Program. (1984b). The Lipid Research Clinics Coronary Primary Prevention Program Trial results: 2. The relationship of reduction in incidence of coronary heart disease to cholesterol lowering. *Journal of the American Medical Association, 251*(3), 365–374.

Little, R. J., & Yau, L. H. Y. (1998). Statistical techniques for analyzing data from prevention trials: Treatment of no-shows using Rubin's causal model. *Psychological Methods, 3*(2), 147–159.

Lloyd, H. M., Paisley, C. M., & Mela, D. J. (1995). Barriers to the adoption of reduced-fat diets in a UK population. *Journal of the American Dietetic Association, 95*(3), 316–322.

Lopreiato, J., & Ottolini, M. (1996). Assessment of immunization compliance among children in the Department of Defense health care system. *Pediatrics, 97*(3), 308–311.

Lord, S. R., Ward, J. A., Williams, P., & Studwick, M. (1995). The effect of a 12 month exercise trial balance, strength, and falls in older women: A randomized controlled trial. *Journal of the American Geriatrics Society, 43*(11), 1198–1206.

Lorenzen, T., Stoehr, A., Weitner, L., Adam, A., Jarke, J., & Plettenberg, A. (1998). Compliance with antiretroviral multidrug therapy in HIV-infected patients and reasons for noncompliance. *International Conference on AIDS, 12,* 596.

Lyon, X. H., Di Vetta, V., Milon, H., Jequier, E., & Schutz, Y. (1995). Compliance to dietary advice directed towards increasing the carbohydrate to fat ratio of the everyday diet. *International Journal of Obesity and Related Metabolic Disorders, 19*(4), 260–269.

Mark, S. D., & Rubins, J. M. (1993). A method for the analysis of randomized trials with compliance information: An application to the Multiple Risk Factor Intervention Trial. *Controlled Clinical Trials, 14,* 79–97.

Martin, E. (1998). Telephone reminders improved compliance with a second dose of hepatitis B vaccine in high risk adults. *Evidence-Based Nursing, 1*(2), 44.

Mason, B. J., Matsuyama, J. R., & Jue, S. G. (1995). Assessment of sulfonylurea adherence and metabolic control. *Diabetes Educator, 21*(1), 52–57.

Matthews, C. E., & Freedson, P. S. (1995). Field trial of a three-dimensional activity monitor: Comparison with self-report. *Medicine and Science in Sports and Exercise, 27,* 1071–1078.

McCarron, D. A., Oparil, S., Chait, A., Haynes, R. B., Kris-Etherton, P., Stern, J. S., Resnick, L. M., Clark, S., Morris, C. D., Hatton, D. C., Metz, J. A., McMahon, M., Holcomb, S., Snyder, G. W., & Pi-Sunyer, F. X. (1997). Nutritional management of cardiovascular risk factors. A randomized clinical trial. *Archives of Internal Medicine, 157*(2), 169–177.

McKee, M., Hull, J. W., & Smith, T. E. (1997). Cognitive and symptom correlates of participation in social skills training groups. *Schizophrenia Research, 23,* 223–229.

Melfi, C. A., Chawla, A. J., Croghan, T. W., Hanna, M. P., Kennedy, S., & Sredl, K. (1998). The effects of adherence to antidepressant treatment guidelines on relapse and recurrence of depression. *Archives of General Psychiatry, 55*(12), 1128–1132.

Meslier, N., Lebrun, T., Grillier-Lanoir, V., Rolland, N., Henderick, C., Sailly, J. C., & Racineux, J. L. (1998). A French survey of 3,225 patients with CPAP for obstructive sleep apnoea: Benefits, tolerence, compliance and quality of life. *European Respiratory Journal, 12*(1), 185–192.

Metz, J. A., Kris-Etherton, P. M., Morris, C. D., Mustad, V. A., Stern, J. S., Oparil, S., Chait, A., Haynes, R. B., Resnick, L. M., Clark, S., Hatton, D. C., McMahon, M., Holcomb, S., Snyder, G. W., Pi-Sunyer, F. X., & McCarron, D. A. (1997). Dietary compliance and cardiovascular risk reduction with a prepared meal plan compared with a self-selected diet. *American Journal of Clinical Nutrition, 66*(2), 373–385.

Moore, S. M., Ruland, C. M., Pashkow, F. J., & Blackburn, G. G. (1998). Women's patterns of exercise following cardiac rehabilitation. *Nursing Research, 47*(6), 318–324.

Moore-Caldwell, S. Y., Werner, M. J., Powell, L., & Greene, J. W. (1997). Hepatitis B vaccination in adolescents: Knowledge, perceived risk, and compliance. *Journal of Adolescent Health, 20*(4), 294–299.

Moran, P. J., Christensen, A. J., & Lawton, W. J. (1998). Social support and conscientiousness in hemodialysis adherence. *Annals of Behavior Medicine, 19*(4), 333–338.

Morisky, D. E., Green, L. W., & Levine, D. M. (1986). Concurrent and predictive validity of a self-reported measure of medication adherence. *Medical Care, 24*(1), 67–74.

Morrell, R. W., Park, D. C., Kidder, D. P., & Martin, M. (1997). Adherence to antihypertensive medications across the life span. *Gerontologist, 37*(5), 609–619.

Morris, A. D., Boyle, D. I., McMahon, A. D., Greene, S. A., MacDonald, T. M., & Newton, R. W. (1997). Adherence to insulin treatment, glycemic control, and ketoacidosis in insulin dependent diabetes mellitus. *Lancet, 350,* 1505–1510.

Morrow, D., Leirer, V., Altieri, P., & Tanke, E. (1991). Elders' schema for taking medication: Implications for instruction design. *Journal of Gerontology, 46,* P378–385.

Morrow, D. G., Hier, C. M., Menard, W. E., & Leirer, V. O. (1998). Icons improve older and younger adults' comprehension of medication information. *Journal of Gerontology, 53,* P240–254.

Morrow, D. G., Leirer, V. O., & Altieri, P. (1995). Explicit formats help older adults understand medication instructions. *Educational Gerontology, 21,* 151–166.

Morrow, D. G., Leirer, V. O., Andrassy, J. M., Hier, C. M., & Menard, W. E. (1998). The influence of list format and category headers on age differences in understanding medication instructions. *Experimental Aging Research, 24,* 231–256.

Morrow, D. G., Leirer, V. O., Andrassy, J. M., Tanke, E. D., & Stine-Morrow, E. A. (1996). Medication instruction design: Younger and older adult schemas for taking medication. *Human Factors, 38,* 556–573.

Mounier-Vehier, C., Bernaud, C., Carre, A., Lequeuche, B., Hotton, J. M., & Charpentier, J. C. (1998). Compliance and antihypertensive efficacy of amlodipine compared with nifedipine slow-release. *American Journal of Hypertension, 11*(4, pt. 1), 478–486.

Muma, R. D., Ross, M. W., Parcel, G. S., & Pollard, R. B. (1995). Zidovudine adherence among individuals with HIV infection. *AIDS Care, 7*(4), 439–447.

Murata, G. H., Kapsner, C. O., Lium, D. J., & Busby, H. K. (1998). Patient compliance with peak flow monitoring in obstructive pulmonary disease. *American Journal of the Medical Sciences, 315*(5), 296–301.

Nadra, W. E., Knight, E. L., Lee, M. B., & Meehan, W. P. (1995). A retrospective study of treatment outcome for patients with non-insulin dependent diabetes at an inner-city hospital. *Diabetes Educator, 21*(2), 113–116.

Nardi, D. A. (1997). Risk factors, attendance, and abstinence patterns of low-income women in perinatal addiction treatment: Lessons from 5-year program. *Issues in Mental Health Nursing, 18*(2), 125–138.

Nelson, K. M., & Talbert, R. L. (1996). Drug-related hospital admissions. *Pharmacotherapy, 16*(4), 701–707.

Newcombe, R. G. (1988). Explanatory and pragmatic estimates of the treatment effect when deviations from allocated treatment occur. *Statistics in Medicine, 7,* 1179–1186.

Oakes, D., Moss, A. J., Fleiss, J. L., Bigger, J. T., Therneau, T., Eberly, S. W., McDermott, M. P., Manatunga, A., Carleen, E., Benhorin, J., & the Multicenter Diltiazem Post-Infarction Trial Research Group. (1993). Use of compliance measures in an analysis of the effect of diltiazem on mortality and reinfarction after myocardial infarction. *Journal of the American Statistical Association, 88,* 44–49.

O'Brien, G., & Lazebnik, R. (1998). Telephone call reminders and attendance in an adolescent clinic. *Pediatrics, 101*(6), E6.

Olivieri, N. F., & Vichinsky, E. P. (1998). Hydroxyurea in children with sickle cell disease: Impact on splenic function and compliance with therapy. *Journal of Pediatric Hematology/Oncology, 20*(1), 26–31.

Pablos-Mendez, A., Knirsch, C. A., Barr, R. G., Lerner, B. H., & Frieden, T. R. (1997). Nonadherence in tuberculosis treatment: Predictors and consequences in New York City. *American Journal of Medicine, 102*(2), 164–170.

Paffenbarger, R. S., Wing, A. L., & Hyde, R. T. (1978). Physical activity as an index of heart attack risk in college alumni. *American Journal of Epidemiology, 108,* 161–175.

Palardy, N., Greening, L., Ott, J., Holderby, A., & Atchison, J. (1998). Adolescents' health attitudes and adherence to treatment for insulin-dependent diabetes mellitus. *Journal of Developmental and Behavioral Pediatrics, 19*(1), 31–37.

Palta, M., & McHugh, R. (1980). Planning the size of a cohort study in the presence of both losses to follow-up and non-compliance. *Journal of Chronic Disease, 33,* 501–512.

Park, D. C., Hertzog, C., Leventhal, H., Morrell, R. W., Leventhal, E., Birchmore, D., Martin, M., & Bennett, J. (1999). Medication adherence in rheumatoid arthritis patients: Older is wiser. *Journal of the American Geriatrics Society, 47,* 172–183.

Park, D. C., Morrell, R. W., Frieske, D., & Kincaid, D. (1992). Medication adherence behaviors in older adults: Effects of external cognitive supports. *Psychology and Aging, 7*(2), 252–256.

Peduzzi, P., Wittes, J., & Detre, K. (1993). Analysis as randomized and the problem of nonadherence: An example from the Veterans Affairs Randomized Trial of Coronary Artery Bypass Surgery. *Statistics in Medicine, 12,* 1185–1195.

Perri, M. G., Martin, A., D., Leermakers, E. A., Sears, S. F., & Notelovitz, M. (1997). Effects of group- versus home-based exercise in the treatment of obesity. Journal of Consulting and Clinical Psychology, 65(2), 278–285.

Piacentini, J., Rotheram-Borus, M. J., Gillis, J. R., Graae, F., Trautman, P., Cantwell, C., Garcia-Leeds, C., & Shaffer, D. (1995). Demographic predictors of treatment attendance among adolescent suicide attempters. *Journal of Consulting and Clinical Psychology, 63*(3), 469–473.

Pierce, J. P., Faerber, S., Wright, F. A., Newman, V., Flatt, S. W., Kealey, S., Rock, C. L., Hryniuk, W., & Greenberg, E. R. (1997). Feasibility of a randomized trial of a high-vegetable diet to prevent breast cancer recurrence. *Nutrition and Cancer, 28*(3), 282–288.

Pocock, S., & Abdalla, M. (1998). The hope and the hazards of using compliance data in clinical trials. *Statistics in Medicine, 17,* 303–317.

Pocock, S. J. (1983). *Clinical trials: A practical approach.* New York: John Wiley & Sons.

Polaneczky, M., & Liblanc, M. (1998). Long-term depot medroxyprogesterone acetate (Depo-Provera) use in inner-city adolescents. *Journal of Adolescent Health, 23*(2), 81–88.

Pollock, M., Kovacs, M., & Charron-Prochownik, D. (1995). Eating disorders and maladaptive dietary/insulin management among youths with childhood-onset insulin-dependent diabetes mellitus. *Journal of the American Academy of Child and Adolescent Psychiatry, 34*(3), 291–296.

Powell, K. M., & Edgren, B. (1995). Failure of educational videotapes to improve medication compliance in a health maintenance organization. *American Journal of Health-System Pharmacy, 52,* 2196–2199.

Probstfield, J. L. (1991). Clinical trial prerandomization compliance (adherence) screen. In J. A. Cramer & B. Spilker (Eds.), *Patient compliance in medical practice and clinical trials* (pp. 323–333). New York: Raven Press.

Rainey, D. Y., Parsons, L. H., Kenney, P. G., & Krowchuk, D. P. (1995). Compliance with return appointments for reproductive health care among adolescent Norplant users. *Journal of Adolescent Health, 16*(5), 385–388.

Rand, C. S., Nides, M., Cowles, M. K., Wise, R. A., & Connett, J. (1995). Long-term metered-dose inhaler adherence in a clinical trial. *American Journal of Respiratory and Critical Care Medicine, 152*(2), 580–582.

Rapoff, M. (1998). Adherence issues among adolescents with chronic diseases. In

S. A. Shumaker & E. Schron (Eds.), *The handbook of health behavior change* (2nd ed., pp. 377–408). New York: Springer Publishing Co.

Razali, S. M., & Yahya, H. (1997). Health education and drug counseling for schizophrenia. *International Medical Journal, 4*(3), 187–189.

Rich, M. W., Gray, D. B., Beckham, V., Wittenberg, C., & Luther, P. (1996). Effect of a multidisciplinary intervention on medication compliance in elderly patients with congestive heart failure. *American Journal of Medicine, 101*(3), 270–276.

Robbins, J. M. (1998). Correction for non-compliance in equivalence trials. *Statistics in Medicine, 17,* 269–302.

Robins, J. M., & Tsiatis, A. A. (1991). Correction for noncompliance in a randomized trial using rank-preserving structural failure time models. *Communications in Statistics: Part A. Theory and Methods, 20,* 2609–2631.

Rohay, J. M., Dunbar-Jacob, J., Sereika, S., Kwoh, K., & Burke, L. E. (1996). The impact of method of calculation of electronically monitored adherence data. *Controlled Clinical Trials, 17*(2S), 82S–83S.

Rohay, J. M., Marsh, G., Sereika, S., Mazumdar, S., & Dunbar-Jacob, J. (1994). The effects of aggregation on medication compliance history in repeated measures ANOVA: A simulation study. *Controlled Clinical Trials, 15*(3S), 98S.

Rost, K., Roter, D., Quill, T., Bertakis, K., & Collaborative Study Group of the Task Force on the Medical Interview. (1990). Capacity to remember prescription drug changes: Deficits associated with diabetes. *Diabetes Research and Clinical Practice, 10,* 183–187.

Roter, D. L., Hall, J. A., Merisca, R., Nordstrom, B., Cretin, D., & Svarstad, B. (1998). Effectiveness of interventions to improve patient compliance: A meta-analysis. *Medical Care, 36*(8), 1138–1161.

Rubin, D. B. (1998). More powerful randomization-based $p$-values in double-blind trials with non-compliance. *Statistics in Medicine, 17,* 371–385.

Schlenker, T., Sukhan, S., & Swenson, C. (1998). Improving vaccination coverage through accelerated measurement and feedback. *Journal of the American Medical Association, 280,* 1482–1483.

Schlundt, D. G., Rea, M., Hodge, M., Flannery, M. E., Kline, S., Meek, J., Kinzer, C., & Pichert, J. W. (1996). Assessing and overcoming situational obstacles to dietary adherence in adolescents with IDDM. *Journal of Adolescent Health, 19*(4), 282–288.

Schmaling, K. B., Afari, N., & Blume, A. W. (1998). Predictors of treatment adherence among asthma patients in the emergency department. *Journal of Asthma, 35*(8), 631–636.

Schneiders, A. G., Zusman, M., & Singer, K. P. (1998). Exercise therapy compliance in acute low back pain patients. *Manual Therapy, 3*(3), 147–152.

Schork, M. A., & Remington, R. D. (1967). The determination of sample size in treatment-control comparisons for chronic disease studies in which drop-out or nonadherence is a problem. *Journal of Chronic Disease, 20,* 233–238.

Schreiber, J. M., Effgen, S. K., & Palisano, R. J. (1995). Effectiveness of parental collaboration on compliance with a home program. *Pediatric Physical Therapy, 7*(2), 59–64.

Schweizer, R. T., Rovelli, M., Palmeri, D., Vossler, E., Hull, D., & Bartus, S. (1990). Noncompliance in organ transplant receipients. *Transplantation, 49,* 374–377.

Sereika, S., Dunbar-Jacob, J., Rand, C., Hamilton, G., Schron, E., Czajkowski, S., Waclawiw, M., Weeks, K., Lew, R., Leveck, M., Huss, K., Farzansar, R., & Friedman, R. (1998, May). *Adherence in clinical trials: A collaborative investigation of self-reported and electronically monitored adherence.* Paper presented at the 19th annual meeting of the Society for Clinical Trials, Atlanta.

Shea, S., Misra, D., Ehrlich, M. H., Field, L., & Francis, C. K. (1992). Correlates of nonadherence to hypertension treatment in a inner-city minority population. *American Journal of Public Health, 82*(12), 1607–1612.

Sheiner, L. B., & Rubin, D. B. (1995). Intention-to-treat analysis and the goals of clinical trials. *Clinical Pharmacology and Therapeutics, 57*(1), 6–15.

Shiffman, S., & Stone, A. A. (1998). Ecological momentary assessment: A new tool for behavioral medicine research. In D. S. Krantz & A. Baum (Eds.), *Technology and methods in behavioral medicine.* Mahwah, NJ: Lawrence Erlbaum Associates.

Shine, D., & McDonald, J. (1997). A computer model for the measurement of compliance using a dual tracer technique. *British Journal of Clinical Pharmacology, 43*(3), 283–290.

Shumway-Cook, A., Gruber, W., Baldwin, M., & Liao, S. (1997). The effect of multidimensional exercises on balance, mobility, and fall risk in community-dwelling older adults. *Physical Therapy, 77*(1), 46–57.

Siegal, B. R., & Greenstein, S. M. (1997). Postrenal transplant compliance from the perspective of African-Americans, Hispanic-Americans, and Anglo-Americans. *Advances in Renal Replacement Therapy, 4*(1), 46–54.

Silva, R. R., Munoz, D. M., Daniel, W., Barickman, J., & Friedhoff, A. J. (1996). Causes of haloperidol discontinuation in patients with Tourette's disorder: Management and alternatives. *Journal of Clinical Psychiatry, 57*(3), 129–135.

Simkin-Silverman, L., Wing, R. R., Hansen, D. H., Klem, M. L., Pasagian-Macaulay, A. P., Meilahn, E. N., & Kuller, L. H. (1995). Prevention of cardiovascular risk factor elevations in healthy premenopausal women. *Preventive Medicine, 24*(5), 509–517.

Simmons, M. S., Nides, M. A., Rand, C. S., Wise, R. A., & Tashkin, D. P. (1996). Trends in compliance with bronchodilator inhaler use between follow-up visits in a clinical trial. *Chest, 109*(4), 963–968.

Simon, P. M., Morse, E. V., & Besch, L. (1995). Barriers to compliance among women co-enrolled in a PCP prophylaxis and compliance protocol. *HIV Infected Women Conference*, P109.

Singh, N., Squier, C., Sivek, C., Wagener, M., Nguyen, M. H., & Yu, V. L. (1996). Determinants of compliance with antiretroviral therapy in patients with human immunodeficiency virus: Prospective assessment with implications for enhancing compliance. *AIDS Care, 8*(3), 261–269.

Singh, R. B., Rastogi, V., Rastogi, S. S., Niaz, M. A., & Beegom, R. (1996). Effect of diet and moderate exercise on central obesity and associated disturbances, myocardial infarction and mortality in patients with and without coronary artery disease. *Journal of the American College of Nutrition, 15*(6), 592–601.

Skelly, A. H., Marshall, J. R., Haughey, B. P., Davis, P. J., & Dunford, R. G. (1995). Self-efficacy and confidence in outcomes as determinants of self-care practices in inner-city, African-American women with non-insulin-dependent diabetes. *Diabetes Educator, 21*(1), 38–46.

Smith, D., & Diggle, P. J. (1998). Compliance in an anti-hypertension trial: A latent process model for binary longitudinal data. *Statistics in Medicine, 17,* 357–370.

Smith, E. O., Hardy, R. J., & Cutter, G. R. (1980). A two-compartment regression model applied to compliance in a hypertension treatment program. *Journal of Chronic Disease, 33,* 645–651.

Smith, M. Y., Rapkin, B. D., Morrison, A., & Kammerman, S. (1997). Zidovudine adherence in persons with AIDS. The relation of patient beliefs about medication to self-termination of therapy. *Journal of General Internal Medicine, 12*(4), 216–223.

Sommer, A., & Zeger, S. L. (1991). On estimating efficacy from clinical trials. *Statistics in Medicine, 10,* 45–52.

Spiers, M. V., & Kutzik, D. M. (1995). Self-reported memory of medication use of the elderly. *American Journal of Health-System Pharmacy, 52*(9), 985–990.

Stetson, B. A., Rahn, J. M., Dubbert, P. M., Wilner, B. I., & Mercury, M. G. (1997). Prospective evaluation of the effects of stress on exercise adherence in community-residing women. *Health Psychology, 16*(6), 515–520.

Straka, R. J., Fish, J. T., Benson, S. R., & Suh, J. T. (1997). Patient self-reporting of compliance does not correspond with electronic monitoring: An evaluation using isosorbide dinitrate as a model drug. *Pharmacotherapy, 17*(1), 126–132.

Swift, C. S., Armstrong, J. E., Campbell, R. K., Beerman, K. A., & Pond-Smith, D. (1997). Current clinical nutrition issues. Dietary habits and barriers among exercising and non-insulin-dependent diabetes mellitus. *Topics in Clinical Nutrition, 12*(2), 45–52.

Switzer, B. R., Stark, A. H., Atwood, J. R., Ritenbaugh, C., Travis, R. G., & Wu, H. M. (1997). Development of a urinary riboflavin adherence marker for a wheat bran fiber community intervention trial. *Cancer Epidemiology, Biomarkers & Prevention, 6*(6), 439–442.

Taylor, A. H., Doust, J., & Webborn, N. (1998). Randomized controlled trial to examine the effects of a GP exercise referral programme in Hailsham, East Sussex, on modifiable coronary heart disease risk factors. *Journal of Epidemiology and Community Health, 52*(9), 595–601.

Taylor, A. H., & May, S. (1996). Threat and coping appraisal as determinants of compliance with sports injury rehabilitation: An application of protection motivation theory. *Journal of Sports Sciences, 14*(6), 471–482.

Thilothammal, N., Krishnamurthy, P. V., Banu, K., & Gandhimathy, S. (1995). Testing compliance of drug taking: A simple bed side method. *Indian Pediatrics, 32*(3), 295–299.

Thompson, S. M., Dahlquist, L. M., Koenning, G. M., & Bartholomew, L. K. (1995). Brief report: Adherence-facilitating behaviors of a multidisciplinary pediatric rheumatology staff. *Journal of Pediatric Psychology, 20*(3), 291–297.

Toh, S. L., Low, C. L., & Goh, S. H. (1998). Drug related visits of geriatrics to the emergency department. *ASHP Annual Meeting, 55*(Jun.), INTL–3.

Toobert, D. J., Glasgow, R. E., Nettekoven, L. A., & Brown, J. E. (1998). Behavioral and psychosocial effects of intensive lifestyle management for women with coronary heart disease. *Patient Education and Counseling, 35*(3), 177–188.

Tracqui, A., Kintz, P., & Mangin, P. (1995). Hair analysis: A worthless tool for therapeutic compliance monitoring. *Forensic Science International, 70*(1–3), 183–189.

Turner, J., Wright, E., Mendella, L., & Anthonisen, N. (1995). Predictors of patient adherence to long-term home nebulizer therapy for COPD. *Chest: The Cardiopulmonary Journal, 108*(2), 394–400.

Turner, M. O., Taylor, D., Bennett, R., & Fitzgerald, J. M. (1998). A randomized trial comparing peak expiratory flow and symptom self-management plans for patients with asthma attending a primary care clinic. *American Journal of Respiratory and Critical Care Medicine, 157*(2), 540–546.

Tynan, M. B., Nicholls, D. P., Maguire, S. M., Steele, I. C., McMaster, C., Moore, R., Trimble, E. R., & Pearce J. (1995). Erythrocyte membrane fatty acid composition as a marker of dietary compliance in hyperlipaemic subjects. *Atherosclerosis, 117*(2), 245–252.

Urban, C., Benesch, M., Lackner, H., Schwinger, W., Kerbl, R., & Gadner, H. (1997). The influence of maximum supportive care on dose compliance and survival: Single-center analysis of childhood acute lymphoblastic leukemia and non-Hodgkin's lymphoma treated within 1984–1993. *Klinische Pädiatrie, 209*(4), 235–242.

Urquhart, J. (1990). Clinical impact of partial patient compliance. *Cardiovascular Review and Reports, 11*, 11–15.

Van Horn, L. V., Dolecek, T. A., Grandits, G. A., & Skweres, L. (1997). Adherence to dietary recommendations in the special intervention group in the Multiple Risk Factor Intervention Trial. *American Journal of Clinical Nutrition, 65*(1S Suppl), 289S–304S.

Van Sciver, M. M., D'Angelo, E. J., Rappaport, L., & Woolf, A. D. (1995). Pediatric compliance and the roles of distinct treatment characteristics, treatment attitudes, and family stress: A preliminary report. *Journal of Developmental and Behavioral Pediatrics, 16*(5), 350–358.

Vanhove, G. F., Schapiro, J. M., Winters, M. A., Merigan, T. C., & Blaschke, T. F. (1996). Patient compliance and drug failure in protease inhibitor monotherapy. *Journal of the American Medical Association, 276*, 1955–1956.

Vrijens, B., & Goetghebeur, E. (1997). Comparing compliance patterns between randomized treatments. *Controlled Clinical Trials, 18*(3), 187–203.

Wadden, T. A., Vogt, R. A., Foster, G. D., & Anderson, D. A. (1998). Exercise and the maintenance of weight loss: One-year follow-up of a controlled clinical trial. *Journal of Consulting and Clinical Psychology, 66*(2), 429–433.

Wadibia, E. C., Lucas, B. D., Stading, J. A., Hilleman, D. E., & Mohiuddin, S. M. (1995). Impact of pharmaceutical counseling on compliance and effectiveness with combination lipid lowering therapy in patients at high risk of recurrent cardiovascular events. *ASHP Midyear Clinical Meeting, 30*(Dec), P–94(E).

Wall, T. L., Sorensen J. L., Batki, S. L., Delucchi, K. L., London, J. A., & Chesney, M. A. (1995). Adherence to zidovudine (AZT) among HIV-infected methadone patients: A pilot study of supervised therapy and dispensing compared to usual care. *Drug and Alcohol Dependence, 37*(3), 261–269.

Wamboldt, F. S., Wamboldt, M. Z., Gavin, L. A., & Roesler, T. A.(1995). Parental criticism treatment outcome in adolescents hospitalized for severe, chronic asthma. *Journal of Psychosomatic Research, 39*(8), 995–1005.

Wang, W., Husan, F., & Chow, S-C. (1996). The impact of patient compliance on drug concentration profile in multiple doses. *Statistics in Medicine, 15*, 659–669.

Watson, D. C., Farley, J. J., Lovelace, S., & Vink, P. (1998). Efficacy and adherence to highly active antiretroviral therapy (HAART) in HIV-1 infected children. *5th Conference on Retroviral Opportunistic Infections* (p. 122).

Watts, R. W., McLennan, G., Bassham, I., & el-Saadi, O. (1997). Do patients with ashtma fill their prescriptions? A primary compliance study. *Australian Family Physician, 26*(Suppl 1), S4–6.

Weaver, T. E., Kribbs, N. B., Pack, A. I., Kline, L. R., Chugh, D. K., Maislin, G., Smith, P. L., Schwartz, A. R., Schubert, N. M., Gillen, K. A., & Dinges, D. F. (1997). Night to night variability in CPAP use over the first three months of treatment. *Sleep, 20*(4), 278–283.

White, I. R., & Goetghebeur, E. (1998). Clinical trials comparing two treatments policies: Which aspects of the treatment policies make a difference? *Statistics in Medicine, 17,* 319–339.

Wiebe, J. S., & Christensen, A. J. (1997). Health beliefs, personality, and adherence in hemodialysis patients: An interactional perspective. *Annals of Behavioral Medicine, 19*(1), 30–35.

Willett, W. C., Sampson, L., & Stampfer, M. J. (1985). Reproducibility and validity of a semi-quantitative food frequency questionnaire. *American Journal of Epidemiology, 122,* 51–65.

Williams, J., Patsalos, P. N., & Wilson, J. F. (1997). Hair analysis as a potential index of therapeutic compliance in the treatment of epilepsy. *Forensic Science International, 84*(1–3), 113–122.

Williams, P., & Lord, S. R. (1995). Predictors of adherence to a structured exercise program for older women. *Psychology and Aging, 10*(4), 617–624.

Williford, S. L., & Johnson, D. F. (1995). Impact of pharmacist counseling on medication knowledge and compliance. *Military Medicine, 160*(11), 561–564.

Wing, R. R., & Anglin, K. (1996). Effectiveness of a behavioral weight control program for blacks and whites with NIDDM. *Diabetes Care, 19*(5), 409–413.

Wing, R. R., Jeffery, R. W., Pronk, N., & Hellerstedt, W. L. (1996). Effects of a personal trainer and financial incentives on exercise adherence in overweight women in a behavioral weight loss program. *Obesity Research, 4*(5), 457–462.

Woodward, J., Wareham, P. S., Grohskopf, L., Madigan, D., & Hooton, T. M. (1998). Protease inhibitor adherence and HIV-1 RNA response. *International Conference on AIDS, 12,* 1066.

Wu, M., Fisher, M., & DeMets, D. (1980). Sample sizes for long-term medical trials with time-dependent drop-out and event rates. *Controlled Clinical Trials, 1,* 111–121.

Zwarenstein, M., Schoeman, J. H., Vundule, C., Lombard, C. J., & Tatley, M. (1998). Randomized controlled trial of self-supervised and directly observed treatment of tuberculosis. *Lancet, 352,* 1340–1343.

## Chapter 4

# Heart Failure Management: Optimal Health Care Delivery Programs

DEBRA K. MOSER

### ABSTRACT

Heart failure is the single most costly health care expenditure in the United States. The major proportion of these costs is attributable to rehospitalizations, and by many estimates the majority of rehospitalizations might be preventable with better health care delivery. The past 5 years have seen an explosion in the number of heart failure disease management programs put in place across the country to try to decrease the economic burden of heart failure and improve patient outcomes. Yet few of these are based on programs tested by researchers, let alone tested in randomized, controlled trials. This chapter summarizes findings from studies of heart failure disease management programs from 1980 to the present, critiques those studies, and offers suggestions for future research in this area.

**Key words: heart failure, quality of life, health care resource utilization, patient and family education, outcomes, disease management**

Heart failure is a clinical syndrome in which progressively deteriorating ventricular function results in the characteristic pathophysiologic changes of vasoconstriction and fluid retention, marked activity intolerance from dyspnea and fatigue, impaired quality of life, and premature death. Heart failure has been called an epidemic (Hoes, Mosterd, & Grobbee, 1998; Massie & Shah, 1996; McMurray, Petrie, Murdoch, & Davie, 1998; O'Connell & Bristow, 1993) because of its increasing prevalence and incidence and is considered "the most important public health problem facing cardiovascular medicine" in this decade (Garg, Packer, Pitt, & Yusuf, 1993, p. 3A). The expected marked increase in incidence and prevalence of heart failure is not unique to the United States. Heart failure is emerging as a growing public health problem in other developed and developing countries (Hoes et al., 1998). For example, the prevalence of heart failure is expected to increase by at least 70% in the Netherlands and Australia by the year 2010 (McMurray et al., 1998).

Heart failure afflicts approximately 5 million people in the United States (American Heart Association, 1997; Goldberg & Konstam, 1999). At least 400,000 to 700,000 new cases are diagnosed each year (American Heart Association, 1997). Morbidity from heart failure is extremely high. It is the primary discharge diagnosis in more than 1 million hospitalizations per year and a secondary diagnosis in another 2 million (Massie & Shah, 1996). Among the elderly, 27% of patients are readmitted within 90 days for recurrent heart failure; 29% of these are readmitted more than once (Vinson, Rich, Sperry, Shah, & McNamara, 1990); and over the past two decades the number of hospital admissions for elderly heart failure patients has more than doubled (Kimmelstiel & Konstam, 1995). Examination of Medicare statistics from Connecticut revealed a 44% readmission rate in 6 months (Krumholz, Parent, et al., 1997). Across the nation the 6-month hospital readmission rate for heart failure is 47% (Starling, 1998). Heart failure is now the most common hospital discharge diagnosis for patients over the age of 65 and is the largest single Medicare hospitalization expenditure (O'Connell & Bristow, 1993). Combined, the inpatient and outpatient care costs for heart failure are estimated at more than $35 billion (O'Connell & Bristow, 1993).

The cost of heart failure is evident not only in terms of the economic toll it exacts but in terms of its negative impact on survival. Heart failure is indicated as the primary cause of death in more than 40,000 patients each year and is implicated as a contributing cause in another 220,000 deaths per year (American Heart Association, 1997; Goldberg & Konstam, 1999). Data from the Framingham study indicate that, within 5 years of being diagnosed with heart failure, only 25% of men and 38% of women are still alive (Ho, Pinsky, & Kannel, 1993).

Further compounding the burden of heart failure is the significant deterioration in quality of life that occurs (Dracup, Walden, Stevenson, & Brecht, 1992; Grady, 1993; Grady, Jalowiec, Grusk, White-Williams, & Robinson, 1992; Stewart et al., 1989). Quality of life is more severely impaired in heart failure than it is in several other common chronic diseases (e.g., hypertension, diabetes, arthritis, chronic lung disease, or angina) (Stewart et al., 1989). Many dimension of quality of life are affected, including physical functioning; family, social, and work roles (Walden et al., 1994); emotional well-being (Dracup et al., 1992; Hawthorne & Hixon, 1994); and sexual activity and satisfaction (Jaarsma, Dracup, Walden, & Stevenson, 1996). Furthermore, recent reports indicate that quality of life may be an independent predictor for subsequent mortality and rehospitalizations (Konstam et al., 1996).

The care of patients with heart failure is challenging because, once diagnosed, recurrent rehospitalization for exacerbation of failure is common (O'Connell & Bristow, 1993). Many of these readmissions may be preventable with better delivery of care (Rich, 1999; Vinson et al., 1990) and with attention to modifiable factors that play a role in the high rate of rehospitalization (Ghali, Kadakia, Cooper, & Ferlinz, 1988; Happ, Naylor, & Roe-Prior, 1997; Jaarsma, Halfens, & Huijer-AbuSaad, 1996; Michalsen, Konig, & Thimme, 1998; Vinson et al., 1990). Investigators specifically examining reasons for rehospitalizations among patients with heart failure have consistently demonstrated that as many as half and, in some cases, up to two-thirds of rehospitalizations could have been prevented (Bennett et al., 1998; Ghali et al., 1988; Michalsen et al., 1998; Vinson et al., 1990). In the majority of cases, failure to adhere to prescribed medication and diet therapy was a major preventable cause of rehospitalization for heart failure exacerbation.

Nonadherence to heart failure treatment plans is common and appears to increase as heart failure progresses (Bennett et al., 1998; Chin & Goldman, 1997; Ghali et al., 1988; Michalsen et al., 1998; Monane, Bohn, Gurwitz, Glynn, & Avorn, 1994; Vinson et al., 1990). Adherence to outpatient digoxin prescription has been reported as low as 10% (Monane et al., 1994). In from 42% to 64% of heart failure readmissions, lack of adherence to prescribed medication and/or diet plans has been implicated as the proximate cause of the readmission (Ghali et al., 1988; Michalsen et al., 1998).

Other important and common preventable factors contributing to heart failure rehospitalization include inadequate patient follow-up after discharge, failed social support systems, and patient failure to obtain medical assistance when symptoms increase (Vinson et al., 1990). Failure to prescribe appropriate recommended drug therapy also contributes substantially to the high rate of rehospitalizations for heart failure. Despite publication of guidelines (American College of Cardiology/American Heart Association, 1995; Konstam et al., 1994; Packer & Cohn, 1999) explicating standards for heart failure medical therapy, as many as 50% to 72% of patients still are not prescribed angiotensin-converting enzyme inhibitors and other drugs demonstrated to be effective in heart failure, do not receive them in adequate doses, and are prescribed drugs such as calcium channel blockers that may have deleterious effects in heart failure (Clinical Quality Improvement Network Investigators, 1996; Nohria et al., 1999; Stafford, Saglam, & Blumenthal, 1997; Sueta et al., 1999). Thus, although there have been some recent improvements in prescription patterns for patients with heart failure, widespread use of appropriate medications for patients with heart failure is not a reality (McDermott et al., 1997; Nohria et al., 1999).

In most cases, patients with heart failure are still treated in traditional health care delivery models that are characterized by episodic care delivered during periods of acute exacerbation of heart failure. Many aspects of this care contribute to rehospitalization. In-hospital patient and family education is limited, and many patients receive little appropriate education and counseling (Krumholz, Wang, et al., 1997; McDermott et al., 1997). In a study of the association between the quality of inpatient care and early readmission, Ashton and associates (Ashton, Kuykendall, Johnson, Wray, & Wu, 1995) demonstrated that approximately one in five unplanned hospital readmissions for heart failure was attributable to substandard inpatient care. Follow-up after hospital discharge usually consists of a few short physician office visits in which there is little time to address the multiple and complex medical, behavioral, psychosocial, environmental, and financial issues that complicate the care of patients with heart failure. The areas of substandard care thought to contribute most to readmissions were lack of patient and family education and failure to organize follow-up care. Recognition that these issues must be addressed to improve heart failure outcomes, along with the increasing incidence, prevalence, and economic costs of heart failure (Croft et al., 1997), have prompted many to call for a change from our current treatment patterns of fragmented acute inpatient care to comprehensive, integrated expert multidisciplinary care patterns (O'Connell & Bristow, 1993).

To meet the many challenges of caring for patients with heart failure, several excellent consensus guidelines have been developed to assist clinicians to provide optimal care (American College of Cardiology/American Heart Association, 1995; Konstam et al., 1994; Packer & Cohn, 1999; Task Force of the Working Group on Heart Failure, 1997; World Health Organization, 1996). These guidelines, developed by expert panels, translate the findings of clinical trials into specific practice recommendations for treating patients with heart failure. In general, these guidelines have focused on evaluation of heart failure and optimization of pharmacologic management. Although diet, activity, and other lifestyle changes and patient and family education and counseling are discussed, none of the guidelines has focused on the organization of health care delivery for the management of heart failure. Although this omission was probably appropriate, given the level of research in this area at the time most guidelines were developed, the recent marked increase in the number of published research studies that report the outcomes of various heart failure disease management programs now warrants examination of this literature.

The purpose of this chapter is to present a review and critique of the available English-language research literature regarding heart failure disease management programs designed to decrease rehospitalization rates, reduce health care costs, and improve patients' quality of life and functional status. Disease management has been defined as "an approach to patient care that emphasizes coordinated, comprehensive care along the continuum of disease and across health care delivery systems" (Ellrodt et al., 1997, p. 1687). Disease management programs are designed to improve the structure of care delivery for a group of patients with a common chronic disease that has associated high costs and complex management needs (Bernard, Townsend, & Sylvestri, 1998).

Studies for review were identified by a computerized search of the MEDLINE database and the Cumulative Index of Nursing and Allied Health Literature (CINAHL). The heading *congestive heart failure* was used with the subcategories of economics, nursing, and therapy. In addition, the term *congestive heart failure* was combined with each of the following subject headings: *disease management, health services research, evaluation studies, patient care planning, treatment outcomes, managed care programs, risk management, hospitalization, readmission,* and *multidisciplinary care team.* The reference lists of studies reviewed were examined for any additional relevant articles.

All heart failure disease management studies from 1980 to the first quarter of 1999 found using these strategies were included in this review if data on at least one of the following outcomes was reported: (1) quality of life; (2) health care resource utilization, including rehospitalizations or emergency department visits; (3) costs of care; (4) functional status; or (5) mortality. Excluded from this review were articles that were not research reports but were simple descriptions of ongoing institutional heart failure disease management programs with mention of program outcomes but no statistical support for their conclusions. Also excluded were studies in which a disease management approach was applied to a variety of patients with different diagnoses and patients with heart failure were not the primary focus of the study (e.g. Naylor et al., 1999). In addition, two studies that were retrospective chart reviews were excluded (Dennis, Blue, Stahl, Benge, & Shaw, 1996; Martens & Mellor, 1997). One study that was excluded was reported as having tested a disease management program but consisted of a one-component intervention (mailed educational materials without contact with health care providers) that does not meet even loose criteria for disease management (e.g., Serxner, Miyaji, & Jeffords, 1998).

## TESTED HEART FAILURE DISEASE MANAGEMENT PROGRAMS

Since 1980, investigators have tested a variety of disease management programs designed to improve outcomes in patients with heart failure, although the largest concentration of studies has been in the past 5 years. This proliferation of studies in recent years is a result of sharply increased awareness of the poor outcomes and high cost associated with care of heart failure patients. Because many of these programs were developed and reported simultaneously, there has been little opportunity for investigators to build on the work of others. As a consequence, although many of the tested heart failure disease management programs have similar components, they also have marked differences. This variety and the multiple components tested make comparison of studies difficult. Even more difficult is determining which components are essential for a successful program.

Although the programs described here reflect a wide variety of approaches, all represent programs in which there was a significant departure from traditional episodic care delivery, in that patients received additional heart failure–specific attention using a disease management approach (Table 4.1). These programs can be categorized broadly and will be described, in three categories: (1) specialty heart failure clinics (Cintron, Bigas, Linares, Aranda, & Hernandez, 1983; Cline, Israelsson, Willenheimer, Broms, & Erhardt, 1998; Fonarow et al., 1997; Hanumanthu, Butler, Chomsky, Davis, & Wilson, 1997; Smith, Fabbri, Pai, Ferry, & Heywood, 1997), (2) specialty care that extends to the home (Kornowski et al., 1995; Rich et al., 1993, 1995; Shah, Der, Ruggerio, Heidenreich, & Massie, 1998; Stewart, Pearson, & Horowitz, 1998; Stewart, Vandenbrock, Pearson, & Horowitz, 1999; West et al., 1997), and (3) increased access to primary care (Weinberger, Oddone, & Henderson, 1996).

*Specialty heart failure clinics* represent disease management programs in which service is provided primarily in an outpatient clinic setting where patients come to the clinic to receive care from practitioners with expertise in heart failure. Those programs offering *specialty care that extends to the home* include a variety of disease management approaches that all have in common heart failure–specific care that is delivered primarily in the patient's home. *Increased access to primary care* is care provided to heart failure patients by primary care providers primarily in an outpatient setting that emphasizes increased vigilance and assessment of problems that contribute to rehospitalization.

## Specialty Heart Failure Clinics

In one of the earliest studies of specialized heart failure care, Cintron and associates (1983) examined the impact of care delivered to patients in a heart failure clinic managed by a nurse practitioner. Heart failure patients from the San Juan Veteran's Administration Hospital were referred to the clinic after stabilization. Care consisted of frequent (every 3 weeks) follow-up visits in the clinic for assessment of status, education about medications, weight control and diet, and assessment of home problems and family support. In addition, the nurse practitioner was available for patients with problems and without appointments. A cardiologist was available for consultation. After an average follow-up of 12 months and compared to the time period before implementation of the clinic, patients experienced a 60% reduction in rehospitalizations and an 85% reduction

**TABLE 4.1   Studies of Heart Failure Programs**

| Reference | Patients<br>• Percentage male<br>• Country in which study conducted | Study design | Intervention | Components of intervention | Outcomes[a] |
|---|---|---|---|---|---|
| *Specialty Heart Failure Clinics* | | | | | |
| Cintron et al., 1983 | • 15, NYHA III–IV, mean age 65 years<br>• Sex of patients not indicated although study conducted at a Veteran's Administration hospital so likely exclusively men<br>• Puerto Rico | Within-subjects preintervention-postintervention comparison with mean follow-up of 24 months | Nurse practitioner heart failure clinic | • Nurse practitioner managed<br>• Frequent follow-up via clinic visits<br>• Education reinforced at each visit: medication, weight control, diet<br>• Assessment of home situation<br>• Family support<br>• Increased availability of nurse practitioner ("walk-ins" encouraged)<br>• Cardiologist consultation for unstable patients | • 60% reduction in rehospitalizations<br>• 85% reduction in hospital days<br>• Reduction in total medical costs of $8,009 per patient |

**TABLE 4.1    Studies of Heart Failure Programs** (*Continued*)

| Reference | Patients • Percentage male • Country in which study conducted | Study design | Intervention | Components of intervention | Outcomes[a] |
|---|---|---|---|---|---|
| Hanumanthu et al., 1997 | • 134, NYHA not indicated, mean age 52 ± 12 years • 71% • United States | Within-subjects preintervention-postintervention comparison with follow-up of 12 months | Physician-directed, nurse-coordinated comprehensive heart failure outpatient program | • Heart failure/ transplant physician directed • Nurse coordinators assist with inpatient and outpatient management • Team exclusively manages heart failure patients • Optimization of medical therapy • Other details not provided • Periodic meetings with home health care agency and hospice program to integrate care | • 53% reduction in annual hospitalization rate • 63% reduction in heart failure rehospitalizations • Increased peak $VO_2$ |
| Fonarow et al., 1997 | • 214, NYHA III and IV, mean | Within-subjects preintervention- | Heart failure cardiologist | • Heart failure cardiologist | • 89% reduction in rehospitalizations |

age 52 ± 10 years
- 81%
- United States

postintervention comparison with follow-up of 6 months

directed, clinical nurse specialist follow-up, comprehensive inpatient and outpatient management program

directed
- Follow-up by heart failure cardiologist, clinical nurse specialist, and referring physician
- Optimization of drug therapy in hospital and during follow-up
- Comprehensive patient and family/caregiver education by heart failure clinical nurse specialist about daily weights and flexible diuretic regimen, diet, medications, smoking and alcohol abstinence, home exercise instruction, warning signs of worsening heart failure, and prognosis

Improvement in functional status
Lower costs

**TABLE 4.1    Studies of Heart Failure Programs (*Continued*)**

| Reference | Patients<br>• Percentage male<br>• Country in which study conducted | Study design | Intervention | Components of intervention | Outcomes[a] |
|---|---|---|---|---|---|
| Fonarow et al., 1997 (*cont.*) | | | | • Weekly follow-up at heart failure clinic until stable, with education reinforced<br>• Phone follow-up after medication changes and if indicated | |
| Smith et al., 1997 | • 21, mean NYHA 2.6 ± 0.5, mean age 61 years<br>• 100%<br>• United States | Within-subjects preintervention-postintervention comparison with follow-up of 6 months | Physician or nurse practitioner comprehensive care in heart failure clinic | • Care provided by physician or nurse practitioner<br>• Optimization of medical therapy<br>• Identification and management of etiology of heart failure<br>• Patient education about diet, medications, | • 86% reduction in heart failure hospitalizations<br>• Improved quality of life<br>• Improved functional status<br>• More patients on optimal medications and doses |

| Cline et al., 1998 | • 190, mean NYHA 2.6 ± 0.7, mean age 75.6 ± 5.3 years<br>• 52.3%<br>• Sweden | Randomized control trial with follow-up of 12 months | Nurse-directed outpatient clinic | |

Intervention:
- compliance, daily weights and flexible diuretic regimen, alcohol abstinence
- Nurse practitioner available by phone
- Increased access to clinic (without appointment) for worsening symptoms or medication needs
- Before hospital discharge, patient and family education about heart failure and pharmacologic and nonpharmacologic aspects of its treatment
- Medication organizer given
- Patients receive guidelines for self-management of diuretics
- One-hour information visits for patient and

Outcomes:
- Time to first admission 33% longer in intervention group
- 59% increase in number of days hospitalized, compared to 12-month period before start of study in control group versus no increase in intervention group
- 36% fewer hospitalizations in intervention group (but nonsignificant

**TABLE 4.1   Studies of Heart Failure Programs (*Continued*)**

| Reference | Patients <br>• Percentage male <br>• Country in which study conducted | Study design | Intervention | Components of intervention | Outcomes[a] |
|---|---|---|---|---|---|
| Cline et al., 1998 (*cont.*) | | | | family at home after discharge <br>• Easy access to a nurse-directed outpatient clinic with one prescheduled visit at 8 months; nurses available by phone and could see patients at short notice <br>• Encouragement to contact nurses at clinic for any problems or questions or concerns | at $p = .08$) <br>• Trend toward mean annual reduction in health care costs ($p = .07$) |

*Specialty care that extends to the home*

| Rich et al., 1993 | • 98, mean NYHA 2.8, all patients > 70 years<br>• 41%<br>• United States | Randomized controlled trial with follow-up of 90 days | Nurse-directed multidisciplinary team with in-hospital education and home follow-up | • Comprehensive daily in-hospital education by experienced geriatric cardiovascular nurse about diagnosis, symptoms, treatment, including medications and diet, follow-up, and prognosis<br>• Individualized dietary assessment and instruction by registered dietitian<br>• Detailed daily weighing instruction<br>• Simplification of medication regimen when possible by a geriatric cardiologist<br>• Discharge planning by social worker and home care with identification and management of | • 27% fewer hospital admissions although not statistically significant<br>• 25% fewer hospital days although not statistically significant |

**TABLE 4.1   Studies of Heart Failure Programs (*Continued*)**

| Reference | Patients • Percentage male • Country in which study conducted | Study design | Intervention | Components of intervention | Outcomes[a] |
|---|---|---|---|---|---|
| Rich et al., 1993 (*cont.*) | | | | economic, social, and transportation problems • Intensive home follow-up visits and phone calls • Increased access to study personnel for problems | |
| Kornowski et al., 1995 | • 42, NYHA III–IV, mean age 78 ± 8 years • 57% • Israel | Within-subjects preintervention-postintervention comparison with follow-up of 12 months | Home care by physician and nurse | • Weekly home visits by physician and nurse • Physical examination • Medication review • Change in medication if needed • Intravenous diuretic therapy as needed | • 62% reduction in total rehospitalizations, with 77% reduction in hospital days • 72% reduction in cardiovascular rehospitalizations, with 83% reduction in hospital days • 50% of patients never hospitalized |

| Study | Sample | Design | Intervention | Outcomes |
|---|---|---|---|---|
| Rich et al., 1995 | • 282, mean NYHA 2.4, median age 79 years<br>• 37%<br>• United States | Randomized, controlled trial (intervention compared to usual care) with follow-up of 90 days for intervention and 12 months for data collection | Nurse-directed multidisciplinary team with in-hospital education and home follow-up<br><br>• Comprehensive daily in-hospital education by experienced geriatric cardiovascular nurse about diagnosis, symptoms, treatment, including medications and diet, follow-up, and prognosis<br>• Individualized dietary assessment and instruction by registered dietitian<br>• Detailed daily weighing instruction<br>• Simplification of medication regimen when possible by a geriatric cardiologist<br>• Discharge planning by social worker and home care, with<br>• Increased availability of physician (extra visits if needed) | • Comprehensive daily in-hospital education during follow-up period<br>• Improvement in functional status<br>• 44% reduction in total readmissions<br>• 36% reduction in hospital days<br>• 56% fewer heart failure hospitalizations<br>• Improved quality of life<br>• Cost of care lower at $460 per patient |

**TABLE 4.1　Studies of Heart Failure Programs (*Continued*)**

| Reference | Patients • Percentage male • Country in which study conducted | Study design | Intervention | Components of intervention | Outcomes[a] |
|---|---|---|---|---|---|
| Rich et al., 1995 (*cont.*) | | | | identification and management of economic, social, and transportation problems • Intensive home follow-up visits and phone calls • Increased access to study personnel for problems | |
| West et al., 1997 | • 51, NYHA I 22%, II 38%, III 28%, IV 12%, mean age 66 ± 10 years • 71% • United States | Within-subjects preintervention-postintervention comparison with follow-up of 138 ± 44 days for intervention and 12 months for data collection | Physician-supervised, nurse-managed, home-based | • Primary physician retained overall responsibility • Nurses managed care and initial visit by nurse was followed by weekly phone calls for 6 weeks • Cardiologist | • 23% reduction in general medical visits • 31% reduction in cardiology visits • 67% reduction in emergency department visits for heart failure • 87% reduction in |

| Shah et al., 1998 | • 27, NYHA II 37%, III–IV 63%, mean age 62 years<br>• Sex of patients not indicated although study conducted at a | Within-subjects preintervention-postintervention comparison with follow-up of 12 months | Nurse-monitored comprehensive education and telemonitoring | • 8 weekly education mailings about causes and manifestations of heart failure, medications, diet<br>• Paging system to | available for consultation to nurse in difficult cases<br>• Implementation of consensus heart failure guidelines<br>• Optimization of drug, specifically angiotensin-converting enzyme inhibitor or isosorbide dinitrate/hydralazine, therapy<br>• Comprehensive education about medications, diet, signs of worsening failure, and techniques for increasing compliance | • 67% reduction in cardiovascular hospitalizations<br>• 92% fewer hospital days | heart failure readmissions<br>• 74% reduction in total hospitalizations<br>• Improved functional status and quality of life<br>• 82% increase in patients receiving target doses of angiotensin-converting enzyme inhibitors |

**TABLE 4.1    Studies of Heart Failure Programs (*Continued*)**

| Reference | Patients<br>• Percentage male<br>• Country in which study conducted | Study design | Intervention | Components of intervention | Outcomes[a] |
|---|---|---|---|---|---|
| Shah et al., 1998 (*cont.*) | • Veterans Administration hospital so likely exclusively men<br>• United States | | | transmit reminders to patients about taking medications, weights, heart rate, and blood pressure<br>• Heart failure nurse phoned weekly<br>• Increased access to nurse (24-hr availability by phone)<br>• Patient data sent to cardiologist monthly or more frequently as required for consultation | |
| Stewart et al., 1998 | • 97, NYHA II 49%, III 43%, IV 4%, mean age 75 years<br>• 49%<br>• Australia | Randomized, controlled trial with follow-up of 6 months | Nurse and pharmacist inpatient and home-based education | • Before hospital discharge, patient education and counseling from nurse about complying with | • 42% fewer unplanned admissions<br>• 43% fewer hospital days<br>• Lower hospital costs |

| Stewart et al., 1999 | • 97, NYHA II 49%, III 43%, IV 4%, mean age 75 years | Randomized, controlled trial, follow-up of | Nurse and pharmacist inpatient and | treatment regimen and reporting signs of worsening heart failure<br>• Home visit 1 week after hospital discharge by nurse and pharmacist<br>• Pharmacist-assessed knowledge about medications and extent of compliance<br>• For those with low knowledge or compliance, remedial counseling, daily medication reminders, medication box given, incremental monitoring by caregivers, medication information and cards, referral to community pharmacist for more regular review<br>• Nurse-assessed signs of clinical deterioration and adverse drug effects<br>• Before hospital discharge, patient education and | • Fewer unplanned readmissions<br>• Lower length of |

**TABLE 4.1   Studies of Heart Failure Programs (*Continued*)**

| Reference | • Patients<br>• Percentage male<br>• Country in which study conducted | Study design | Intervention | Components of intervention | Outcomes[a] |
|---|---|---|---|---|---|
| Stewart et al., 1999 (*cont.*) | • 49%<br>• Australia | Stewart et al., 1998, at 18 months | Home-based education | counseling from nurse about complying with treatment regimen and reporting signs of worsening heart failure<br>• Home visit 1 week after hospital discharge by nurse and pharmacist<br>• Pharmacist-assessed knowledge about medications and extent of compliance<br>• For those with low knowledge or compliance, remedial counseling, daily medication reminders, | hospital stay<br>• Fewer out-of-hospital deaths |

*Increased access to primary care*

| Study | Sample | Design | | Intervention | Outcomes |
|---|---|---|---|---|---|
| | | | medication box given, incremental monitoring by caregivers, medication information and cards, referral to community pharmacist for more regular review<br>• Nurse-assessed signs of clinical deterioration and adverse drug effects | | • More readmission in the intervention group<br>• Greater number of hospital days in the intervention group<br>• No difference in quality of life between the two groups<br>• Greater satisfaction with care in the intervention group |
| Weinberger et al., 1996 | • 1396 total, 504 with heart failure, NYHA I 13%, II 38%, III 33%, IV 16%, mean age 63 years<br>• 98%–99%<br>• United States | Randomized, controlled trial with follow-up for 6 months | Increased access to primary care | • Care directed by primary care physician and nurse teams<br>• Assessment by primary care nurse prior to patient discharge of postdischarge needs, provision of relevant education materials, assignment of primary care physician, and card | |

**TABLE 4.1   Studies of Heart Failure Programs** *(Continued)*

| Reference | Patients • Percentage male • Country in which study conducted | Study design | Intervention | Components of intervention | Outcomes[a] |
|---|---|---|---|---|---|
| Weinberger et al., 1996 *(cont.)* | | | | given to patient with names and numbers of primary care team<br>• Visit by primary care physician prior to discharge to discuss postdischarge regimen<br>• Clinic appointment within 1 week of discharge<br>• Phone call by primary care nurse within 2 days of discharge to assess problems<br>• Revision of therapeutic plan by physician and nurse at clinic visit | |

[a] Results are statistically significant unless otherwise indicated; NYHA = New York Heart Association functional class.

in number of hospital days. Costs for outpatient care increased but were offset by a substantial reduction in inpatient care costs.

Hanumanthu and associates (1997) compared outcomes in 134 patients before and after referral to their heart failure program. The program consisted of long-term follow-up by three physicians and two nurse coordinators who worked exclusively with heart failure patients. Physicians used cardiopulmonary exercise testing and hemodynamic monitoring to manage patients. After referral to the program, patients' functional status and quality of life increased significantly, and rehospitalizations were reduced by 53% compared to a similar time period before referral.

In the same year, Fonarow and colleagues (1997) reported outcomes of 214 patients referred to their heart failure program as potential heart transplant candidates. In this study, outcomes 6 months earlier were compared to those 6 months after referral to the program. The program consisted of management and follow-up by cardiologists with heart failure expertise and a heart failure clinical nurse specialist; optimization of pharmacologic therapy, using hemodynamic monitoring; comprehensive patient education and counseling regarding diet, risk factor modification, warning symptoms of worsening heart failure, and flexible diuretic regimen; and recommendations to walk for 30–45 minutes four times weekly. The team managed patients both in the hospital and as outpatients. Compared to 6 months before referral, patients demonstrated improved functional status and an 89% reduction in hospitalizations.

Smith and associates (1997) compared New York Heart Association (NYHA) functional class, exercise time, peak oxygen consumption, quality of life, rehospitalizations, and emergency room visits 6 months before and after referral to a cardiomyopathy clinic among 21 male symptomatic heart failure patients. Care was provided by a heart failure cardiologist and nurse practitioner and consisted of optimization of pharmacologic therapy; aggressive treatment of hypertension and ischemia; risk factor modification; education about medications, diet, and importance of compliance; daily weight and prn diuretic dosing instruction; and increased access to a nurse practitioner by telephone. Improved NYHA functional class, exercise time, and quality of life were reported after referral. Emergency department visits and hospitalizations were both reduced by at least 80% compared to the period before referral.

In the only published randomized controlled trial of a heart failure specialty clinic, Cline and associates (1998) reported their experience with 190 Swedish patients. These patients were randomized to either usual care or a program of hospital and outpatient education, flexible patient-managed diuretic regimen, and referral to an easy-access, nurse-directed outpatient clinic. Compared to the control group, intervention patients demonstrated 33% longer time to first hospital readmission; no increase in number of hospital days, compared to 12 months prior to intervention, versus a 59% increase in control patients; and trends toward 36% fewer hospitalizations and reduced health care costs.

*Summary.* Together, a total of 574 patients were enrolled in these five studies of heart failure disease management clinics, and in two of them only men were studied (Cintron et al., 1983; Smith et al., 1997). Hanumanthu and associates (1997) enrolled 71% men, and Fonarow and associates (1997) enrolled 81% men. In only the Swedish study (Cline et al., 1998) were equal numbers of men and women enrolled. These five studies of heart failure specialty clinics include only one randomized, controlled trial (Cline et al., 1998). That study was conducted in Sweden, which limits generalizability to the United States with its different health care system. In the remaining studies, data after implementation of the program were compared to data prior to implementation (Cintron et al., 1983; Fonarow et al., 1997; Hanamanthu et al., 1997; Smith et al., 1997). Nonetheless, the consistent findings from this group of studies demonstrates that selected heart failure patients who receive care in a heart failure specialty clinic experience improved outcomes in terms of reduction in number of subsequent hospitalizations, hospital days, and improvement in quality of life and functional status. Furthermore, this care appears to be cost-effective, the increased costs of specialty heart failure clinic care being offset by reductions in rehospitalizations (Cintron et al., 1983; Cline et al., 1998; Fonarow et al., 1997).

Each of these disease management programs contained several components that likely contributed to their success. Common components of these five approaches include the following: (1) comprehensive care (i.e., attention to multiple important aspects of heart failure care), including patient and family education; (2) care under direction of experienced heart failure cardiologist (Fonarow et al., 1997; Hanumanthu et al., 1997; Smith et al., 1997) or one available for consultation (Cintron et al., 1983; Cline et al., 1998); (3) care either directed/managed (Cintron et al., 1983; Cline et al., 1998; Smith et al., 1997) or coordinated/assisted (Fonarow et al., 1997; Hanamanthu et al., 1997) by a nurse practitioner or clinical nurse specialist; (4) optimization of medical therapy and/or attention to improving compliance to prescribed medications; and (5) increased patient access to health care providers and vigilant patient follow-up. In three of these studies, patients received instruction on self-managed, flexible use of diuretics in response to changes in weight (Cline et al., 1998; Fonarow et al., 1997; Smith et al., 1997).

## Specialty Care That Extends to the Home

In a study conducted in Israel, Kornowski and associates (1995) targeted elderly patients with heart failure for an intensive home surveillance program. A physician and nurse made once-weekly home visits for purposes of patient assessment, alterations in therapy, and administration of intravenous diuretics if needed. At 12 months follow-up, compared to the preintervention period, there was a 62% reduction in the number of total rehospitalizations with a 77% reduction in hospital days, a 72% reduction in hospitalizations for cardiovascular causes with an 83% reduction in associated hospital days, and a significant improvement in functional status.

In the first randomized controlled trials of comprehensive, multidisciplinary heart failure care, Rich and associates (1993, 1995) demonstrated positive outcomes of their program. Testing the intervention piloted and reported in 1993 (Rich et al., 1993), these investigators studied the impact of their intervention on outcomes in 282 elderly heart failure patients randomized to receive either usual care or the heart failure program after a hospitalization for heart failure (Rich et al., 1995). The program consisted of inpatient medication analysis and adjustment by a geriatric cardiologist, intensive inpatient heart failure education by a cardiovascular nurse, diet assessment and instruction by a registered dietitian, social services consultation and discharge planning, intensive follow-up by home health services, and follow-up by the study nurse, using home visits and telephone contact. At follow-up, the intervention group demonstrated 56% fewer rehospitalizations for heart failure, 61% fewer multiple admissions, 36% reduction in hospital days, significantly improved quality of life, and lower costs, compared to the control group.

Comparable outcomes have been reported from a physician supervised home-based program that was administered by nurses (West et al., 1997). These investigators studied 51 heart failure patients; they demonstrated improved functional status and quality of life and an 87% reduction in heart failure rehospitalizations after referral to their program. The program consisted of an initial clinic visit followed by weekly telephone calls for 6 weeks; intensive education to promote adherence to diet and drug regimens, and self-monitoring of symptoms; risk factor modification; and promotion of activity. Care for patients remained under the control of primary physicians, but study nurses contacted them to promote optimization of drug therapy according to published guidelines that were adapted to local practice. Doses of angiotensin-converting enzyme inhibitors increased significantly after referral to the program.

Shah and associates (1998) used educational mailing combined with phone contact by a nurse and reminders to patients by pager to take medications, weigh themselves, and measure their heart rate and blood pressure. Patients' cardiologists were given monthly reports of data collected and were notified immediately of signs of worsening heart failure. These investigators compared rehospitalizations and hospital days for the period before and after the intervention. Following the intervention, the number of hospitalizations for cardiovascular causes significantly decreased, as did hospital days and hospitalizations for all causes. The greatest benefit from the program was evident in those patients with the most severe heart failure.

In Australia, Stewart and associates (1998) conducted a randomized, controlled trial of a home-based nurse-pharmacist intervention. In the intervention group, hospitalized heart failure patients received an educational visit from a nurse prior to discharge and then a home visit 1 week after discharge from a pharmacist and nurse to assess knowledge, compliance, and physical status. If patients demonstrated poor medication knowledge or nonadherence (evidenced by pill count) at this visit, they received a combination of remedial counseling, a daily reminder routine to increase adherence to medication prescription, a pill box, incremental monitoring by caregivers, medication information and reminder cards, and referral to a community pharmacist for regular review. At 6 months follow-up, compared to the usual care group, patients in the intervention group experienced 42% fewer hospitalizations and hospital days. These investigators continued follow-up for 18 months and reported that the effects of the intervention were sustained (Stewart et al., 1999). Intervention patients had significantly fewer readmissions, hospital days, and out-of-hospital deaths and lower hospital costs than did usual care patients (Stewart et al., 1999).

*Summary.* In this group of studies, a total of 597 patients was studied. In the two studies by Rich and associates (1993, 1995), approximately 60% of patients enrolled were women. In one study only men were enrolled (Shah et al., 1998). In the remainder, the proportion of women enrolled ranged from 29% to 51%. Both the study conducted in Israel (Kornowski et al., 1995) and the one conducted in Australia (Stewart et al., 1998, 1999) have components of care that are not transferable to the United States. Only the pilot study by Rich and associates (1993), their subsequent larger clinical trial (Rich et al., 1995), and the study by Stewart and associates (1998, 1999) were randomized, controlled clinical trials. In all of the six studies reviewed in this section, the disease management approach tested produced positive outcomes. Patients receiving care in these programs experienced significantly fewer total and heart failure rehospitalizations, fewer hospital days when hospitalized, improved quality of life, and lower health care costs.

There was even more diversity in the components included in these six disease management programs than was seen with the heart failure clinics. Identification of common components among these programs assists others in trying to implement a similar program to determine the components that should be included to produce positive outcomes. Common components among the approaches described in this section include the following, which were also common to the heart failure clinics: (1) comprehensive care; (2) care either directed/managed (Rich et al., 1993, 1995;

West et al., 1997) or coordinated/assisted (Kornowski et al., 1995; Shah et al., 1998; Stewart et al., 1998, 1999) by a nurse; (3) optimization of medical therapy and/or attention to improving compliance to prescribed medications; and (4) increased patient access to health care providers and vigilant patient follow-up. Unlike the studies of heart failure clinics, the educational preparation of nurses involved in the care of heart failure patients in the studies described in this section was not specified, and it is unclear if these nurses were advanced practice nurses. A physician was involved (Kornowski et al., 1995) or a cardiologist available for consultation in many of the studies in this section (Rich et al., 1993, 1995; Shah et al., 1998; West et al., 1997). However, with the exception of the study conducted in Israel (Kornowski et al., 1995), physician involvement was less intensive, and more of the responsibility for patient management fell to nurses in the studies in this section where specialty care extended into the home.

### Increased Access to Primary Care

Weinberger and associates (1996) investigated the impact of increased access to primary care providers. Although not an example of comprehensive specialty care of the previously described studies, this study will be discussed because it has been cited several times as an example of failure of the disease management model. In a randomized, controlled clinical trial, the investigators reported significantly greater numbers of rehospitalizations, hospital days, and multiple admissions for heart failure patients randomized to a program of increased access to a primary care provider team that consisted of a physician and nurse. Outcomes in this group were compared to outcomes from a usual-care group. There was no difference in quality of life between the intervention and control groups, but the intervention group did report greater satisfaction with care.

*Summary.* This intervention lacks several components of other successful programs, which may explain the negative findings. A major missing component was failure to provide disease-specific education and counseling. Furthermore, despite the opportunity for increased access to primary care, in-hospital contact and outpatient follow-up of these high-risk patients (49% were NYHA classes III and IV) by the primary care team was minimal. Finally, the team had no plan in place for optimization of medical therapy or management of worsening heart failure.

## CRITIQUE AND SUMMARY

Taken together, these studies offer evidence that it is possible to reduce rehospitalization rates and costs substantially and improve functional status and quality of life by using specialized heart failure disease management programs. However, there are a number of limitations that must be considered when determining their clinical implications and their wholesale adoption into practice. These limitations include the following: (1) design and generalizability issues; (2) lack of attention to behavior change theory in designing programs; (3) disease management programs consisting of multiple components; and (4) difficulty in translating findings into routine practice.

## Design Issues

In only a few of these investigations was a randomized controlled clinical trial used to test the impact of the intervention (Rich et al., 1995; Stewart et al., 1998, 1999; Weinberger et al., 1996). In the majority of these studies, outcomes after the intervention were compared to those before institution of the intervention (Cintron et al., 1983; Fonarow et al., 1997; Hanumanthu et al., 1997; Kornowski et al., 1995; Shah et al., 1998; Smith et al., 1997; West et al., 1997). In most cases, when a preintervention-postintervention comparison design is used, the magnitude of the impact on outcomes is inflated. This phenomenon is evident in the group of studies reviewed here. For example, rehospitalization rates were reduced by 60% to 89% among the studies when postintervention outcomes were compared to preintervention outcomes. In studies in which a control group was used and patients were randomized, rehospitalization rates were reduced by 43% to 56%. Although the reductions were substantial when both types of designs were used, the smaller reductions evident in the randomized, controlled trials provide better estimates on which to base cost-benefit analyses and make decisions regarding implementation into practice.

Another limitation of the studies reviewed related to their generalizability. As can be seen when examining sample composition (Table 4.1), sample sizes were relatively small, and women were underrepresented in most studies. Heart failure is equally prevalent in women and men (Moser, 1997), and further attention to enrolling similar numbers of women and men and examining the impact of interventions tested between them is warranted.

Further limiting generalizability was the lack of attention to race or ethnicity. Among the studies reviewed, reference to patients' race or ethnicity was found only in the studies by Rich and associates (1993, 1995), Smith and associates (1997), Stewart and associates (1998, 1999), West and associates (1997), and Weinberger and associates (1996). With the exception of Rich and associates (1995), who enrolled similar numbers of African Americans and Caucasians, most investigators enrolled predominantly Caucasians. However, the finding by Stewart and associates (1999) of greater mortality in non-English-speaking patients suggests the importance of examining the impact of race and ethnicity on outcomes in studies of heart failure disease programs and of enrolling greater numbers of non-Caucasians.

Another important threat to generalizability is the selection of patients into the majority of studies on the basis of rather stringent criteria that do not reflect the characteristics of many (possibly most) patients in the community. The consequence of this is that we are left unsure of the impact of these programs on the usual heart failure patient. It is possible that a program may be more effective in patients encountered in everyday practice, or (and this is more likely) the program may be significantly less effective.

## Lack of Attention to Behavior Change Theory in Designing Programs

A number of behaviors must be adopted or changed for heart failure patients to successfully adhere to the typical prescribed regimen. Despite the importance of behavior change and the recognition that it can be extremely difficult, in none of the reviewed heart failure disease management programs is a behavior change theory explicated. A number of health behavior change theories have been used to design successful interventions and programs to address needed lifestyle changes for a variety of medical conditions (Glanz, Lewis, & Rimer, 1997). Use of a tested behavior change theory to guide program development helps ensure attention to details necessary to successful programs. Theories that have guided successful programs in other medical conditions include the Health Belief Model and its modifications, Social Cognitive Theory, the Transactional Model of Stress and Coping, the Theory of Planned Behavior, and the Transtheoretical Model and Stages of Change (Glanz et al., 1997). Future researchers in the area of heart failure disease management should incorporate and explicate appropriate health behavior change models.

Despite these limitations that should be addressed in future studies, the similarity in results among these studies lends credence to the validity of their findings. This group of studies demonstrated that it is possible to improve patient outcomes and reduce health care resource utilization when specialized care delivery models are used. There are, however, two major challenges to translating these interventions into routine clinical practice.

## Multicomponent Nature of Disease Management Programs Tested

The first challenge is to determine which intervention or combination of interventions to institute. The range of interventions tested was striking— from intensive, multidisciplinary, combined inpatient and home-care programs to heart failure specialty clinics to telemanagement systems. Within the tested interventions there were a number of components, each of which could possibly have the desired effects. There have been no studies comparing the relative effectiveness of different interventions or comparing components of interventions. Future research is needed to examine which components of these interventions are necessary to produce positive outcomes in terms of decreased hospitalizations, reduced costs, and improved quality of life.

Until such research is available, however, identification of components common to successful programs can offer guidance to clinicians planning heart failure programs (Table 4.2). These components can be adapted to a wide variety of communities and settings. It seems important to insure that the planned program include intensive guideline-based education about diet, medications, weighing, symptoms heralding worsening failure, the importance of seeking early treatment for these symptoms, and the importance of compliance (Cintron et al., 1983; Rich et al., 1995; West et al., 1997; Fonarow et al., 1997; Smith et al., 1997; Shah et al., 1998; Stewart et al., 1998). Frequent follow-up in some form and increased access to health care providers also appear to be vital components (Cintron et al., 1983; Fonarow et al., 1997; Kornowski et al., 1995; Rich et al., 1995; West et al., 1997). Optimization of medical therapy is an important aspect (Fonarow et al., 1997; Hanamanthu et al., 1997; Rich et al., 1995; Smith et al., 1997; West et al., 1997). Since the majority of rehospitalizations for exacerbation are the result of fluid overload (Bennett et al., 1998), some mechanism for addressing early signs of fluid overload is essential. In many programs, educating patients about flexible diuretic regimens is very successful (Fonarow et al., 1997; Smith et al., 1997). Other options, when patients or their families or caregivers are unable or unwilling to assume this degree of responsibility, include home visits by a nurse to give a diuretic or drop-in visits to a heart failure clinic. It seems clear that increasing access to primary care without attention to heart failure–specific education and intensive follow-up will not produce the desired outcomes (Weinberger et al., 1996).

## Translating Findings into Practice

A second challenge is determining how to implement a heart failure program outside of an academic medical center. The programs reviewed were conducted in such centers, where there is greater access to specialized heart failure professionals and other resources. How, then, does one implement a heart failure program in a typical community setting? Experienced cardiovascular advanced practice nurses (i.e., nurse practitioners or clinical nurse specialists) who have access to a cardiologist for consultation manage many successful heart failure programs on a day-to-day basis. This option for heart failure specialty programs is a viable one in most communities. Routine care and follow-up is done by the nurse on the basis of

**TABLE 4.2    Components of Successful Heart Failure Disease Management Programs**

Care managed by an experienced cardiovascular nurse with access to a cardiologist for consultation

Vigilant, frequent follow-up after hospital discharge

Increased access to health care professional

Optimization of medical therapy; patients prescribed appropriate drugs in appropriate doses using published guidelines based on large-scale randomized, controlled clinical trials

Intensive, comprehensive patient and family/caregiver education about heart failure, emphasizing low-salt diet, medications, symptoms signaling worsening failure, weighing, and management strategies for problems

Early attention to signs and symptoms of fluid overload (e.g., flexible diuretic regimen)

Supplementation of in-hospital education with outpatient education

Emphasis on addressing barriers to compliance

published practice guidelines and protocols or clinical pathways developed in conjunction with the cardiologist consultant (Brass-Mynderse, 1996; Venner & Seelbinder, 1996). Nurses provide direct care and also function as case managers as they provide patient follow-up. A team that includes nurses and the consulting physician typically sets up these programs, and the program ideally is designed with the unique needs of the heart failure population in a given community in mind.

Another unresolved issue in implementing a heart failure disease management program is reimbursement of nurses who coordinate the program. Many institutions are reluctant to fund such programs because nurses' salaries are the major expense and reimbursement is still difficult or impossible to obtain from many federal agencies and private insurance companies for nursing care. Changing federal policy regarding reimbursement of advanced practice nurses and the approval of proposals, by some insurance companies, from institutions for reimbursement that document the cost-effectiveness of their nurse-managed disease management programs may begin to resolve this issue. However, despite the ultimate cost-effectiveness of heart failure disease management programs (Rich & Nease, 1999), reimbursement of nurses who manage care for patients with heart failure remains a major impediment to setting up disease management programs.

Patients with heart failure are at considerable risk for frequent rehospitalization due to a variety of often modifiable factors. Evidence from a small but growing number of studies of specialized heart failure programs demonstrates that it is possible to reduce rehospitalization rates and health care costs and improve patient quality of life in a cost-effective fashion.

However, these programs represent a significant departure from traditional health care delivery models, and there are still many unanswered questions that must be addressed before widespread adoption of any of these programs is recommended. Nonetheless, the study of specialized heart failure programs is a fruitful area for nursing research and one that is will undoubtedly result in improved patient outcomes.

## REFERENCES

Ashton, C. M., Kuykendall, D. H., Johnson, M. L., Wray, N. P., & Wu, L. (1995). The association between the quality of inpatient care and early readmission. *Annals of Internal Medicine, 122,* 415–421.

American College of Cardiology/American Heart Association Task Force on Practice Guidelines. (1995). Guidelines for the evaluation and management of heart failure. *Circulation, 92,* 2764–2784.

American Heart Association. (1997). *1998 heart and stroke statistical update.* Dallas, TX: American Heart Association.

Bennett, S. J., Huster, G. A., Baker, S. L., Milgrom, L. B., Kirchgassner, A., Birt, J., & Pressler, M. L. (1998). Characterization of the precipitants of hospitalization for heart failure decompensation. *American Journal of Critical Care, 7,* 168–174.

Bennett, S. J., Milgron, L. B., Champion, V., & Huster, G. A. (1997). Beliefs about medication and dietary compliance in people with heart failure: An instrument development study. *Heart and Lung, 26,* 273–279.

Bernard, D. B., Townsend, R. R., & Sylvestri, M. F. (1998). Health and disease management: What is it and where is it going? What is the role of health and disease management in hypertension? *American Journal of Hypertension, 11,* 103S–108S.

Brass-Mynderse, N. J. (1996). Disease management for chronic congestive heart failure. *Journal of Cardiovascular Nursing, 11,* 54–62.

Chin, M. H., & Goldman, L. (1997). Factors contributing to hospitalization of patients with congestive heart failure. *American Journal of Public Health, 87,* 643–648.

Cintron, G., Bigas, C., Linares, E., Aranda, J. M., & Hernandez, E. (1983). Nurse practitioner role in a chronic congestive heart failure clinic: In-hospital time, costs, and patient satisfaction. *Heart and Lung, 12,* 237–240.

Cline, C. M. J., Israelsson, B. Y. A., Willenheimer, R. B., Broms, K., & Erhardt, L. R. (1998). Cost effective management programme for heart failure reduces rehospitalization. *Heart, 80,* 442–446.

Clinical Quality Improvement Network Investigators. (1996). Mortality risk and patterns of practice in 4606 acute care patients with congestive heart failure. The relative importance of age, sex, and medical therapy. *Archives of Internal Medicine, 56,* 1669–1673.

Croft, J. B., Giles, W. H., Pollard, R. A., Casper, M. L., Anda, R. F., & Livengood, J. R. (1997). National trends in the initial hospitalization for heart failure. *Journal of American Geriatrics Society, 45,* 227–275.

Dennis, L. I., Blue, C. L., Stahl, S. M., Benge, M. E., & Shaw, C. J. (1996). The relationship between hospital readmissions of Medicare beneficiaries with chronic illnesses and home care nursing interventions. *Home Healthcare Nurse, 14,* 303–309.

Dracup, K., Walden, J. A., Stevenson, L. W., & Brecht, M. L. (1992). Quality of life in patients with advanced heart failure. *Journal of Heart and Lung Transplantation, 11,* 273–279.

Dunbar, S. B., Jacobson, L. H., & Deaton, C. (1998). Heart failure: strategies to enhance patient self-management. *AACN Clinical Issues in Critical Care, 9,* 244–256.

Ellrodt, G., Cook, D. J., Lee, J., Cho, M., Hunt, D., & Weingarten, S. (1997). Evidence-based disease management. *Journal of the American Medical Association, 278,* 1687–1692.

Fonarow, G. G., Stevenson, L. W., Walden, J. A., Livingston, N. A., Steimle, A. E., Hamilton, M. A., Moriguchi, J., Tillisch, J. H., & Woo, M. A. (1997). Impact of a comprehensive heart failure management program on hospital readmission and functional status of patients with advanced heart failure. *Journal of the American College of Cardiology, 30,* 725–732.

Garg, R., Packer, M., Pitt, B., & Yusuf, S. (1993). Heart failure in the 1990's: Evolution of a major public health problem in cardiovascular medicine. *Journal of the American College of Cardiology, 22*(Suppl A), 3A–5A.

Gattis, W. A., Larsen, R. L., Hasselblad, V., Bart, B. A., & O'Connor, C. M. (1998). Is optimal angiotensin-converting enzyme inhibitor dosing neglected in elderly patients with heart failure? *American Heart Journal, 136,* 43–48.

Ghali, J. K., Kadakia, S., Cooper, R., & Ferlinz, J. (1988). Precipitating factors leading to decompensation of heart failure. Traits among urban Blacks. *Archives of Internal Medicine, 148,* 2013–2016.

Glanz, K., Lewis, F. M., & Rimer, B. K. (1997). *Health behavior and health education. Theory, research, and practice.* San Francisco: Jossey-Bass.

Goldberg, R. J., & Konstam, M. A. (1999). Assessing the population burden from heart failure. Need for sentinel population-based surveillance systems. *Archives in Internal Medicine, 159,* 15–17.

Grady, K. L. (1993). Quality of life in patients with chronic heart failure. *Critical Care Nursing Clinics of North America, 5,* 661–670.

Grady, K. L., Jalowiec, A., Grusk, B. B., White-Williams, C., & Robinson, J. A. (1992). Symptom distress in cardiac transplantation. *Heart and Lung, 21,* 434–439.

Hanumanthu, S., Butler, J., Chomsky, D., Davis, S., & Wilson, J. R. (1997). Effects of a heart failure program on hospitalization frequency and exercise tolerance. *Circulation, 96,* 2842–2848.

Happ, M. B., Naylor, M. D., & Roe-Prior, P. (1997). Factors contributing to rehospitalization for elderly patients with heart failure. *Journal of Cardiovascular Nursing, 11*(4), 75–84.

Hawthorne, M. H., & Hixon, M. E. (1994). Functional status, mood disturbance and quality of life in patients with heart failure. *Progress in Cardiovascular Nursing, 9,* 22–32.

Ho, K. K. L., Pinsky, J. L., & Kannel, W. B. (1993). The epidemiology of heart failure: The Framingham study. *Journal of the American College of Cardiology, 22*(4, Suppl A), 6A–13A.

Hoes, A. W., Mosterd, A., & Grobbee, D. E. (1998). An epidemic for heart failure? Recent evidence from Europe. *The European Society of Cardiology, 19*(Suppl L), L2–L8.

Jaarsma, T., Dracup, K., Walden, J., & Stevenson, L. W. (1996). Sexual function in patients with advanced heart failure. *Heart and Lung, 25,* 262–270.

Jaarsma, T., Halfens, R. J., & Huijer-AbuSaad, H. (1996). Readmission of older heart failure patients. *Progress in Cardiovascular Nursing, 11,* 15–20, 48.

Kimmelstiel, C. D., & Konstam, M. A. (1995). Heart failure in women. *Cardiology, 86,* 304–309.

Konstam, M. A., Dracup, K., Baker, D. W., Bottorff, M. B., Brooks, N. H., Dacey, R. A., Dunbar, S. A., Jackson, A. B., Jessup, M., Johnson, J. C., Jones, R. H., Luchi, R. J., Massie, B. M., Pitt, B., Rose, E. A., Rubin, L. J., Wright, R. F., & Hadorn, D. C. (1994). Heart failure: Evaluation and care of patients with left-ventricular systolic dysfunction. *Clinical Practice Guideline,* no. 11. (AHCPR Publication no. 94-0612). Rockville, MD: U.S. Department of Health and Human Services, Agency for Health Care Policy and Research, Public Health Service.

Konstam, V., Salem, D., Pouleur, H., Kostis, J., Gorkin, L., Shumaker, S., Mottard, I., Woods, P., Konstam, M. A., & Yusuf, S. (1996). Baseline quality of life as a predictor of mortality and hospitalization in 5,025 patients with congestive heart failure. *American Journal of Cardiology, 78,* 890–895.

Kornowski, R., Zeeli, D., Averbuch, M., Finkelstein, A., Schwartz, D., Moshkovitz, M., Weinrub, B., Hershkovitz, Eyal, D., Miller, M., Levo, Y., & Pines, A. (1995). Intensive home-care surveillance prevents hospitalization and improves morbidity rates among elderly patients with severe congestive heart failure. *American Heart Journal, 129,* 762–766.

Krumholz, H. M., Parent, E. M., Tu, N., Vaccarino, V., Wang, Y., Radford, M. J., & Hennen, J. (1997). Readmission for hospitalization for congestive heart failure among Medicare beneficiaries. *Archives of Internal Medicine, 157,* 99–104.

Krumholz, H. M., Wang, Y., Parent, E. M., Mockalis, J., Petrillo, M., & Radford, M. J. (1997). Quality of care for elderly patients hospitalized with heart failure. *Archives of Internal Medicine, 157,* 2242–2247.

Martens, K. H., & Mellor, S. D. (1997). A study of the relationship between home care services and hospital readmission of patients with congestive heart failure. *Home Healthcare Nurse, 15,* 123–129.

Massie, B. M., & Shah, N. B. (1996). The heart failure epidemic. *Current Opinions in Cardiology, 11,* 221–226.

McDermott, M. M., Feinglass, J., Lee, P., Mehta, S., Lefevre, F., Puppala, J., & Gheorghiade, M. (1997). Heart failure between 1986 and 1994: Temporal trends in drug-prescribing practices, hospital admissions, and survival at an academic medical center. *American Heart Journal, 134,* 901–909.

McMurray, J. J., Petrie, M. C., Murdoch, D. R., & Davie, A. P. (1998). Clinical epidemiology of heart failure: Public and private health burden. *European Heart Journal, 19*(Suppl), 9–16.

Michalsen, A., Konig, G., & Thimme, W. (1998). Preventable causative factors leading to hospital admission with decompensated heart failure. *Heart, 80,* 437–441.

Monane, M., Bohn, R. L., Gurwitz, J. H., Glynn, R. J., & Avorn, J. (1994). Noncompliance with congestive heart failure therapy in the elderly. *Archives of Internal Medicine, 154,* 433–437.

Moser, D. K. (1997). Heart failure in women. *Critical Care Nursing Clinics of North America, 9,* 511–519.

Naylor, M. D., Brooten, D., Campbell, R., Jacobsen, B. S., Mezey, M. D., Pauly, M. V., & Schwartz, J. S. (1999). Comprehensive discharge planning and home follow-up of hospitalized elders. *Journal of the American Medical Association, 281,* 613–620.

Nohria, A., Chen, Y., Morton, D. J., Walsh, R., Vlases, P. H., & Krumholz, H. M. (1999). Quality of care for patients hospitalized with heart failure at academic medical centers. *American Heart Journal, 137,* 1028–1034.

O'Connell, J. B., & Bristow, M. R. (1993). Economic impact of heart failure in the United States: Time for a different approach. *Journal of Heart and Lung Transplantation, 13,* S107–S112.

Packer, M., & Cohn, J. N., on behalf of the Steering Committee and Membership of the Advisory Council to Improve Outcomes Nationwide in Heart Failure. (1999). Consensus recommendations for the management of chronic heart failure. *American Journal of Cardiology, 83,* 2A–38A.

Rich, M. W. (1999). Heart failure disease management: A critical review. *Journal of Cardiac Failure, 5,* 64–75.

Rich, M. W., Beckham, V., Wittenberg, C., Leven, C. L., Freedland, K. E., & Carney, R. M. (1995). A multidisciplinary intervention to prevent readmission of elderly patients with congestive heart failure. *New England Journal of Medicine, 333,* 1190–1195.

Rich, M. W., & Nease, R. F. (1999). Cost-effectiveness analysis in clinical practice. The case of heart failure. *Archives of Internal Medicine, 159,* 1690–1700.

Rich, M. W., Vinson, J. M., Sperry, J. C., Shah, A. S., Spinner, L. R., Chung, M. K., & Davila-Roman, V. (1993). Prevention of readmission in elderly patients with congestive heart failure: Results of a prospective, randomized pilot study. *Journal of General Internal Medicine, 8,* 585–590.

Serxner, S., Miyaji, M., & Jeffords, J. (1998). Congestive heart failure disease management: A patient education intervention. *Congestive Heart Failure, 4,* 23–28.

Shah, N. B., Der, E., Ruggerio, C., Heidenreich, P. A., & Massie, B. M. (1998). Prevention of hospitalizations for heart failure with an interactive home monitoring program. *American Heart Journal, 135,* 373–378.

Smith, L. E., Fabbri, S. A., Pai, R., Ferry, D., & Heywood, J. T. (1997). Symptomatic improvement and reduced hospitalization for patients attending a cardiomyopathy clinic. *Clinical Cardiology, 20,* 949–954.

Stafford, R. S., Saglam, D., & Blumenthal, D. (1997). National patterns of angiotensin-converting enzyme inhibitor use in congestive heart failure. *Archives of Internal Medicine, 157,* 2460–2464.

Starling, R. (1998). The heart failure pandemic: Changing patterns, costs, and treatment strategies. *Cleveland Clinic Journal of Medicine, 65,* 351–358.

Stewart, A. L., Greenfield, S., Hays, R. D. Wells, K., Rogers, W. H., Berry, S. D., & McGlynn, E. A. (1989). Functional status and well-being of patients with chronic conditions: Results from the medical outcomes study. *Journal of the American Medical Association, 262,* 907–913.

Stewart, S., Pearson, S., & Horowitz, J. D. (1998). Effects of a home-based intervention among patients with congestive heart failure discharged from acute hospital care. *Archives of Internal Medicine, 158,* 1067–1072.

Stewart, S., Vandenbroek, A. J., Pearson, S., & Horowitz, J. D. (1999). Prolonged beneficial effects of a home-based intervention on unplanned readmissions and mortality among patients with congestive heart failure. *Archives of Internal Medicine, 159,* 257–261.

Sueta, C. A., Chowdhury, M., Boccuzzi, S. J., Smith, S. C., Alexander, C. M., Londhe, A., Lulla, A., & Simpson, R. J., Jr. (1999). Analysis of the degree of undertreatment of hyperlipidemia and congestive heart failure secondary to coronary artery disease. *American Journal of Cardiology, 83,* 1303–1307.

Task Force of the Working Group on Heart Failure of the European Society of Cardiology (1997). The treatment of heart failure. *European Heart Journal, 18,* 736–753.

Venner, G. H., & Seelbinder, J. S. (1996). Team management of congestive heart failure across the continuum. *Journal of Cardiovascular Nursing, 10,* 71–84.

Vinson, J. M., Rich, M. W., Sperry, J. C., Shah, A.S., & McNamara, T. (1990). Early readmission of elderly patients with congestive heart failure. *Journal of the American Geriatrics Society, 38,* 1290–1295.

Walden, J. A., Stevenson, L. W., Dracup, K., Hook, J. F., Moser, D. K., Hamilton, M., & Fongrow, G. C. (1994). Extended comparison of quality of life between stable heart failure patients and heart transplant recipients. *Journal of Heart and Lung Transplantation, 13,* 1109–XX.

Weinberger, M., Oddone, E. Z., & Henderson, W. G., for the Veterans Affairs Cooperative Study Group on Primary Care and Hospital Readmission. (1996). Does increased access to primary care reduce hospital readmissions? *New England Journal of Medicine, 333,* 1190–1195.

West, J. A., Miller, N. H., Parker, K. M., Sennaca, D., Ghandour, G., Clark, M., Greenwald, G., Heller, R. S., Fowler, M. B., & DeBusk, R. F. (1997). A comprehensive management system for heart failure improves clinical outcomes and reduces medical resources. *American Journal of Cardiology, 79,* 58–63.

World Health Organization Council on Geriatric Cardiology. (1996). Task force on heart failure education: Concise guide to the management of heart failure. *Journal of Cardiac Failure, 2,* 153–154.

## Chapter 5

# Cancer Care: Impact of Interventions on Caregiver Outcomes

JEANNIE V. PASACRETA AND RUTH MCCORKLE

### ABSTRACT

The purpose of this review is to examine the research literature on interventions aimed at caregivers who, in the current health care environment, are assuming increasing responsibility for the complex care of significant others experiencing cancer. The general aim of the review is to synthesize the literature on interventions targeted to cancer caregivers and to summarize outcomes associated with the various intervention strategies described. Three broad categories of interventions were described in the literature: (1) educational, (2) counseling/psychotherapeutic, and (3) hospice and palliative home care. The review included studies that met the following criteria: data-based studies that described an intervention aimed at assisting caregivers to care for patients with cancer, studies published between 1975 and January 1999, and studies published in English. A total of 29 published papers was included.

Although the original intent was to limit the review to studies that associated interventions with outcomes, a lack of well-delineated outcome variables was revealed as a major gap in the literature. Thus, some studies that did not include outcome variables were reviewed and the following conclusions made: (1) there is a dearth of data-based literature describing interventions aimed at caregivers; interventions that are described often lack well-defined effects due to a lack of or poor operationalization of outcomes; (2) of the small number of studies in this area, many used small samples and lacked randomization; and (3) studies often revealed selection bias to well-adjusted caregivers who were accepting of support, able to obtain respite care in order to participate, and often willing to avail themselves of a group-style intervention.

**Key words: caregiver, caregiving, family, cancer, outcomes, interventions, quality of life, coping, psychological stress**

## OVERVIEW OF CONTEXTUAL ISSUES

Although individuals and families have been living with cancer and its consequences for years, it wasn't until the National Cancer Act was signed by President Nixon in 1971 that cancer became recognized as a major public health problem. Following passage of the National Cancer Act, research and clinical resources focused primarily on finding novel discoveries to treat different types of cancers and on developing comprehensive cancer centers to house clinical and basic scientific efforts. As cancer treatments that prolonged life expectancy became available, cancer was more and more associated with chronicity, remissions, and exacerbations; thus, its impact on patients and families became increasingly evident. Gradually, a body of literature evolved that documented the impact of cancer on patients and demonstrated that the diagnosis was a time of crisis (Krouse & Krouse, 1982; McCorkle & Benoliel, 1983; Weisman & Worden, 1976).

Simultaneously, there were scientific developments that documented that families also experienced a crisis associated with a cancer diagnosis, its subsequent treatment, and in some cases premature death (Benoliel & McCorkle, 1978; Giaquinta, 1977; Hampe, 1975; MacVicar & Archbold, 1976; Vachon, 1982; Wellisch, Mosher, & VanScoy, 1978). As research regarding the psychosocial impact of cancer has evolved, there have been parallel and pervasive changes in health care delivery, as well as dramatic scientific advances that have continued to highlight the chronic as opposed to the terminal nature of a cancer diagnosis.

Recent years have seen an escalating trend toward early discharge of hospitalized patients and a shift to high utilization of ambulatory care services. As a result, increasing numbers of patients with cancer are being cared for at home by family members (Cawley & Gerdts, 1988; Conkling, 1989; McCorkle & Given, 1991; McCorkle et al., 1993). This demand on families is not new, although the caregiver role has changed dramatically from promoting convalescence to providing high-technology care and psychological support in the home. Members of the patient's family are of vital importance in meeting the patient's physical and psychosocial needs and accomplishing treatment goals (Ganz, 1990; Mor, Guadagnoli, & Wool, 1987).

The burden of caring for patients with a diagnosis of cancer, however, may adversely affect families who lack adequate resources or that are insufficiently prepared for this new, complex role. There is mounting evidence that changes in family roles and the burden placed on family caregivers may have negative effects on the quality of life of both cancer patients and their caregivers (McCorkle et al., 1993), particularly during advanced stages of cancer. Despite growing evidence that significant others are assuming increasing responsibility for cancer care and that this responsibility has detrimental effects, there are few data that document the efficacy of standardized intervention strategies specifically for cancer caregivers.

The period spanning the middle of the 20th century, during which patients were routinely cared for in acute care hospitals, may turn out to be but a brief period in medical history. Before this time, patients were cared for primarily at home by their families. Today, social and economic forces are interacting to remove patients from the hospital and quickly return them home once again. Although at face value these changes seem positive, they have highlighted gaps and deficiencies in the current health care delivery system.

Scientific advances have allowed us to keep patients with cancer alive increasingly longer despite complex and chronic health problems. The burden of their care usually falls on families, which often are not adequately prepared to handle the physically and emotionally demanding needs for care that are inherent in chronic illnesses such as cancer. In addition, family members have increasingly become primary care providers, within the context of other demands such as employment outside the home and competing family roles. The necessity among most of our nation's family members to assume employment outside the home and to alter those arrangements when faced with a sick relative has created an as yet immeasurable strain on physical, emotional, and financial resources. The increasing responsibilities of the family in providing care, in the face of limited external support, and the consequences of that caregiving for patient and family raise important challenges for clinicians and provide unique opportunities for researchers (Sarna & McCorkle, 1996).

The purpose of this review is to provide a comprehensive synthesis of the literature on interventions and associated outcomes designed for those who care for cancer patients. For the review, a combination of computerized and manual searches was used. Because both interdisciplinary and nursing intervention studies were of interest, diverse databases were searched, using the following key words: *caregiver, caregiving, family, cancer, outcomes, interventions, quality of life, coping,* and *psychological stress.* Initially, the search sought articles from 1976, and a large number of articles (562) on family and caregiving were found; but the majority of these articles were descriptive in nature and documented the need for caregiver interventions. Articles were retrieved through computerized databases— MEDLINE, CINAHL (Cumulative Index to Nursing and Allied Health Literature), and PsychInfo. For the final review, data-based studies that described interventions aimed at cancer caregivers were selected.

Although the original intent was to limit the review to studies that associated interventions with outcomes, a lack of well-delineated outcome variables was revealed as a major gap in the literature. Thus, some studies that did not include outcome variables were included in the review. The search yielded a total of 29 published papers for inclusion, studies that met the following criteria: (1) data-based studies that described an intervention aimed at assisting caregivers to care for patients with cancer, (2) studies published between 1976 and January 1999, and (3) studies published in English.

The questions to be addressed by this review were as follows: What are the needs of cancer caregivers, and what intervention strategies have been used to address those needs? What is the methodological adequacy of the research, including the adequacy of outcome variables used? What are the major findings and gaps in the literature, and how should they guide future research efforts in this important area?

## CAREGIVER NEEDS AND THE IMPACT OF CAREGIVING

A number of studies have identified the needs of family members providing care to patients with cancer (Gotay, 1984; Wellisch, Jamison, & Pasnau, 1978). Recognition of the burden that the diagnosis and treatment of cancer places on family members has appeared in the cancer literature since the early 1980s. A study by Grobe and colleagues (Grobe, Istrup, & Ahmann, 1980) identified methods of education that were provided for 87 patients in the advanced stages of cancer and their homebound caregivers. This study revealed that families perceived that little if any education was provided to them. Hinds (1985) conducted a study examining the perceived needs of 83 family caregivers. Findings indicated that family members felt inadequately prepared to provide care for their sick relatives in the home and identified numerous informational and skill deficits.

Oberst and colleagues (Oberst, Gass, & Ward, 1989) assessed the demands on cancer caregivers, including their perceptions of providing care in the home environment. Subjects reported that the majority of their time was spent providing transportation and emotional support and maintaining the household. More than one third of subjects reported a lack of assistance from health professionals in providing care. In addition, caregiver demands escalated as the treatment regimen progressed. Another study (Perry & Roades de Menses, 1989) lent support to the isolative and stressful nature of caregiving in that 85% of a sample of cancer caregivers failed to utilize available resources to assist them in caregiving activities. In addition, 77% of the sample reported increased stress, and 28% required medication to help them cope with the burden associated with caregiving.

As the body of literature has grown, there have been a number of review articles to describe the impact of cancer on the family and family caregivers (Cooley & Moriarty, 1997; Hull, 1989; Kristjanson & Ashcroft, 1992; Laizner, Shegda, Barg, & McCorkle, 1993; Lewis, 1986; Northouse, 1984). These accounts present persuasive documentation that caring for a person with cancer is a stressful experience and can have major emotional and physical consequences for caregivers. In their review of caregiver research, Sales, Schultz, and Biegel (1990) concluded that a significant number of cancer caregivers exhibit psychological distress and physical symptoms. Predictors of distress included a number of illness-related variables, including more advanced stages of cancer, disability, and complex care needs. McCorkle and colleagues (1993) followed a sample of cancer patients and their caregivers at hospital discharge and at 3 and 6 months. Findings indicated that patients were being discharged from the hospital with ongoing acute care needs. By 3 and 6 months posthospitalization, patients' conditions had stabilized or improved, but their caregivers continued to report unchanging levels of burden. Study results highlight the importance of developing interventions to reduce caregiver burden in providing posthospital care for patients with complex care requirements.

Weitzner and colleagues (Weitzner, Moody, & McMillan, 1997) noted the presence of increased symptoms of depression, anxiety, psychosomatic symptoms, restrictions of roles and activities, strain in marital relationships, and poorer physical health among family caregivers. Various dimensions of caregiver reactions have been identified by previous researchers (Given et al., 1992; Stetz, 1987, 1989). Mor and colleagues (1987) divided caregiving tasks into categories of personal care, instrumental tasks, and transportation. Each of these areas was associated with greater demands as patient physiological factors worsened or if their caregivers associated their care with a high level of burden (Siegel, Raveis, Houts, & Mor, 1991; Siegel, Raveis, Mor, & Houts, 1991). Foxall and Gaston-Johansson (1996) described objective versus subjective burden in family caregivers of hospitalized bone marrow transplant (BMT) patients. In their study, objective burden was linked to all health outcomes and occurred during critical time periods post-BMT. Wallhagen (1992) studied caregiver perception of caregiving demands and concluded that caregivers view personal demands as more difficult than task demands. Given and colleagues (Given, Helms, Stommel, & Devoss, 1992, 1997) reported that patients' symptoms and symptom distress, mobility, and dependency with instrumental activities were linked to significant burden in family caregivers.

In general, the literature on caregivers of cancer patients highlights (1) the increasing number of complex tasks assumed by cancer caregivers; (2) the high proportion of unmet caregiver needs; (3) the subjective nature of the caregiving experience, which encompasses both positive and negative elements; and (4) the conceptualization of caregiver burden as positively linked to negative reactions to caregiving.

## Framework

Although two major frameworks were selected a priori to review the literature regarding interventions for cancer caregivers: (the cancer illness trajectory and the categories of interventions tested), they did not always provide a useful context for the analysis. Prior to delving into the review of intervention studies and particularly after reviewing the literature on caregiver needs, the authors thought that the cancer illness trajectory would be the most useful framework for categorizing the literature on clinical interventions targeted at enhancing outcomes of cancer caregivers. Unfortunately, the state of the science has not evolved to the point where the body of literature reflects the illness phases: early diagnostic, acute care, curative, recurrence, chronic, terminal, and bereavement (Holland, 1989; Kristjanson & Ashcroft, 1994).

The second framework (categories of interventions) has been used previously by Northouse and Peters-Golden (1993) and, given the paucity of research, made the best fit in light of the low number of intervention studies located to review. Their categories included information and support. For this review, a third category was added, hospice and palliative home care services; despite the fact that many interventions described in these studies were informal and nonstandardized, they represent important directions for future research in this area. Thus, the final three categories used to examine the cancer caregiver intervention literature were (1) educational; (2) support, counseling, and psychotherapy; and (3) hospice and palliative home care services.

## EDUCATIONAL INTERVENTIONS

The value of providing information to cancer caregivers has been reported consistently in the research literature (Wilson & Morse, 1991; Zahlis & Shands, 1991). Reported in the literature with equally consistent frequency, however, is the difficulty that caregivers have in obtaining information from health care professionals, particularly physicians and nurses (Wilson & Morse, 1991; Wright & Dyke, 1984; Zahlis & Shands, 1991). Despite the fact that it is often difficult to obtain, caregivers report that information is a critical element in helping them to cope with the patient's illness (Gotay, 1984; Northouse, 1989).

In addition to providing information about the physical aspects of the illness, caregivers need to learn more about the emotional aspects of illness and recovery (Northouse & Peters-Golden, 1993). According to Oberst and Scott (1988), caregivers should be informed about what to expect regarding the emotional aspects of the illness for both themselves and the patient. In this manner, caregivers can be reassured proactively that their own and the patient's psychological distress is to be expected and not a sign of poor coping.

The times when caregivers appear to be in the greatest need of information are at the time of diagnosis (Northouse, 1989); during the hospital period, especially at the time of surgery (Northouse, 1989; Northouse & Swain, 1987); at the start of new treatments (Wilson & Morse, 1991); and at the time of recurrence (Wilkerson, 1991). Despite the documented importance of providing information to caregivers, only a few intervention programs have been reported that demonstrated how and what information should be provided. Outcomes associated with educational interventions were not clearly described, nor were consistent variables and measures used to describe relevant outcomes. This makes replication of studies in this area difficult at best and undermines the importance of conducting research in an effort to bolster caregiver supports.

Carmody and colleagues (Carmody, Hickey, & Boakbinder, 1991) developed a program in which specific nurses were linked with families during and after a patient's surgery to provide information about the patient's status. Caregivers responded favorably to this program although specific outcome variables were not well delineated. In this age of cost constraints and streamlining of services it is of critical importance to document the tangible benefits of caregiver interventions, especially in terms of quality of life, productivity, and health care costs.

Derdiarian (1989) conducted an intervention with a group of men and their wives immediately following the man's cancer diagnosis. The experimental group received individualized information, standard written information from the American Cancer Society and the National Cancer Institute, and resources to contact with questions. Findings revealed fewer informational needs and greater satisfaction with care in the group that received the intervention. Well-known group interventions such as "I Can Cope," developed by Johnson (1982), were initially developed to teach patients over a series of eight sessions about cancer, its treatment, and its physical and psychological management strategies. Although not initially developed for them, caregivers often attended I Can Cope meetings. On the basis of this observation, Johnson and Norby (1981) expanded the program and developed the "We Can Weekend," which focused primarily on families. One study that followed participants in the program after it was initially developed (Johnson, 1982) found the program to be effective in that participants who completed it reported significantly reduced anxiety, increased knowledge, and improved perception of purpose in life. A follow-up study by Diekmann (1988) reported a significant decline in attendance at I Can Cope programs. The fact that many potential participants were intimidated by the group format and the fear associated with cancer were identified as two significant reasons for nonattendance. As a result, the addition of a psychological support component to the I Can Cope program was suggested.

Reele (1993) built on this recommendation and examined the effect of a revised I Can Cope program that incorporated both group and individual counseling components on the quality of life of cancer patients and their caregivers. Three groups studied included Group 1, which participated in a revised I Can Cope Program for 8 sessions ($n = 12$); Group 2, which attended the eight sessions and then elected to participate in an ongoing support group ($n = 8$); and Group 3, which did not participate in either intervention ($n = 12$). Unfortunately, the investigator did not include caregiver psychological distress as an outcome. Following the intervention, there were no significant differences among groups on variables that included quality of life and coping, although attendees reported group attendance to be a positive experience. Possible explanations for the lack of significant findings included small sample size, lack of randomization to study groups, lack of sensitivity of the outcomes to the intervention delivered, heterogeneity of the groups in that attendees may have had very different information and support needs, and the self-selected nature of the sample.

Two international studies found in the literature addressed caregiver education interventions, although limitations were similar to those already described. Grahn (1996) developed an education and support program in Sweden called Learning to Live with Cancer, which focused on education about cancer and its treatment and on the adaptation process, particularly how to live with the uncertainty associated with the disease. Seventy-three cancer patients and 54 caregivers (125 patients and 125 caregivers were invited) attended eight 2-hour group sessions. The authors interviewed participants about their group experiences, using an open-ended format that focused on experiences of increased knowledge and decreased confusion and anxiety. Interviews were analyzed by using a grounded theory approach, and it was concluded that groups reinforced confidence in evolving appropriate coping strategies for dealing with cancer (Grahn & Danielson, 1996). Two major methodologic issues revealed in this study relate to the self-selected nature of the sample and the likelihood that those who attended were the most likely to benefit. Also, the follow-up interviews seemed to be leading respondents to provide information that supported the positive nature of the programs; outcomes associated with the intervention are nebulous at best.

A study by Natvig (1982) examined the impact of pre- and postoperative education on a convenience sample of 189 Norwegian laryngectomy patients and their spouses. Seventy percent of spouses felt that they had not been offered adequate information and believed that the problems they encountered at home could have been relieved by improved education and counseling. Outcome variables were not clearly defined in this study although patient and spouse satisfaction with the intervention could be loosely implied. In addition, the investigators report grave mental trauma, anxiety, and depression postoperatively in patients and spouses. They suggest that this could have been improved with adequate pre- and postoperative education, but the manner in which these psychological variables were measured was not clear.

The description of a psychoeducational curriculum by Barg and colleagues (1998) was designed as a one-group intervention, with a structured educational program developed specifically for caregivers, and included standardized outcome measures. Despite a clear program description and the delineation of measurable outcomes, the researchers reported that a lack of willingness by many cancer caregivers to attend group meetings posed a major obstacle to its successful evaluation. Group-style interventions clearly lend themselves to the study of a self-selected sample. In fact, caregivers who attend groups may possibly be those who are least in need of intervention because they demonstrate an ability to utilize social support and/or have respite care available, making group attendance feasible.

Ferrell and colleagues (Ferrell, Grant, Chan, Ahn, & Ferrell, 1995) examined the impact of cancer pain education on family caregivers of elderly cancer patients. Fifty family caregivers of elderly patients who were at home and experiencing cancer-related pain were recruited for participation in this quasi-experimental study. Caregiver outcomes examined as a result of the intervention included quality of life, knowledge about pain, and caregiver burden. Findings demonstrated the significant burden to caregivers associated with pain management, particularly in the psychological realm. The pain education program proved efficacious in terms of improving caregiver knowledge and quality of life. This study highlights the nature of many nursing studies in terms of describing interventions that teach caregivers to become proficient in the physical aspects of patient care. As demonstrated, this type of intervention often has the effect of indirectly improving the caregiver's well-being. This type of educational intervention is in contrast to those outlined in several nonnursing studies that provide direct psychological services such as group or individual counseling to caregivers.

## SUPPORT, COUNSELING, AND PSYCHOTHERAPY

The sources of support available to cancer patients are many and varied, ranging from one-to-one interactions to a myriad of formal support groups and networks. Sources of support for family caregivers have lagged far behind those provided for patients (Northouse & Golden-Peters, 1993). Spouses in particular report little support from health professionals, often because of limited contact with physicians and nurses in hospital and outpatient settings (Northouse, 1988; Northouse & Northouse, 1987).

There is a dearth of information regarding the effectiveness of supportive and counseling interventions with cancer caregivers despite the implications from studies of educational interventions that may seem to be inadequate. Sabo, Brown, and Smith (1986) developed a support program for husbands of women with breast cancer. Despite the fact that only 6 of 24 husbands chose to participate, attendees reported significantly more communication with their wives about the mastectomy than did husbands in the control group. It was also determined that the support group promoted increased communication between couples regarding discussions about intimacy, recurrence, and death. Based on other studies, described earlier, that imply a self-selected group of individuals who are amenable to group interventions, the testing of individual interventions that utilize principles from successful group interventions is clearly in order.

Houts and colleagues (Houts, Nezu, Nezu, & Bucher, 1996) described a prescriptive problem-solving model for how care should be managed at home and for the kind of information and training family caregivers should receive. The Prepared Family Caregiver model, which is summarized in the acronym COPE (creativity, optimism, planning, and expert information), teaches caregivers how to develop and implement plans that address both medical and psychosocial problems and are coordinated with care plans of health professionals. The model is based on extensive research regarding unmet needs of caregivers and problem-solving training and therapy. According to the authors, the program empowers family members and patients to cope with illness and can help to moderate caregiver stress, although there are no outcomes used in the research design to document the program's effectiveness.

Blanchard and colleagues (Blanchard, Toseland, & McCallion, 1997) reported on the effect of a six-session intervention with spouses of cancer patients. They used a problem-solving intervention to help spouses solve individually identified problems. Results at 6-month follow-up showed no significant impact associated with the intervention, even for those spouses who were most distressed. Interestingly, patients of spouses who received the intervention showed significant decline in depression. It could not be determined whether this was related to altered communication between spouses and patients following the intervention or relief on the part of patients that spouses were receiving help. Findings suggested the importance of studying the spouse/patient dyad as opposed to each person individually.

Heinrich and Schag (1985) developed the Stress and Activity Management (SAM) intervention for cancer patients and their spouses. The intervention consisted of structured small-group meetings that met weekly for 2 hours over a 6-week period. Groups were designed to educate patients and spouses about cancer and its impact; teach specific skills that could be used to manage stress and daily problems, such as relaxation techniques and physical and recreational activities; and promote problem solving. Of 92 patients who met eligibility criteria, 51 participated in the study, along with 25 of their spouses. Twenty-six patients and 12 spouses were randomized to the treatment group and 25 patients and 13 spouses to the control group. The primary outcome variables included psychological adjustment, depression, and anxiety, which improved for both treatment and control groups, supporting the notion of natural improvement in psychological status that occurs over time. The SAM patients and spouses reported high satisfaction with the intervention, although due to the self-selected nature of the treatment and control groups, it is likely that the control subjects also would have been satisfied.

Support for the unique and positive impact of the SAM treatment intervention came from the improvement in scores on the Cancer Information Test, indicating that the program increased participants' knowledge about cancer and coping. This finding is noteworthy because most patients and spouses had been living with cancer for about 2 years and demonstrated minimal knowledge about their illness. SAM spouses in particular were more satisfied with the education and support they received than were the control spouses, who received the usual care and were not routinely included in physician office visits. Despite the small number of subjects studied and the self-selected nature of the sample, this study is noteworthy in several respects: it is a well-described replicable intervention, randomization, and clear delineation of outcome variables.

Goldberg and Wool (1985) provided a counseling support intervention to lung cancer patients and their spouses. The intervention consisted of 12 sessions that were geared toward specific goals, such as maintaining support systems, promoting feeling expression, and facilitating negotiation of the health care system. Following intervention, no difference was found between psychological functioning of the control and intervention groups. The authors suggested that the lack of intervention effect may be due to the relatively positive adjustment of couples in both groups, reported before the start of the program. This again highlights the possibility that caregiver studies may be recruiting subjects who are accessible and available and thus least in need of intervention. Innovative recruitment strategies must be developed to target caregivers with limited resources, who need respite services and have poor coping abilities, to name just a few problems, to ascertain whether interventions would prove effective if directed toward those who need them most. In this vein, Pfefferbaum and colleagues (Pfefferbaum, Pasnan, & Jamison, 1977) described a comprehensive program for breast cancer patients and their families that followed families pre- and postoperatively and had a positive impact on coping outcomes. In this program, a mental health professional worked with the surgical team to provide counseling to patients and family members who were identified ahead of time as being in need of assistance. This notion of identifying caregivers who are at high risk for problems in specific areas and tailoring interventions to their special needs seems to be an important direction for research as implied by the lack of positive findings in some of the studies reviewed.

## HOSPICE AND PALLIATIVE HOME CARE SERVICES

When cancer has advanced to the extent that a change in management strategy ensues, from cure to palliation, new issues and stressors emerge for both patient and caregiver. These stressors may be particularly evident if the dying person is cared for at home, where there may be inadequate financial, physical, and emotional resources to manage the complex needs that are involved in the care. If caregivers are unable to deal satisfactorily with the multiple demands and have overwhelming feelings and affect associated with them, the potential exists for deterioration of the caregivers' psychological and physical health (Axelsson & Sjoden, 1988; Hull, 1992). Institutional and home hospice services have been used to help patients and caregivers deal with the insults to physical and emotional well-being that are imposed by terminal illness. They have also incorporated caregivers into patient care by educating them and supporting their caring efforts. In this sense, recent studies have shown an increase in hospice-supported home care, with an emphasis on supporting the primary caregiver role (Schachter, 1992).

Jepson, McCorkle, Adler, Nuamah, and Lusk (1999) designed a randomized clinical trial to examine changes in the psychosocial status of caregivers of postsurgical patients with cancer at the patients' discharge and 3 months and 6 months later. Within a week after discharge from the hospital, patients were randomly assigned to either the treatment or the control condition. Patients in the treatment group received a Standardized Nursing Intervention Protocol (SNIP) over a 4-week period between discharge and the second interview. The intervention was provided by advance practice nurses and consisted of three home visits and six telephone calls. The nursing interventions included problem assessment and monitoring of the patient's condition, symptom management, and teaching caregivers how to problem-solve, administer medications, and provide self-care behaviors. Psychosocial status was measured by the Caregiver Reaction Assessment (Given et al., 1992) and the CES-Depression Scale. Overall, the caregiver's psychosocial status improved from baseline to 3 months and stabilized thereafter; but among caregivers with physical problems, the psychosocial status of those in the treatment group declined over time, compared to those in the control group. The researchers concluded that caregivers of cancer patients who have physical problems of their own are at risk for psychological morbidity as they assume the caregiving role.

Systematic research that has quantified the effects of palliative care services on specific caregiver outcomes has primarily focused on the hospice paradigm. Unfortunately, in these studies, specific caregiver intervention strategies are not clearly delineated and can best be described as informal services that integrate the caregiver into the patient's overall plan of care. According to Neal and Clark (1992), hospice and palliative care services recognize the "dying triad" of patient, informal (nonprofessional) caregiver, and professional. Hospice services, whether hospital- or home-based, have had an explicit aim of treating families as the unit of care although the literature reveals that there is a pressing need to operationalize interventions and document standard outcomes across studies.

McMillan and Mahon (1994) evaluated the effectiveness of institutional and home care hospice services on the quality of life of 68 primary caregivers. Caregivers' quality-of-life scores remained constant from the initiation of hospice services to Week 4. In light of the extreme stress that is often associated with the transition to terminal care, this constancy in quality of life is noteworthy. McMillan (1996) also studied the effectiveness of hospice home care programs on 118 cancer caregivers' quality of life. She reported that caregivers' quality-of-life scores remained constant from the start of home care to Week 4, with a slight increase in caregivers' emotional well-being scores. The relationship of 55 caregiver outcomes were examined. Relationship of outcomes to the duration of time spent in the caregiving role and length of time in hospice were examined. Findings revealed that the length of time caregivers were involved with hospice was positively related to the number of communication tasks reported and consistent with the hospice approach to management of the terminally ill. There were no significant findings for the effect of duration of caregiving and length of time in hospice on caregivers' outcomes (Yang & Kirschling, 1992).

Distress for cancer caregivers carries on after the death of the patient and into the bereavement phase. Specifically at the time of death and beyond, caregivers are burdened with the loss of a loved one and unresolved negative caregiver experiences. Bereavement-related adjustments are influenced by the survivor's psychological, physical, cultural, and social traits. Evidence exists that maladaptive bereavement may place the survivor at risk for psychiatric and medical illness; therefore, interventions are recommended during this time to encourage positive survivor health outcomes (Kurtz, Kurtz, Given, & Given, 1997).

Studies that link interventions to bereaved-survivor outcomes are more descriptive in delineating standardized interventions used than the hospice literature, which, as stated, associates the hospice philosophy and its intrinsic involvement of caregivers in the overall plan of care with its caregiver outcomes. Categories of bereavement interventions described in the literature include home care services by nurses specifically trained in oncology care, bereavement support groups, and formalized bereavement follow-up services.

McCorkle and colleagues (McCorkle, Robinson, Nuamah, Lev, & Benoliel, 1998) conducted a secondary analysis to test the effects of oncology home care for terminally ill lung cancer patients on spousal distress during the bereavement period. Forty-six lung cancer patients and spouse dyads were entered into the study 2 months after diagnosis and remained until the patients' deaths. Follow-up continued for 25 months after the death. Advance practice nurses developed Oncology Transition Services to assist dying patients and their families through the living-dying transition (Tornberg, McGrath, & Benoliel, 1984). The intervention consisted of personalized care in the home that focused on advanced symptom management. The nurse served as central coordinator for care, and 24-hour access was provided. Psychological distress was the primary outcome variable (Derogatis & Spencer, 1982) and initially was significantly lower among the spouses cared for in the oncology home care group, although there were no significant differences at 25 months. Findings suggest that the bereaved's psychological distress was positively influenced by specialized nursing interventions provided during the terminal phase of illness. This study also supports the notion that nursing interventions that incorporate caregivers into the patient's care should be operationalized and linked with specific outcomes in future studies.

Fakhoury and colleagues (Fakhoury, McCarthy, & Addington-Hall, 1997) surveyed 1,858 bereaved caregivers in 20 health care districts in England 10 months after the death of the patient. Results indicated that half of the respondents rated their physical and psychological health as good after the death and felt that they were adjusting well. About one third of respondents reported bereavement-related health problems. There was a statistically significant association between positive reports of health and adjustment and ratings of high satisfaction with specialized care provided by community-based nurses and physicians. Again, this study supports the notion that bereaved individuals have specialized needs that, when managed by professionals who are adept at addressing them, lead to better individual outcomes and as yet untold benefits for society in terms of the resources that are used to compensate for the diminished productivity and the psychological and physical sequelae associated with bereavement.

Levy, Derby, and Martinowski (1993) examined whether membership in a bereavement support group influenced adaptation. During the first 18 months following the patient's death, group members and nonmembers both exhibited significant reductions in depression, anger, anxiety, subjective stress, and psychotropic medication reliance. In another study, the effectiveness of a psychoeducational bereavement-support group was studied at an outpatient cancer center. The bereaved caregiver participants reported increased knowledge about the grieving process and development of new coping strategies, particularly the ability to share thoughts and feelings with individuals experiencing a similar loss (Goldstein, Alter, & Axelrod, 1996). Bromberg and Higginson (1996) conducted a study to describe the activities of five palliative care support teams responsible for following 215 cancer caregivers after the patient's death. The investigators concluded that the team's main activity was to maintain contact with the family versus employing specific interventions to resolve grief. Again, research that clearly delineates intervention strategies with well-defined outcomes is in order.

As is the case with other caregiver intervention research, efforts to describe and standardize interventions must be undertaken so that interventions can be successfully replicated across studies. In addition, outcomes must be clearly described and measured in several areas, including physical health, psychological health, utilization of costly health care services, and functional productivity. Only when bereavement interventions are clearly linked to societal benefit will their merits and utility be fully recognized.

## DESIGN AND METHODOLOGICAL LIMITATIONS

There is a dearth of data-based literature describing interventions aimed at caregivers. Interventions described often lacked clear description. Lack of or poor operationalization of the intervention was often due to an assumption that there was an implicit understanding of the intervention, such as the caregiver being included in conceptualization of hospice care.

Of the small number of studies in this area, many used small convenience samples that lacked randomization. Although convenience samples are often used in caregiver research, their use makes it difficult to generalize results. Small sample size may not reveal hypothesized relationships because statistical power is low. Future studies should attempt to employ strategies to maximize sample size such as multisite studies and secondary analysis of large data sets. Many studies used a cross-sectional design. The use of longitudinal designs would greatly enhance our understanding of caregiver responses to interventions over time, including the potential preventive nature of caregiver interventions over time and the optimal timing of interventions. Recruitment and retention of caregivers in longitudinal studies is an important area needing further attention. Difficulties retaining subjects in family research has been outlined (Cooley & Moriarty, 1997; Moriarty, 1990). Creative strategies are needed for recruiting and retaining caregivers who are experiencing the unique stresses associated with caring for a loved one with cancer.

Attrition was noted as a problem in several studies. The use of statistical techniques to determine whether a remaining sample differs from the initial sample is important in terms of assessing the internal validity of the study (Cook & Campbell, 1979). Given, Kielman, Collins, and Given (1990) proposed strategies to minimize attrition in research with cancer caregivers. Data collectors should be prepared to deal with high subjective distress. Ongoing communication by the researchers with the subjects, continuity of subject contact with consistent data collectors, and creation of a positive interpersonal relationship between research team and subjects are essential to minimize subject attrition.

Many studies revealed selection bias, often to well-adjusted caregivers who were accepting of support, able to obtain respite care in order to participate, and often willing to avail themselves of a group-style intervention.

Efforts to recruit the most vulnerable caregivers, such as those who are homebound or have chronic medical conditions themselves, must be developed and described.

A lack of well-delineated outcome variables was revealed as a major gap in the literature. Outcomes, or the results of care, are frequently viewed as indicators of the quality of service provided. Globally, outcomes can be categorized into those related to the quality and need for services, the cost of care, and access to care issues. In this age of soaring health care costs and diminishing nonessential services, the documentation of outcomes associated with interventions, especially those geared toward vulnerable individuals, is paramount.

Overall, interventions targeted at caregivers of cancer patients have been developed by nurse and nonnurse researchers. In general, nurses tend to develop interventions that are geared toward increasing the proficiency of caregivers to address the physical and psychosocial needs of the patient. Nonnurse researchers tend to develop a greater abundance of individual and group psychological interventions directed specifically at caregivers. As research examining the efficacy of caregiver interventions is clearly in its infancy, the field would be greatly enhanced by an emphasis on interdisciplinary efforts that capitalize on each discipline's theoretical orientation and clinical strengths.

## CONCLUSIONS AND DIRECTIONS FOR FUTURE STUDY

Despite the fact that a cancer diagnosis causes major changes in family roles and functioning, in addition to increased responsibility for complex care being absorbed by family caregivers, data supporting the effectiveness of caregiver interventions are limited at best. In fact, most studies show that interventions have little if any effect. A seminal review by Blanchard and colleagues (1997) reported that between 20% and 30% of partners suffered from psychological impairment and mood disturbance as a result of a spouse's cancer. The review goes on to describe factors that may predict high levels of caregiver distress. The authors highlighted the need to explore the mediating role of suggested risk factors on specific outcome variables such as family functioning and psychological distress and suggested that interventions be targeted to high-risk individuals. Factors suggested to affect distress levels in caregivers are summarized below:

- *Disease stage:* advanced disease is often accompanied by higher distress.
- *Patient's emotional adjustment:* correlated with caregiver adjustment.
- *Gender:* female family members more distressed than males.

- *Age:* inversely related to emotional distress.
- *Socioeconomic status and other life stressors:* lower SES and more life stressors correlated with higher distress.
- *Personality traits:* caregiver optimism may predict caregiver reactions.
- *Coping and social support:* perceived coping efficacy may mediate effect between caregiver strain and depression. Social support may mediate relationship between functioning and caregiver depression.
- *Marital adjustment:* good communication correlated with ability to meet demands.
- *Family functioning:* (measured by the FACES [Family Adaptability and Cohesion Evaluation Scales]); lower distress is found in spouses and children if families are not rigid or chaotic.

Clearly, additional work is needed with regard to the identification of factors that predict those at highest risk for distress. The demands of the illness and thus stage of disease seem to be important factors, although, as suggested, their impact may be mediated by variables such as gender, personality, and family functioning. Interventions in those experiencing high levels of distress also should be tested at different points in the cancer trajectory to determine, for example, if interventions are most effective at certain points in the illness, whether interventions can be preventive across illness stages, and whether different types of caregiver interventions should be implemented at different stages of the cancer.

Other areas for future research include the impact of ethnic differences and nontraditional family styles on caregiver needs and intervention response. A family's social and ethnic background may influence relationships with and perceptions of health care professionals, access to care issues, and roles in caring for the patient. To date, little attention has been paid to social and cultural issues in cancer caregiver research.

Another notable gap in the cancer caregiver research relates to variation in family structure. Most research is done from the perspective of the traditional marriage dyad or a two-parent family structure (Kristjanson & Ashcroft, 1994). There are many other types of families, which may have needs different from those of traditional couples and may warrant the development and testing of innovative intervention strategies. For example, remarried and blended families, gay and lesbian couples with and without children, and unmarried partners may have unique needs and properties that require definition. Errors in the development of interventions may occur if research findings generated from other family forms are applied inappropriately. Further research to address these gaps is needed.

Current trends in health care focus on cutting costs in acute care settings, resulting in a shift of care from the hospital to the home. Despite what may seem to some to be societal cost savings and enhanced efficiency of the health care system, the locus of the financial, physical, and emotional burden of cancer care is often shifted to families that may incur emotional, economic, and physical consequences. Intervention initiatives underscore the need for caregiver advocacy in these changing times.

The development of interventions that have firm theoretical grounding based on the well-documented needs of cancer caregivers and are well described is in order to allow for replication. Interventions targeted to those at high risk for problems with the caregiving role will also maximize the impact of selected interventions. Innovative recruitment strategies are critical to promote adequate sample size and determination of intervention effect, randomization, and standardization of consistent outcome measures across studies that are theoretically linked to study variables. Careful attention to these issues will document the characteristics of individuals most amenable to caregiver interventions, as well as the efficacy of various intervention models. These measures are critical so that programs to assist caregivers can be adopted through policy initiatives as changes in the health care system continue to evolve.

## REFERENCES

Axelsson, B., & Sjoden, P. (1998). Quality of life of cancer patients and their spouses in palliative home care. *Journal of Palliative Medicine, 12,* 29–39.

Barg, F. K., Pasacreta, J. V., Nuamah, I. F., Robinson, K. D., Angeletti, K., Yasko, J. M., & McCorkle, R. (1998). A description of a psychoeducational intervention for family caregivers of cancer patients. *Journal of Family Nursing, 4,* 394–413.

Benoliel, J. Q., & McCorkle, R. (1978). A holistic approach to terminal illness. *Cancer Nursing, 1,* 143–149.

Blanchard, C. G., Toseland, R. W., & McCallion, P. (1997). The effects of a problem solving intervention with spouses of cancer patients. *Journal of Psychosocial Oncology, 14,* 1–21.

Bromberg, M. H., & Higginson, I. (1996). Bereavement follow-up: What do palliative support teams actually do? *Journal of Palliative Medicine, 12,* 12–17.

Carmody, S., Hickey, P., & Boakbinder, M. (1991). Preoperative needs of families. *American Operating Room Nurses Journal, 54,* 561–567.

Cawley, M. M., & Gerdts, E. K. (1988). Establishing a cancer care givers program: An interdisciplinary approach. *Cancer Nursing, 11,* 267–273.

Conkling, V. K. (1989). Continuity of care issues for cancer patients and families. *Cancer, 64,* 290–294.

Cook, T. D., & Campbell, D. T. (1979). *Quasi-experimentation: Design and analysis issues for field settings.* Chicago: Rand-McNally.

Cooley, M. E. , & Moriarty, H. J. (1997). An analysis of empirical studies examining the impact of the cancer diagnosis and treatment of an adult on family functioning. *Journal of Family Nursing, 3,* 318–347.

Derdiarian, A. (1989). Effects of information on recently diagnosed cancer patients' and spouses' satisfaction with care. *Cancer Nursing, 12,* 285–292.

Derogatis, L., & Spencer, P. M. (1982). *The Brief Symptom Inventory (BSI): Administration, scoring and procedures, Manual I.* Towson, MD: Clinical Psychometric Research.

Diekmann, J. M. (1988). An evaluation of selected "I Can Cope" prognosis by registered participants. *Cancer Nursing, 11,* 274–282.

Fakhoury, W. K. H., McCarthy, M., & Addington-Hall, J. (1997). Carers' health status: Is it associated with their evaluation of the quality of palliative care? *Scandinavian University Press, 25,* 297–301.

Ferrell, B. R., Grant, M., Chan, J., Ahn, C., & Ferrell, B. A. (1995). The impact of cancer pain education on family caregivers of elderly patients. *Oncology Nursing Forum, 22,* 1211–1218.

Foxall, M. J., & Gaston-Johansson, F. (1996). Burden and health outcomes of family caregivers of hospitalized bone marrow transplant patients. *Journal of Advanced Nursing, 24,* 915–923.

Ganz, P. A. (1990). Current issues in cancer rehabilitation. *Cancer, 65,* 742–751.

Giaquinta, B. (1977). Helping families face the crisis of cancer. *American Journal of Nursing, 12,* 1585.

Given C. W., Given, B., Stommel, M., Collins, C., King, S., & Franklin, S. (1992). The caregiver reactions assessment (CRA) for caregivers to persons with chronic physical and mental impairments. *Research in Nursing and Health, 15,* 271–283.

Given, B., Helms, C. W., Stommel, M., & Devoss, D. N. (1997). Determinants of family caregivers reaction: New and recurrent cancer. *Cancer Practice, 5,* 17–24.

Given, B. A., Keilman, L. J., Collins, C., & Given, C. W. (1990). Strategies to minimize attrition in longitudinal studies. *Nursing Research, 39,* 184–186.

Goldberg, R. J., & Wool, M. S. (1985). Psychotherapy for the spouses of lung cancer patients: Assessment of an intervention. *Psychotherapy Psychosomatic, 43,* 141–150.

Goldstein, J., Alter, C. L., & Axelrod, R. (1996). A pychoeducational bereavement-support group for families provided in an outpatient cancer center. *Journal of Cancer Education, 11,* 233–237.

Gotay, C. C. (1984). The experience of cancer during early and advanced stages: The views of patients and their mates. *Social Science and Medicine, 18,* 605–613.

Grahn, G. (1996). Coping with the cancer experience: 1. Developing an education and support programme for cancer patients and their significant others. *European Journal of Cancer Care, 5,* 176–181.

Grahn, G., & Danielson, M. (1996). Coping with the cancer experience: 2. Evaluating an education and support programme for cancer patients and their significant others. *European Journal of Cancer Care, 5,* 182–187.

Grobe, M. E., Istrup, S. M., & Ahmann, E. L. (1980). Skills needed by family caregivers to maintain the care of an advanced cancer patient. *Cancer Nursing, 4,* 371–375.

Hampe, S. (1975). Needs of the grieving spouse in a hospital setting. *Nursing Research, 24,* 113–119.

Heinrich, R. L., & Schag, C. C. (1985). Stress activity management: Group treatment for cancer patients and spouses. *Journal of Consulting and Clinical Psychology, 43,* 439–446.

Hinds, C. (1985). The needs of families who care for patients with cancer at home: Are we meeting them? *Journal of Advanced Nursing, 10,* 575–581.

Holland, J. C. (1989). Clinical course of cancer. In J. C. Holland & J. H. Rowland (Eds.), *Handbook of psychooncology: Psychological care of the patient with cancer* (pp. 75–100). New York: Oxford University Press.

Houts, P. S., Nezu, A. M., Nezu, C. M., & Bucher, J. A. (1996). The prepared family caregiver: A problem-solving approach to family caregiver education. *Patient Education and Counseling, 27*(1), 63–73.

Hull, M. M. (1989). Family needs and supportive nursing behaviors during terminal cancer: A review. *Oncology Nursing Forum, 16,* 787–792.

Hull, M. M. (1992). Coping strategies of family caregivers in hospice home care. *Oncology Nursing Forum, 19,* 1179–1187.

Jepson, C., McCorkle, R., Adler, D., Nuamah, I., & Lusk, E. (1999). Effects of home care on caregivers' psychosocial status. *Image: Journal of Nursing Scholarship, 31,* 115–120.

Johnson, J. (1982). The effects of a patient education course on persons with a chronic illness. *Cancer Nursing, 2,* 117–120.

Johnson, J. L., & Norby, P. A. (1981). We can weekend: A program for cancer families. *Cancer Nursing, 4,* 23–27.

Kristjanson, L., & Ashcroft, B. (1994). The family's cancer journey: A literature review. *Cancer Nursing, 17,* 1–17.

Krouse, H., & Krouse, J. (1982). Cancer as crisis: The critical elements of adjustment. *Nursing Research, 31,* 96–101.

Kurtz, M. E., Kurtz, J. C., Given, C. W., & Given, B. (1997). Predictors of postbereavement depressive symptomatology among family caregivers of cancer patients. *Support Care Center, 5,* 53–60.

Laizner, A., Shedga, L., Bard, F., & McCorkle, R. (1993). Needs of family caregivers of persons with cancer: A review. *Seminars in Oncology Nursing, 9,* 114–120.

Levy, L. H., Derby, J. F., & Martinowski, K. S. (1993). Effects of membership in bereavement support groups on adaptation to conjugal bereavement. *American Journal of Community Psychology, 21,* 361–381.

Lewis, F. M. (1986). The impact of cancer on the family: A critical analysis of the research literature. *Patient Education and Counseling, 8,* 269–289.

MacVicar, M., & Archbold, P. (1976). A framework for family assessment in chronic illness. *Nursing Forum, 15,* 180–194.

McCorkle, R., & Benoliel, J. Q. (1983). Symptom distress, current concerns and mood disturbance after diagnosis of life threatening disease. *Social Science and Medicine, 17,* 431–438.

McCorkle, R., & Given, B. (1991). Meeting the challenge of caring for chronically ill adults. In P. Chin (Ed.), *Health policy: Who cares?* (pp. 2–7). Kansas City, MO: American Academy of Nursing.

McCorkle, R., Robinson, L., Nuamah, I., Lev, E., & Benoliel, J. Q. (1998). The effects of home nursing care for patients during terminal illness on the bereaved's psychological distress. *Nursing Research, 47,* 2–10.

McCorkle, R., Yost, L. S., Jepson, C., Malone, D., Baird, S., & Lusk, E. (1993). A cancer experience: Relationship of patient psychosocial responses to caregiver burden over time. *PsychoOncology, 2,* 21–32.

McMillan, S. C. (1996). Quality of life of primary caregivers of hospice patients with cancer. *Cancer Practice, 4,* 191–198.

McMillan, S. C., & Mahon, M. (1994). The impact of hospice services on the quality of life of primary caregivers. *Oncology Nursing Forum, 21,* 1189–1195.

Mor, V., Guadagnoli, E., & Wool, M. (1987). An examination of the concrete service needs of advanced cancer patients. *Journal of Psychosocial Oncology, 5,* 1–17.

Moriarty, H. J. (1990). Key issues in the family research process: Strategies for nurse researchers. *Advances in Nursing Science, 12,* 1–14.

Nativg, K. (1983). Laryngectomies in Norway. Study no. 2. Pre-operative counseling and post-operative training evaluated by patients and their spouses. *Journal of Otolaryngology, 12,* 249–254.

Neal, B., & Clark, D. (1992). Informal care of people with cancer: A review of research on needs and services. *Journal of Cancer Care, 1,* 193–198.

Northouse, L. (1984). The impact of cancer on the family: An overview. *International Journal of Psychiatry in Medicine, 14,* 215–243.

Northouse, L. L. (1988). Social support in patients' and husbands' adjustment to breast cancer. *Nursing Research, 37,* 91–95.

Northouse, L. (1989). A longitudinal study of the adjustment of patients and husbands to breast cancer. *Oncology Nursing Forum, 16,* 511–516.

Northouse, L., & Golden-Peters, H. (1993). Cancer and the family: Strategies to assist spouses. *Seminars in Oncology Nursing, 9,* 74–82.

Northouse, L. L., & Swain, M. A. (1987). Adjustment of patients and husbands to the initial impact of breast cancer. *Nursing Research, 36,* 221–225.

Northouse, P. G., & Northouse, L. L. (1987). Communication and cancer: Issues confronting patients, health professionals, and family members. *Journal of Psychosocial Oncology, 5,* 17–46.

Oberst, M. T., Gass, K. A., & Ward, S. E. (1989). Caregiving demands and appraisal of stress among family caregivers. *Cancer Nursing, 12,* 209–215.

Oberst, M. T., & Scott, D. W. (1988). Postdischarge distress in surgically treated cancer patients and their spouses. *Research in Nursing and Health, 11,* 223–233.

Perry, G. R., & Roades de Menses, M. (1989). Cancer patients at home. Needs and coping styles of primary caregivers. *Home Healthcare Nurse, 7,* 27–30.

Pfefferbaum, B., Pasnan, R. O., & Jamison, K. (1977). A comprehensive program for psychosocial care for mastectomy patients. *International Journal of Psychiatry Medicine, 8,* 63–71.

Reele, B. (1994). Effect of counseling on quality of life for individuals with cancer and their families. *Cancer Nursing, 17,* 101–112.

Sabo, D., Brown, J., & Smith, C. (1986). The male role and mastectomy: Support groups and men's adjustment. *Journal of Psychosocial Oncology, 4,* 19–31.

Sales, E., Schultz, R., & Biegel, D. (1990). Predictors of strain in families of cancer patients: A review of the literature. *Journal of Psychosocial Oncology, 10,* 1–26.

Sarna, L., & McCorkle, R. (1996). Burden of care and lung cancer. *Cancer Practice, 4*(5), 245–251.

Schachter, S. (1992). Quality of life for families in the management of homecare patients with advanced cancer. *Journal of Palliative Care, 8,* 61–66.

Siegel, K., Raveis, V. H., Houts, P., & Mor, V. (1991). Caregiver burden and unmet patient needs. *Cancer, 68,* 1131–1140.

Siegel, K., Raveis, V. H., Mor, V., & Houts, P. (1991). The relationship of spousal caregiver burden to patient disease and treatment related conditions. *Annals of Oncology, 2,* 511–516.

Stetz, K. M. (1987). Caregiving demands during advanced cancer: The spouse's needs. *Cancer Nursing, 10,* 260–268.

Stetz, K. M. (1989). The relationship among background characteristics, purpose in life and caregiving demands on perceived health of spouse caregivers. *Scholarly Inquiry for Nursing Practice, 3,* 133–153.

Tornberg, M. J., McGrath, B. B., & Benoliel, J. Q. (1984). Oncology transition service: Partnerships of nurses and families. *Cancer Nursing, 7*(2), 131–137.

Vachon, M. L. S. (1982). Grief and bereavement: The family's experience before and after death. In I. Gontlos (Ed.), *Care for the dying and the bereaved* (pp. 142–174). Toronto: Anglican Book Centre.

Wallhagen, M. (1992). Caregiving demands: Their difficulty and effects on the well-being of elderly caregivers. *Scholarly Inquiry for Nursing Practice, 6,* 111–127.

Weisman, A., & Worden, J. (1976). The existential plight in cancer: Significance of the first 100 days. *International Journal of Psychiatry in Medicine, 7,* 1–15.

Weitzner, M. A., Moody, L. N., & McMillan, S. C. (1997). Symptom management issues in hospice care. *American Journal of Hospice and Palliative Care, 14*(4), 190–195.

Wellisch, D. K., Jamison, K. R., & Pasnau, R. O. (1978). Psychosocial aspects of mastectomy: 2. The man's perspective. *American Journal of Psychiatry, 135*(5), 543–546.

Wellisch, D., Mosher, M. B., & VanScoy, C. (1978). Management of family emotional stress: Family group therapy in a private oncology practice. *International Journal of Group Psychotherapy, 28*(2), 225–231.

Wilkerson, S. (1991). Factors which influence how nurses communicate with cancer patients. *Journal of Advanced Nursing, 16,* 677–688.

Wilson, S., & Moore, J. M. (1991). Living with a wife undergoing chemotherapy. *Image, 23,* 78–84.

Wright, K., & Dyck, S. (1984). Expressed concerns of adult cancer patients' family members. *Cancer Nursing, 7*(5), 371–374.

Yang, C. T., & Kirschling, J. M. (1992). Exploration of factors related to direct care and outcomes of caregiving: Caregiving of terminally ill older persons. *Cancer Nursing, 15,* 173–181.

Zahlis, E., & Shands, M. E. (1991). Breast cancer: Demands of one illness on the patient's partner. *Journal of Psychosocial Oncology, 9,* 75–93.

# Chapter 6

# Interventions for Children with Diabetes and Their Families

MARGARET GREY

## ABSTRACT

The purpose of this review is to examine the research literature on interventions for children with type 1 diabetes and their families, with a specific focus on three types of intervention (educational and psychosocial/behavioral interventions that focus on individuals with diabetes and family interventions for families, usually parents, of individuals with diabetes). The aim of the review is to determine what interventions produce what outcomes in what populations of children and families. The review includes articles that met the following criteria: (a) empirical study reporting the impact of an intervention on such outcomes as knowledge, behavior, self-care, and metabolic control; (b) children with type 1 diabetes and/or their families as primary subjects; (c) publication between 1980 and January 1, 1999; and (d) publication in English. A total of 41 published papers were included. On the basis of this review, conclusions are as follows: (a) Educational interventions are useful in improving diabetes knowledge but not consistently helpful in improving metabolic control; (b) psychosocial interventions, especially coping skills training and peer support, assist primarily adolescents to improve adjustment and sometimes metabolic control; and (c) family interventions may be helpful in reducing parent-child conflict about diabetes management and care.

**Key words: type 1 diabetes, interventions, education, children, adolescents**

Diabetes is the fifth leading cause of death in the United States, and type 1 diabetes is a major health problem affecting over 140,000 American children and adolescents (National Institute of Diabetes, Digestive and Kidney Diseases [NIDDK], 1995). Type 1 diabetes, or insulin-dependent diabetes, is characterized by alterations in carbohydrate, protein, and fat metabolism due to the absolute lack of insulin production (American Diabetes Association, 1999). Management is complex and demanding and consists of daily injections of insulin, self-monitoring of blood glucose, and careful regulation of dietary intake and exercise. Nonetheless, the life expectancy of a child with diabetes at the age of 10 is 44 years, whereas his or her age mates without diabetes have a life expectancy of 72 years (NIDDK, 1995). This early mortality is related to the long-term complications of the disease. The findings of the Diabetes Control and Complications Trial (DCCT) demonstrate that intensive therapy and better metabolic control, as measured by glycosylated hemoglobin (Hb $A_{1c}$) can reduce such complications by 27% to 76% (DCCT Research Group, 1993). Hb $A_{1c}$ is an index of the glycosylation of the hemoglobin molecule that reflects the degree of metabolic control of diabetes over the most recent 2 months (Grey & Boland, 1996).

Because of the complexity of diabetes management and the necessity for most of this intensive management to be provided at home, education of children and parents regarding care of diabetes has long been a mainstay of treatment (Travis, Brouhard, & Schreiner, 1987). In addition, nurses have often been responsible for such interventions, making their evaluation important to improving knowledge for clinical practice. Unfortunately, the majority of these educational and supportive interventions have not been scientifically evaluated. Thus, the purpose of this review is to examine the research literature on interventions for children with type 1 diabetes and their families. The aim of the review is to determine what interventions produce what outcomes in what populations of children and families.

Specifically, this review focuses on three types of interventions (educational, psychosocial or behavioral, and family interventions). Articles were divided for the review according to the main purpose of the intervention. This distinction was made by the author, using the description of the intervention provided in the paper to categorize the paper. Educational interventions were defined as those focusing on increasing knowledge about diabetes and its care and increasing competence to perform self-care behaviors. Psychosocial/psychological interventions included those that focused primarily on improving adjustment or adaptation to diabetes in children and adolescents. Finally, family interventions were defined as those whose primary target was the family of the child or adolescent with diabetes. Outcomes of family interventions might be at either the individual level (e.g., metabolic control) or the family level (family conflict).

To conduct the review, computerized databases (CINAHL, MEDLINE, PsychInfo, ERIC) were searched, using the following key words: *diabetes, insulin dependent, limit to children and adolescents; education, psychosocial/psychological;* and *family therapy.* The focus was on published literature from 1980 to the present. No attempt was made to search for unpublished works.

This search yielded a total of 48 potential papers for inclusion. Authors known to have contributed to this literature (Grey, Wysocki, Anderson, Delamater, Pichert, and Marrero) also were searched by author, yielding a total of 10 new papers for review. Finally, a hand search of relevant journals *(Diabetes Educator, Diabetes Care, Patient Counseling and Education)* was conducted to assure that no important papers were missed; this search yielded only one additional article. Articles were retrieved and reviewed for inclusion using the following criteria: (a) empirical study reporting results of an intervention; (b) children with type 1 diabetes and/or their families as primary subjects; (c) publication between 1980 and January 1, 1999; and (d) publication in English. A total of 59 articles were identified for inclusion, and after review, 41 were included. No articles were identified that could not be located for review.

The questions to be answered by this review included the following: What intervention strategies have been used with children with type 1 diabetes and their families? What is the methodological adequacy of these studies? What outcomes have been studied, and how reliable and valid are they? What are the substantive findings of these studies?

## EDUCATIONAL INTERVENTIONS

In diabetes care, patient education is the standard approach. The American Diabetes Association (ADA) guidelines suggest the importance of education for patients with type 1 diabetes and their families (ADA, 1999). Indeed, because so much of diabetes care is performed by children and their families (Grey & Boland, 1996), treatment goals cannot be accomplished without sufficient patient education. Nonetheless, there have been relatively few studies that have carefully examined structure and content of diabetes education programs for children and families.

Reviews specifically focused on interventions for children and adolescents with type 1 diabetes could not be found in the literature. Two recent reviews (Brandt, 1998; Deatrick, 1998) focused on children, but neither was specific to the topic of this review. Brandt (1998) conducted a review of behavioral research in children and adolescents with diabetes, but the focus was not on interventions. In contrast, Deatrick (1998) reviewed the intervention literature for children with chronic illnesses and their families but included only two studies of children with diabetes. Thus, this review is timely and appropriate.

For this analysis, educational programs were divided into programs as follows: (a) general education was provided; (b) structured education was provided without new educational technology; and (c) structured education was provided with some new educational technology. There were four articles dealing with general education, seven with structured education without educational technology, and six on structured education with new educational technology.

## General Education

Epstein, Figueroa, Farkas, and Beck (1981) reported the results of a study of the use of feedback training versus extended practice and its effect on accuracy of urine testing for glucose concentration in 35 children (age 6–16 years; diabetes duration over 1 year). Once determination was made that children had difficulty in accurately testing urine for glucose, they were randomly assigned to receive feedback training, consisting of testing 20 tubes of urine and receiving immediate feedback on accuracy of results; those assigned to the control condition of more practice tested 20 more tubes of urine but without feedback. Errors were determined by a standardized procedure developed in a previous study. Results demonstrated that children in the feedback group had significantly fewer errors than those in the practice-only group. Although urine testing is not a prominent task in diabetes treatment today, these results may have relevance for other forms of self-monitoring, such as blood glucose testing.

Similarly, Wolanski, Sigman, and Polychonakos (1996) studied the effectiveness of feedback instruction on self-monitoring of blood glucose in an experimental study conducted at a diabetes camp over two summers. As with the urine testing study, potential subjects were screened to determine if they made substantial errors in blood glucose testing. Errors were determined by observation of several behavioral skills associated with blood glucose testing, and the systematic and random errors were calculated. Those with difficulty were randomly assigned to routine camp education or to routine education plus individualized feedback on technique. A total of 20 subjects (age, 8–16 years) were randomized, but only marginal differences were found between the two groups on errors in technique after the intervention.

The two other studies that dealt with general education focused on evaluation of overall diabetes education programs in two foreign countries. Both studies used preexperimental designs. K. Anderson (1997) conducted an evaluation of a diabetes education program for children and adolescents in Canada. Of 100 eligible subjects, 22 (age 13–17) returned satisfaction questionnaires designed for this study, and chart audits were conducted on all 100 subjects. Aspects of the program that respondents liked the most included learning, problem solving, interacting with staff, and support. Chart audits demonstrated that most had received appropriate screenings for complications (eye referral, 24-hour urine testing for microalbumin), but only 17.5% had reached metabolic treatment goals. Only 6% had a foot examination recorded in the chart. No data are presented on the reliability of the tools used in this study.

To investigate whether a diabetes education program was successful in creating awareness and imparting knowledge about diabetes in children in India, Shobhana, Rao, Vijay, Snehalatha, and Ramachandran (1997) involved 37 children (age 8–18) in a 2-day program consisting of didactic group content on general diabetes and individual sessions on injections, monitoring, and dietary counseling. Using a one-group, pretest-posttest design, they demonstrated improvement in knowledge over 3 months, using a self-prepared tool in the areas of general knowledge about diabetes, insulin, injections, hypoglycemia, and total knowledge score. They found no differences in diet, exercise, or monitoring knowledge.

## Structured Education Without New Educational Technology

A number of studies have been reported that examined structured educational programs that did not involve the use of new educational technology. Some of these programs focused on specific aspects of diabetes care, such as exercise, whereas others were more general.

Huttunen et al. (1989) studied the effects of exercise training in children ($N = 34$; 17 matched pairs; 20 males, 14 females; age $M = 11.9$, 8–16 years; duration M = 4.7, .6–13 years) over a 3-month period. Exercise training consisted of structured, monitored exercise, including jogging, running, gymnastics, and other active games. The results demonstrated that fitness, as measured by $VO_2$ and pedaling time, improved in the experimental group but that metabolic control, as measured by blood and urine glucose, was not improved. Glycosylated hemoglobin, measured by hemoglobin $A_{1c}$ (Hb $A_{1c}$), worsened in the exercise group but improved in those who attended the most exercise sessions.

A retrospective chart review designed to evaluate the impact of a comprehensive diabetes management program for children on inpatient hospitalizations for diabetic ketoacidosis (DKA) and length of stay for DKA was conducted (Drozda, Dawson, Long, Freson, & Sperling, 1990). The educational program, recognized by ADA, offered a combination of medical and support services and daily telephone contact. The program was evaluated by comparing medical records of children hospitalized before the program began (1978–1986) and after the program (1978–1987). Results indicated that fewer admissions for DKA and shorter length of stay were positive outcomes of the program.

Delamater and colleagues (1990) conducted a randomized trial of evaluation of a structured program designed to teach decision making in insulin adjustments and compared this program to supportive counseling focusing on psychosocial adjustment issues and conventional follow-up. The Self-Management Training (SMT) program consisted of seven sessions held over the 4 months immediately after discharge at diagnosis. The emphasis was on blood glucose monitoring technique, reinforcement of accurate monitoring and recording, and use of the blood glucose data in making appropriate behavioral changes. Subjects were 36 children (age, $M = 9.3$, 3–16 years; 50% male) with new-onset type 1 diabetes, who were followed for 2 years postdiagnosis. The major outcome was metabolic control as measured by Hb $A_1$ levels, and results demonstrated that self-management training significantly improved metabolic control at 1 and 2 years compared to conventional follow-up, but not compared to supportive counseling.

Similarly, McNabb, Quinn, Murphy, Thorp, and Cook (1994) conducted an experimental study to test the hypothesis that school-age children can learn to become more independent in their diabetes self-management without compromising metabolic control. A total of 22 children (age, $M = 9.7$, 8–12 years; duration, at least 3 months) were matched for age and race, then one of each pair was randomized to the In Control program, consisting of six small group sessions (1 hour/week) to teach self-care concepts and skills of self-management to children and parents. After 3 months of follow-up, scores on the Children's Diabetes Inventory (a scale developed for this study for which reliability and validity were assessed) showed that children who received the experimental program had higher responsibility in insulin administration, responding to symptoms of hypo- and hyperglycemia, record keeping, and communication but not in glucose monitoring, caring for equipment and supplies, meal planning, adjusting regimen, and modifying care during illness. Metabolic control (Hb $A_{1c}$) was not significantly different between the two groups after 3 months.

Some studies focus on a particular age group. For example, Court (1991) studied the provision of transition services for youth who were graduating from pediatric programs to adult programs. They surveyed 70 youth (32 male; age, $M = 20.5$, 17–27 years; 100% White) who had left pediatric services between the ages of 17 and 19 years, using a questionnaire developed for this study. They found that the educational services most valued in transition were information about diabetes and complications, access to emergency services, and assistance with personal or social problems and that such programs in outpatient settings are important in transition but may not improve metabolic control.

A study of the impact of an educational program for school-age children and their mothers used a one-group prospective evaluation (Brandt & Magyary, 1993). A total of 17 mother-child pairs participated in the educational program, which consisted of 5 days and 11 sessions designed to improve knowledge and skills as well as improve the child's feelings of competence and the parent's supportive network. A number of well-established tools were used to collect data on the outcomes, including the Diabetes Knowledge Questionnaire (S. B. Johnson et al., 1982), Diabetes Skills Tests (Pollak & Johnson, 1979), and the Perceived Competence Scale (Harter, 1979) for the children and the Personal Resource Questionnaire

(Brandt & Weinert, 1981), Life Experience Survey (Sarason, Johnson, & Seigel, 1978), and the Parent Acceptance/Rejection Questionnaire (Rohner, 1981) for the mothers. Findings indicated that both children and mothers had immediate improvement in knowledge and skills, but these gains were not maintained to 3 months. Child competence was not affected by the program, as indicated by the Harter scales, nor were the mothers' supportive networks, as measured by the Personal Resource Questionnaire.

Mitchell (1996) developed a booklet, *Improving Compliance with Treatment for Diabetes,* that identified issues in adherence, discussed causes and interpretations, and offered basic management techniques for children after discharge from hospitalization for newly diagnosed diabetes. She evaluated the impact of this booklet in an experimental pilot study. A total of 32 children (age, $M = 10.6$, 8–16 years; 18 males) with newly diagnosed diabetes were enrolled and randomized to routine care or routine care plus the booklet. Results indicated that there were no differences in the identification of diabetes-related problems as measured by the Problem Situations Questionnaire (Gillis, 1990) at 1 month. However, at 3 months, the experimental group did better than the control group. There were no differences on the Child Behavior Checklist (Achenbach & Edelbrock, 1983) or in metabolic control (Hb $A_{1c}$).

## Structured Education with New Educational Technology

Several investigators have recently begun to assess the use of new educational technologies in diabetes education for children. Studies have been conducted using computer-assisted management, anchored instruction using videodiscs, and telecommunication to assist in outpatient management.

Horan, Yarborough, Besigel, and Carlson (1990) investigated the effects of a microcomputer-based system on control, adherence, and behavioral change in adolescents. The *Diabetes in Self-Control (DISC)* is a three-component system: (1) data management and review—storing, compiling, and reviewing blood glucose and other data; (2) computer-assisted factual and applied diabetes education; and (3) problem solving and goal setting to improve control compared to written modules for education. Twenty teens ($N = 20$, age, 12–19 years; 14 females, 80% White) were matched on grade, gender, race, Hb $A_{1c}$, and knowledge, then randomized to use the *DISC* or to receive written materials. The education program lasted 15 weeks, with 16–18 contacts per subject, involving diabetes education, goal setting and problem solving, and posttesting with and without the *DISC* program. Results showed that there were no differences between the two groups on Hb $A_{1c}$, but there were differences in blood glucose levels at lunch and dinner. The *DISC* group performed significantly more tests, but there were no differences between the groups in either general or problem solving knowledge, as measured by the Test of Diabetes Knowledge

(Johnson, Pollack, et al., 1982). Subjects in the *DISC* group self-reported more changes in behaviors than did the control group in response to a question asking if they had changed their diabetes management behaviors.

Pichert and colleagues (Murkin, Snyder, Pichert, & Boswell, 1990; Pichert et al., 1994a; Pichert, Snyder, Kinzer, & Boswell, 1992, 1994) have conducted a number of studies using anchored instruction, an approach in which the study of many concepts and skills is situated in a single, graphically presented interface. Using diabetes campers ranging in age from 9 to 15 years as subjects, they examined the effectiveness of two anchored instruction videodiscs, *Sydney Meets the Ketone Challenge* and *The Grade, the Date, and the Race,* to teach problem solving for sick-day management and dietary adherence. In all studies they found that the experimental groups performed better on tests of knowledge recall and self-management behavior developed for these studies. Long-term follow-up was conducted with the sick-day management study (Pichert et al., 1994). Results indicated that differences in knowledge persisted and the experimental group self-reported more sharing of management responsibilities during sick days than did the control group. Effects on metabolic control were not reported.

An experimental evaluation of the efficacy of using a telecommunication system (Data-Link® modem with meters, biweekly transmission of results, protocol for telephone follow-up to achieve mean blood glucose level of 140 mg/dl) was conducted by Marrero et al. (1995). In a comparison of outcomes after 1 year, the authors found that, in general, there were few differences between the group that used the new system and the conventional system of telephone follow-up in the following areas: Hb $A_{1c}$, hospitalizations and emergency room use documented by chart audit, psychological status as measured by the Offer Self-Image questionnaire (Offer, Ostrove, & Howard, 1977), family dynamics as measured with the Family Assessment Device (Bishop, Epstein, Keitner, Miller, & McMaster, 1983), quality of life as measured by the Diabetes Quality of Life for Youth scale (Ingersoll & Marrero, 1991), responsibility for diabetes care as measured by the Parent-Child Responsibility Scale (Anderson, Auslander, Jung, Miller, & Santiago, 1990) or attitudes about diabetes as assessed by a structured interview. In terms of efficacy, however, nurse practitioners spent less time per call with those in the experimental group to achieve the same outcomes, so the system may be more efficient than usual telephone follow-up.

In summary, educational studies have been conducted with a broad range of children with diabetes, but the majority focus on adolescents. This focus on adolescents is not surprising considering that, in general, adolescents are more difficult to manage than younger children (Grey & Boland, 1996). The majority of studies are experimental in design, and several use samples large enough for confidence in the findings. For the most part, these studies have tested a simple cause-and-effect relationship, without consideration of a range of antecedent and intervening variables. A range of outcomes has been studied, including knowledge, metabolic control, psychosocial status, and health care utilization, but interestingly, many studies are atheoretical and fail to use reliable and valid measures of outcomes. Results have been generally positive with regard to changes in knowledge but mixed in other outcomes.

## PSYCHOSOCIAL INTERVENTIONS

There have been a number of studies on the effects of psychosocial interventions for children and adolescents with diabetes. Such studies are important because of the potential for chronic conditions such as type 1 diabetes to have a negative impact on psychosocial outcomes in children (Brandt, 1998). Studies in this group were categorized as intervention studies if the target of the intervention was the child with diabetes rather than the family and if the primary goal was a psychosocial outcome rather than a knowledge or self-care behavior outcome. As with educational interventions, reviews of this literature have not previously been published. Several authors (Bauman, Drotar, Leventhal, Perrin, & Pless, 1997; Deatrick, 1998; LaMontagne, 1993) have published reviews of interventions with children, but these have not focused specifically on diabetes. Thus, these reviews included fewer of the studies reported here. Reports on psychosocial interventions were further divided in to the following categories: (a) coping skills training ($N = 8$), (b) psychotherapy ($N = 2$), (c) stress management and relaxation ($N = 2$), and (d) social support in groups or camps ($N = 7$).

### Coping Skills Training

A series of studies using coping skills training for children and adolescents with diabetes has been conducted. Coping skills training is designed to increase competence and mastery by retraining inappropriate or nonconstructive coping styles and patterns of behavior into more constructive behaviors. Coping skills training for youth with diabetes is based on the hypothesis that improving coping skills will improve the ability of youth to cope with the problems faced on a day-to-day basis in managing diabetes.

In the early 1980s a number of preexperimental studies (Gross, Heiman, Shapiro, & Schultz, 1983; Gross, Johnson, Wildman, & Mullett, 1982; Johnson, Gross, & Wildman, 1982) were conducted with 5 to 10 school-age children and preadolescents. These studies suggested that the coping skills training approach had merit, with increases in appropriate verbalization in assertiveness and appropriate performance in social situations (Bornstein, Bellack, & Herson, 1977) but no differences in metabolic control.

Massouh, Steele, Alseth, and Diekmann (1989) conducted an experimental study of a single-session social learning intervention with 34 adolescents at a diabetes camp. The social learning intervention involved a 40-minute session with a psychological therapist who guided the campers in role modeling behaviors to deal with peer pressure against self-care. The outcome was metabolic control measured 3 months after camp completion. Unfortunately, the intervention was found to have no effect.

In an experimental study that combined both instruction in blood glucose management and coping skills training, called Stress Management Training in Adolescents, Boardway, Delameter, Tomakowsky, and Gutai (1993) found that although diabetes-specific stress was decreased in the experimental group, there were no differences in Hb $A_{1c}$, coping styles (Folkman & Lazarus, 1980), self-efficacy (Grossman, Brink, & Hauser, 1987), life events (Sarason et al., 1978), or adherence (Johnson, Pollack, et al., 1982) over 9 months. However, as with the earlier studies, only 19 subjects were studied, so the statistical power to determine these effects was limited.

In contrast, Grey and colleagues (Davidson, Boland, & Grey, 1997; Grey, Boland, Davidson, & Tamborlane, 1999; Grey et al., 1998) reported on the results of a larger randomized clinical trial with a sufficient sample to achieve statistical power in determining both metabolic and psychosocial effects of coping skills training. These studies focused on adolescents initiating intensive insulin therapy after the results of the Diabetes Control and Complications Trial (DCCT) were released (DCCT Research Group, 1994) . In their study of 77 youth (age, 13–21, $M = 16.2$; duration, $M = 8.4$ years), they found significant improvements in metabolic control, general self-efficacy (Grossman et al., 1987), and quality of life (Ingersoll & Marrero, 1991), compared to the control group over 6 months of follow-up (Grey et al., 1999).

## Psychotherapy

Another approach to working with young people with diabetes is psychotherapy. This approach is based on previous studies that have suggested that youth with poorer diabetes control may have more depression and psychiatric problems than those in better control (Grey, Cameron, Lipman, & Thurber, 1995; Kovacs, Mukerji, Iyengar, & Drash, 1996). Two studies were found that examined the effectiveness of psychotherapy in adolescents and adults with diabetes. Both of these studies were conducted primarily with adults, but since adolescents were included in the samples, they are included here for completeness.

Both studies enrolled subjects who were having difficulty in diabetes control as perceived by their physicians. Viinamaki, Niskanen, and Tynkkynen

(1991) examined the records of nine patients who were referred for psychiatric treatment and compared outcomes to those who did not receive treatment ($N = 54$). Psychotherapy was psychodynamically and phase-specifically oriented and was provided in the outpatient area of the psychiatric clinic an average of two times per week over 1 year. They found that there were no differences in metabolic control, but they noted clinical improvement in psychiatric symptoms after 1 year. Similarly, in another study (Fosbury, Bosley, Ryle, Sonksen, & Judd, 1997), 26 patients with clinically poorly controlled diabetes were randomized to receive cognitive analytic therapy or education. Cognitive analytic therapy is a time-limited psychotherapy that integrates techniques from psychoanalytic and cognitive/behavior therapy to alleviate individual problems. As in the previous study, there were no differences between groups, but Hb $A_{1c}$ improved over 3 months and 9 months in the cognitive therapy group, and improvement was noted in interpersonal difficulties as measured by the Inventory of Interpersonal Problems (Fosbury et al., 1997). Thus, psychiatric intervention appears to be helpful in adolescents and young adults who are having difficulty in achieving metabolic treatment goals.

## Stress Management or Relaxation

Two studies were found that used meditation and other forms of stress reduction as a method to improve diabetes care and outcomes. Because stress has been found to be associated with alterations in metabolic control, it is hypothesized that such interventions will assist those with diabetes to have better metabolic control. Mendez and Belendez (1997) conducted a quasi-experiment of stress management in 37 adolescents (age, 11–18 years, $M = 13.5$; duration, $M = 4.1$ years; 50% female) and compared this program to routine medical care. The program consisted of 12 sessions that included review, information, and practicalities of diabetes management, with a focus on stress and coping with stress, including problem solving. This project might have been included in the coping skills training group or the education group but was included here because the main focus was on stress reduction and management, rather than on coping skills or education.

Nonetheless, results are similar to education programs described above, with posttest improvements in diabetes information (unpublished tool), adherence (Glascow, McCaul, & Schafer, 1986), daily hassles (unpublished tool), social responses (unpublished tools), skills, frequency of testing and errors in blood glucose testing (as measured by observation), and negative family support (Schafer, McCaul, & Glasgow, 1986). There were no effects on self-reported dietary and physical exercise behavior or Hb $A_{1c}$. When retested at 13 months after the intervention, knowledge, barriers to adherence, hassles, and social interactions remained better in the stress management group.

Smith and colleagues (Smith, Schreiner, Brouhard, & Travis, 1991) examined the effect of a stress management program, provided at a diabetes camp, on coping strategies in adolescents in a pretest-posttest, one-group evaluation design. This program focused on helping adolescents to identify stressors in their own lives and to increase awareness of techniques that could be used to manage stress; it was provided in small-group sessions lasting about 1 hour. A total of 108 subjects (age, 13–17 years, $M$ = 14.5; duration, $M$ = 53.7 months; 96% White; 56% female) participated. At posttest, campers reported an intent to use more problem-focused and fewer detachment strategies as assessed with the Ways of Coping Checklist (Folkman & Lazarus, 1980). Additionally, those with more diabetes-related stressors, measured with a visual analog scale, had larger effects than those with fewer diabetes-related stressors.

## Social Support Groups

Over the years a number of studies have suggested that social support is associated with adherence and metabolic control in adolescents with diabetes (Burroughs, Harris, Pontious, & Santiago, 1997). A recent review of this literature concluded that despite the understanding that social support is important, there have been relatively few investigations of socially supportive interventions (Burroughs et al., 1997). These interventions differ from group approaches used to teach coping skills and other approaches in that the goal is to improve the supportiveness of the environment rather than to attain specific skills. Interventions that focus on the family as the unit of social support are discussed below under family interventions. Seven studies met the criteria to be included in this section.

Three research groups (Siminerio, 1980; Templeton, Burkhart, Anderson, & Bacon, 1988; Warren-Boulton, Anderson, Schwartz, & Drexler, 1981) conducted early studies using preexperimental designs to describe and evaluate support groups for young people with diabetes. Siminerio (1980) described the effect of a diabetes youth support group on two preadolescents. Warren-Boulton et al. (1981) evaluated, in a pretest-posttest design, a monthly support group for five inner-city African American older teenagers. Both described improvements in self-reported compliance or adherence and better psychosocial adjustment. Finally, Templeton et al. (1988) used a group approach for nutritional problem solving with similar results.

Anderson and colleagues (Anderson, Wolf, Burkhart, Cornell, & Bacon, 1989) examined the effectiveness of a peer group intervention for young adolescents to attempt to prevent the usual decline in metabolic control associated with adolescents. They hypothesized that providing peer support and education in making adjustments in the diabetes regimen according to self-monitored blood glucose results would prevent this decline. In this intervention, small groups of adolescents met at each of their clinic visits. Emphasis was placed on the use of blood glucose data and peer support to improve control. Results indicated that Hb $A_1$ was significantly better in the experimental group, which reported more adjustments for exercise, diet, and insulin dose based on blood glucose testing than did those who received routine follow-up care.

Others are interested in social support provided over the telephone or by adult mentors for younger youth. Farquhar (1989) described the use of a telephone support tree to provide social support for 180 adolescents with diabetes in England. He notes that the results were "positive," but he provides no data on outcomes. A different approach to social support was described by Daley (1992). She paired adults with type 1 diabetes with adolescents with newly diagnosed diabetes to improve adolescents' adjustment to diabetes. The sample for this study differs from most of the intervention studies, in that it is approximately 44% minority (Hispanic and African American). The 54 subjects ranged in age from 12 to 16 years, and the sponsor intervention was provided for 10 months. Results indicated that, for the most part, there were no differences (metabolic control, Child Behavior Checklist [Achenbach & Edelbrock, 1983], Diabetes Adjustment Scale [Sullivan, 1979], State Trait Anxiety Inventory [Spielberger, 1983]) between the sponsorship group and the control group, but on the Harter Self-Perception Profile for Adolescents (Harter, 1988), subjects in the sponsorship group had an increase in social acceptance and romantic appeal. Further, in qualitative interviews, subjects in the experimental group reported that the sponsors provided an important source of previously unavailable support.

Blake (1997) described a case study of a similar approach (i.e., providing mentorship for adolescents with diabetes) and suggests the use of similar measures for evaluation (metabolic control, Diabetes Adjustment Scale). Data on outcomes are not provided, however.

In summary, there have been a number of psychosocial approaches studied for children and adolescents with diabetes. Many of these reports are not rigorous experimental designs but case control studies or one-group, pretest-posttest preexperimental designs. Unlike the traditional education studies, however, the instruments used are usually known, reliable, and valid. Nonetheless, where adequate controlled studies have been done, interventions such as coping skills training and peer support have been demonstrated to lead to improved adjustment or quality of life as well as improved metabolic control.

## FAMILY INTERVENTIONS

The final category of intervention study is family interventions. To be included in this category, the target of the intervention had to be the family members of a child or adolescent with diabetes rather than the index child. Reviews of the literature on family aspects of chronic illness reinforce the view that although there have been methodological problems in studying families of individuals with chronic illness, families have an important influence on children and adolescents with diabetes (Anderson & Auslander, 1980; Auslander, Bubb, Rogge, & Santiago, 1993; Glascow & Anderson, 1995). Four studies of family intervention and one on parental relaxation training were included in the review.

Studies of family intervention include those whose intervention was targeted on family members, primarily parents, and did not focus on outcomes in children, adolescents, or parents alone. Compared with the other categories of interventions reviewed for this chapter, this category is relatively recent in the literature. Outcomes may reflect families as a whole or they may also be collected on individuals.

Satin, LaGreca, Zigo, and Skyler (1989) conduced an experimental study of a multifamily group intervention of support and guidance and a multifamily group intervention plus parent simulation of diabetes and compared outcomes with a control group of adolescents and families who received routine care. A total of 32 families (child age, $M = 14.6$ years; duration, $M = 5.9$ years; 20 females) participated and were randomly assigned to the three groups. The interventions consisted of six weekly sessions that included adolescents and their parents, in which guidance and support were provided by using principles of group therapy. For the group who received the multifamily intervention plus simulation, the parents simulated having diabetes and doing all of the self-care for 1 week. Controls received routine care. Results indicated that the group who received the multifamily intervention with simulation had the best improvement in Hb $A_{1c}$. Parents in both intervention groups had more positive perceptions of teens with diabetes as measured by semantic differential scales (Osgood, Suci, & Tannenbaum, 1957). No differences, however, were found on estimates of self-care when using a one-item scale and scores on the Family Environment Scale (Moos, 1974).

Smith, Dickerson, Saylor, and Jones (1989) examined the use of a multifamily group intervention provided during an overnight retreat—a posttest-only preexperimental design. This intervention was designed to provide an opportunity for children with diabetes to be with other children with diabetes in a relaxed, fun-filled environment and for the family members to exchange concerns and ideas with others in a similar situation and discuss current issues related to diabetes care with each other and the diabetes care team. Eleven families participated in the retreat, and they reported that the discussions were helpful, but they did not believe that their diabetes management would change as a result of the intervention. The authors reported qualitatively that the opportunity to be with other families and discuss common concerns and issues was the most helpful aspect of the program.

Wysocki and colleagues (Wysocki, Greco, et al., 1997; Wysocki, Harris, et al., 1997) have conducted an experimental study of the effectiveness of behavioral family systems therapy as compared to education and support groups for families of adolescents in reducing parent-adolescent conflict in diabetes management. Unlike other family studies, this intervention focused on families with pretest scores demonstrating at least moderate general or diabetes-specific family conflict. Behavioral family systems therapy targets parent-adolescent conflict by focusing on family problem solving and communication skills, the degree to which family members hold extreme beliefs about one another's behavior, and the extent of family structural or systemic anomalies.

The experimental treatment consisted of 10 sessions, with parents and adolescents emphasizing problem solving for conflict resolution, communication skills training for parent-adolescent communications, cognitive restructuring for family members' beliefs and attributions, and functional or structural family therapy to target maladaptive characteristics of family functioning. Further, the sample was adequate for the effects studied. A total of 119 families, with adolescents with diabetes (age, $M = 14.5$ years; duration, $M = 5$ years; 50% female; 80% White) participated in these studies. Using scales developed and validated for this study, results demonstrated that the behavioral family systems therapy showed more improvement in parent-adolescent relationships, diabetes-specific family conflicts, treatment adherence, metabolic control (in boys and younger girls only), and treatment evaluation, compared to education and support groups. By 6 months the improvements in parent-adolescent relationships were maintained, but those related to adherence or metabolic control were not.

Finally, the effect of parental relaxation training with biofeedback on their child's blood glucose control was studied (Guthrie, Sargent, Speelman, & Parks, 1990). Guthrie et al. selected only parents who scored highly on a standardized measure of stress and alternately assigned them to participate in the experimental or control group. Although the intervention group was found to be not statistically better than the control group, the within-group improvement in metabolic control was statistically significant in the experimental group.

In summary, studies of interventions that target families of youth with diabetes are just beginning to appear in the literature. Results suggest that parent-child conflict may be amenable to intervention. Nonetheless, the measures used in these studies focus on individual functioning and outcomes, rather than overall family functioning.

## SUMMARY AND CONCLUSIONS

The questions to be answered by this review included the following: What intervention strategies have been used with children with type 1 diabetes and their families? What is the methodological adequacy of those studies? What outcomes have been studied, and how reliable and valid are they? What are the substantive findings of those studies?

The interventions for children and adolescents and their families that have been studied have focused primarily on those with established diabetes and have been provided in outpatient settings. It is interesting that essentially no studies of the impact of diabetes education provided at diagnosis were found in the period of time covered by this review. It may be that the importance of education at the time of diagnosis is so well established that no need for further research is perceived as necessary (Travis et al., 1987). Further, the great majority of the interventions are focused on adolescents or preadolescents, because they have more difficulty in control than younger children.

Interventions fell into three general categories: education, psychosocial, and family. Education studies tended to focus on improving knowledge through standard one-to-one or group techniques; more recently, they have used innovative technologies to provide information. All educational methods were reported to be relatively successful in improving knowledge, but for the most part, newer technologies were more effective than traditional methods.

A number of studies involving psychosocial interventions were conducted. Few of these studies were methodologically adequate, so it is difficult to draw conclusions across types of studies. Nonetheless, coping skills training and peer group support appear to be the most effective of these approaches.

There were few well-controlled studies of family interventions, but those that were found appear to hold promise for decreasing parent-child conflict about diabetes, if not metabolic control. As more investigators begin to focus on issues related to families of children with diabetes and the sophistication in methods for conducting family-centered research increases, more of these studies should be encouraged. Most especially, outcomes that assess family functioning rather than individual outcomes should be assessed.

Very few researchers presented an explicit theoretical basis for the intervention or the hypothesized outcomes. In general, the psychosocial interventions were more likely to include the framework than other interventions. This finding is interesting because there are a number of models of behavioral change that could guide this body of research.

The distribution of methods was bimodal. Approximately one half of the studies reviewed used rigorous experimental designs, but many of these had samples that were too small to detect meaningful differences between experimental and control groups. The remaining studies used quasi-experimental or preexperimental designs, usually with small samples, to assess the effects of new interventions. Thus, it is difficult to draw conclusions across studies. It is also worth noting that the great majority of studies included few non-White subjects, often fewer than would be expected given the distribution of type 1 diabetes in minority youth. It is difficult, then, to assess the relevance of these interventions for minority youth with diabetes. Only one study of the usefulness of sponsorship of inner-city youth with diabetes targeted African American youth. Given that minority youth with diabetes have more difficulty with metabolic control than do nonminority youth (Golden, 1998), emphasis must be placed on designing and evaluating interventions for these youth.

Two outcomes are common to nearly all studies. Metabolic control, as measured by Hb $A_{1c}$, was the most consistently reported outcome. This finding is important, because the ultimate efficacy of an intervention may be determined by whether the intervention leads to improved metabolic control. Other studies examined intermediate outcomes to metabolic control, such as compliance or adherence, but there was no consistently reliable measure of adherence to self-care behaviors. The second most common outcome was, of course, knowledge. Knowledge gains were most often measured by the Diabetes Knowledge Test, a reliable and valid indicator of knowledge of type 1 diabetes and self-care management.

Psychosocial outcomes varied across studies. The studies that focused on coping skills and stress management examined outcomes related to stress, coping, and overall psychosocial adjustment, in addition to metabolic control. Two measures of psychosocial adjustment specific to diabetes, the Diabetes Adjustment Scale and the Diabetes Quality of Life for Youth Scale, are reliable and valid as well as sensitive to changes associated with treatment programs. Several studies also include more general assessments of child adjustment, such as the Child Behavior Checklist and the Harter Self-Perception Profile for Children or Adolescents.

On the basis of this review of the available literature on interventions for children with diabetes and their families, it can be concluded that educational interventions are useful in improving diabetes knowledge but not consistently helpful in improving metabolic control. Psychosocial interventions, especially coping skills training and peer support, assist adolescents primarily to improve adjustment and sometimes metabolic control. Family interventions may be helpful in reducing parent-child conflict about diabetes management and care. Despite the relatively large number of studies, there is much to be accomplished in this field. Few interventions have been subject to replication studies, so there is little evidence of the stability of the outcomes across populations. Newer interventions must be tested in studies with adequate samples so that they are not rejected on the basis of inadequate data. Finally, more studies of minority youth should be conducted.

## ACKNOWLEDGMENTS

The author is grateful to Kimberly Lacey, MSN, and Sheri Kanner, MSN, doctoral students who provided library and search assistance in the preparation of this chapter.

# REFERENCES

Achenbach, T., & Edelbrock, C. (1983). *Manual for the Child Behavior Checklist and Revised Child Behavior Profile.* Burlington: University of Vermont.

American Diabetes Association. (1999). Clinical practice recommendations. *Diabetes Care, 22*(Suppl. 1), S88–S90.

Anderson, B. J., & Auslander, W. F. (1980). Research on diabetes management and the family: A critique. *Diabetes Care, 3,* 696–702.

Anderson, B. J., Auslander, W. F., Jung, K. C., Miller, J. P., & Santiago, J. V. (1990). Assessing family sharing of diabetes responsibilities. *Journal of Pediatric Psychology, 15,* 477–492.

Anderson, B. J., Wolf, F. M., Burkhart, M. T., Cornell, R. G., & Bacon, G. E. (1989). Effects of peer-group intervention on metabolic control of adolescents with IDDM: Randomized outpatient study. *Diabetes Care, 12,* 179–183.

Anderson, K. (1997). An evaluation of an adolescent diabetes education program. *Canadian Journal of Diabetes Care, 21,* 28–33.

Auslander, W. F., Bubb, J., Rogge, M., & Santiago, J. V. (1993). Family stress and resources: Potential areas of intervention in children recently diagnosed with diabetes. *Health and Social Work, 18,* 101–113.

Bauman, L. J., Drotar, D., Leventhal, J. M., Perrin, E. M., & Pless, I. B. (1997). A review of psychosocial interventions with children with chronic health conditions. *Pediatrics, 100,* 244–251.

Bishop, D. S., Epstein, N. B., Keitner, G. I., Miller, I. W., & McMaster, J. (1983). Family Assessment Device and its use in rehabilitation, psychiatric, and normal populations. *Archives of Physical Medicine and Rehabilitation, 64,* 504.

Blake, J. E. (1997). A mentoring program for adolescents with diabetes. *Diabetes Educator, 23,* 681–684.

Boardway, R. H., Delamater, A. M., Tomakowsky, J., & Gutai, J. P. (1993). Stress management training for adolescents with diabetes. *Journal of Pediatric Psychology, 18,* 29–45.

Bornstein, M. R., Bellack, A. S., & Herson, M. (1977). Social skills training for unassertive children: A multiple baseline analysis. *Journal of Applied Behavior Analysis, 10,* 183–195.

Brandt, P. (1998). Childhood diabetes: Behavioral research. In J. J. Fitzpatrick (Ed.), *Annual review of nursing research* (vol. 16, pp. 63–82). New York: Springer Publishing Co.

Brandt, P., & Weinert, C. (1981). The PRQ: A social support measure. *Nursing Research, 30,* 277–280.

Brandt, P. A., & Magyary, D. L. (1993). The impact of a diabetes education program on children and mothers. *Journal of Pediatric Nursing, 8,* 31–40.

Burroughs, T. E., Harris, M. A., Pontious, S. L., & Santiago, J. V. (1997). Research in social support in adolescents with IDDM: A critical review. *Diabetes Educator, 23,* 438–448.

Court, J. M. (1991). Outpatient based transition services for youth. *Pediatrician, 18,* 150–156.

Daley, B. J. (1992). Sponsorship for adolescents with diabetes. *Health and Social Work, 17,* 173–182.

Davidson, M., Boland, E. A., & Grey, M. (1997). Teaching teens to cope: Coping skills training for adolescents with diabetes mellitus. *Journal of the Society of Pediatric Nurses, 2*, 65–72.

Deatrick, J. (1998). Integrative review: Intervention models for children who have chronic conditions and their families. In M. E. Broome, S. Feetham, K. Knafl, & K. Pridham (Eds.), *State of the science in nursing of children and families* (pp. 221–235). Thousand Oaks, CA: Sage.

Delamater, A. M., Bubb, J., Davis, S. G., Smith, J. A., Schmidt, L., White, N. H., & Santiago, J. V. (1990). Randomized, prospective study of self-management training with newly diagnosed diabetic children. *Diabetes Care, 13*, 492–498.

Diabetes Control and Complications Trial (DCCT) Research Group. (1994). Effect of intensive insulin treatment on the development and progression of long-term complications in adolescents with insulin-dependent diabetes mellitus: Diabetes Control and Complications Trial. *Journal of Pediatrics, 125*, 177–188.

Drozda, D. J., Dawson, V. A., Long, D. J., Freson, L. S., & Sperling, M. A. (1990). Assessment of the effect of a comprehensive diabetes management program on hospital admission rates of children with diabetes mellitus. *Diabetes Educator, 16*, 389–393.

Epstein, L. H., Figueroa, J., Farkas, G. M., & Beck, S. (1981). The short-term effects of feedback on accuracy of urine glucose determinations in insulin dependent diabetic children. *Behavior Therapy, 12*, 560–564.

Farquhar, J. W. (1989). Use of a teleport system in parent and adolescent support. *Diabetic Medicine, 6*, 635–637.

Folkman, S., & Lazarus, R. S. (1980). An analysis of coping in a middle-aged community sample. *Journal of Health and Social Behavior, 21*, 219–239.

Fosbury, J. A., Bosley, C. M., Ryle, A., Sonksen, P. H., & Judd, S. L. (1997). A trial of cognitive analytic therapy in poorly controlled type 1 patients. *Diabetes Care, 20*, 959–964.

Gillis, B. (1990). *The role of family psychosocial variables in glucose control of children and adolescents with insulin-dependent diabetes mellitus: A six month study.* Unpublished PhD dissertation, University of Toronto.

Glascow, R., & Anderson, B. J. (1995). Future directions for research on pediatric chronic disease management: Lessons from diabetes. *Journal of Pediatric Psychology, 20*, 389–402.

Glascow, R. E., McCaul, K. D., & Schafer, L. C. (1986). Barriers to regimen adherence among persons with insulin-dependent diabetes. *Journal of Behavioral Medicine, 9*, 65–77.

Golden, M. P. (1998). Incorporation of quality-of-life considerations into intensive diabetes management protocols in adolescents. *Diabetes Care, 21*, 885–886.

Grey, M., & Boland, E. A. (1996). Diabetes mellitus (Type I). In P. L. Jackson (Ed.), *Primary care of the child with a chronic condition* (2nd ed., pp. 350–370). St. Louis: C. V. Mosby.

Grey, M., Boland, E. A., Davidson, M., & Tamborlane, W. V. (1999). Coping skills training as adjunct for youth on intensive therapy. *Applied Nursing Research, 12*, 3–12.

Grey, M., Boland, E. A., Davidson, M., Yu, C., Sullivan-Bolyai, S., & Tamborlane, W. V. (1998). Short-term effects of coping skills training as adjunct to intensive therapy in adolescents. *Diabetes Care, 21*, 902–908.

Grey, M., Cameron, M. E., Lipman, T. H., & Thurber, F. W. (1995). Psychosocial status of children with diabetes over the first two years. *Diabetes Care, 18,* 1330–1336.

Gross, A. M., Heiman, L., Shapiro, R., & Schultz, R. M. (1983). Children with diabetes: Social skills training and hemoglobin A1c levels. *Behavior Modification, 7,* 151–165.

Gross, A. M., Johnson, W. G., Wildman, H., & Mullett, N. (1982). Coping skills training with insulin-dependent pre-adolescent diabetics. *Child Behavioral Therapy, 3,* 141–153.

Grossman, H. Y., Brink, S., & Hauser, S. T. (1987). Self-efficacy in adolescent girls and boys with insulin-dependent diabetes mellitus. *Diabetes Care, 10,* 324–329.

Guthrie, D. W., Sargent, L., Speelman, D., & Parks, L. (1990). Effects of parental relaxation training on glycosylated hemoglobin of children with diabetes. *Patient Education and Counseling, 16,* 247–253.

Harter, S. (1979). *Perceived competence scale for children.* Unpublished manuscript, University of Denver.

Harter, S. (1988). *Manual for the Self-Perception Profile for Adolescents.* Unpublished manuscript, University of Denver.

Horan, P. P., Yarborough, M. C., Besigel, G., & Carlson, D. R. (1990). Computer-assisted self-control of diabetes by adolescents. *Diabetes Educator, 16,* 205–211.

Huttunen, N., Lankela, S., Knip, M., Lautala, P., Kaar, M., Laasonen, K., & Puukka, R. (1989). Effect of a once-a-week training program on physical fitness and metabolic control in children with IDDM. *Diabetes Care, 12,* 737–740.

Ingersoll, G. M., & Marrero, D. G. (1991). A modified Quality of Life Measure for youths: Psychometric properties. *Diabetes Educator, 17,* 114–118.

Johnson, S. B., Pollak, R., Silverstein, J., Rosenbloom, A., Spillar, R., McCallum, M., & Harkavy, J. (1982). Cognitive and behavioral diabetes among children and parents. *Pediatrics, 69,* 708–713.

Johnson, W. G., Gross, A. M., & Wildman, H. E. (1982). Developing coping skills in adolescent diabetics. *Corrective Social Psychology Journal and Behavioral Techniques, Methods, and Theory, 28,* 116–120.

Kovacs, M., Mukerji, P., Iyengar, S., & Drash, A. (1996). Psychiatric disorder and metabolic control among youths with IDDM. *Diabetes Care, 19,* 318–323.

LaMontagne, L. L. (1993). Bolstering personal control in child patients through coping interventions. *Pediatric Nursing, 19,* 235–237.

Marrero, D. G., Vandagriff, J. L., Kronz, K., Fineberg, N. S., Golden, M. P., Gray, D., Orr, D. P., Wright, J. C., & Johnson, N. B. (1995). Using telecommunication technology to manage children with diabetes: The Computer-Linked Outpatient Clinic (CLOC) study. *Diabetes Educator, 21,* 313–319.

Massouh, S. R., Steele, T. M., Alseth, E. R., & Diekmann, J. M. (1989). The effect of social learning intervention on metabolic control of insulin-dependent diabetes in adolescents. *Diabetes Educator, 15,* 518–521.

McNabb, W. L., Quinn, M. T., Murphy, D. M., Thorp, F. K., & Cook, S. (1994). Increasing children's responsibility for self-care: The In-Control study. *Diabetes Educator, 20,* 121–124.

Mendez, F. J., & Belendez, M. (1997). Effects of a behavioral intervention on treatment adherence and stress management in adolescents with IDDM. *Diabetes Care, 20,* 1370–1375.

Mitchell, B. (1996). The effects of an early intervention strategy in improving the adjustment to diabetes in children. *Canadian Journal of Diabetes Care, 20,* 21–27.

Moos, R. (1974). *Family Environment Scale.* Palo Alto, CA: Consulting Psychologists.

Murkin, S. A., Snyder, G. M., Pichert, J. W., & Boswell, E. J. (1990). Anchored instruction enhances diabetes problem solving. *Diabetes, 39,* 17A.

National Institute of Diabetes, Digestive, and Kidney Diseases (NIDDK). (1995). *Diabetes in America* (NIH publication No. 95-1468). Bethesda, MD: Author.

Offer, D., Ostrove, E., & Howard, K. (1977). *The Offer self-image questionnaire for adolescents: A manual.* Unpublished manuscript, Michael Reese Hospital and Medical Center, Chicago.

Osgood, C., Suci, G., & Tannenbaum, P. (1957). *The measurement of meaning.* Unpublished manuscript, University of Illinois, Urbana.

Pichert, J. W., Meek, J. M., Schlundt, D. G., Flannery, M. E., Kline, S. S., Hodge, M. B., & Kinzer, C. K. (1994). Impact of anchored instruction on problem-solving strategies of adolescents with diabetes. *Journal of the American Dietetic Association, 94,* 1036–1038.

Pichert, J. W., Snyder, G. M., Kinzer, C. K., & Boswell, E. J. (1992). Sydney Meets the Ketone Challenge: A videodisc for teaching diabetes sick day management through problem solving. *Diabetes Educator, 18,* 476–477.

Pichert, J. W., Snyder, G. M., Kinzer, C. K., & Boswell, E. J. (1994). Problem-solving anchored instruction about sick days for adolescents with diabetes. *Patient Education and Counseling, 23,* 115–124.

Pollak, R. T., & Johnson, S. B. (1979). *Administration and scoring manual for diabetic knowledge, problem solving, and skills demonstration test.* Unpublished manuscript, University of Florida, Department of Clinical and Health Psychology, Gainesville.

Rohner, R. (1981). *Handbook for the study of parental acceptance and rejection.* Storrs: University of Connecticut.

Sarason, I., Johnson, J., & Seigel, J. (1978). Assessing the impact of life changes: Development of the Life Experiences Survey. *Journal of Consulting and Clinical Psychology, 46,* 932–946.

Satin, W., LaGreca, A. M., Zigo, M. A., & Skyler, J. S. (1989). Diabetes in adolescence: Effects of a multifamily group intervention and parent simulation of diabetes. *Journal of Pediatric Psychology, 14,* 259–275.

Schafer, L. C., McCaul, K. D., & Glasgow, R. E. (1986). Supportive and nonsupportive family behaviors: Relationships to adherence and metabolic control in persons with Type I diabetes. *Diabetes Care, 9,* 179–185.

Shobhana, R., Rao, R., Vijay, V., Snehalatha, C., & Ramachandran, A. (1997). Diabetes education session for young IDDM probands and their family members in a developing country: An evaluation. *Practical Diabetes International, 14,* 123–125.

Siminerio, L. M. (1980). Establishment of a diabetes youth group. *Diabetes Educator, 6,* 22–23.

Smith, K. E., Dickerson, P., Saylor, C. F., & Jones, C. (1989). Issues of managing diabetes in children and adolescents: A multifamily group approach. *Child Health Care, 18,* 49–52.

Smith, K. E., Schreiner, B.-J., Brouhard, B. H., & Travis, L. B. (1991). Impact of a camp experience on choice of coping strategies by adolescents with insulin dependent diabetes mellitus. *Diabetes Educator, 17,* 49–53.

Spielberger, C. D. (1983). *Manual for the State-Trait Anxiety Inventory*. Palo Alto, CA: Consulting Psychologists Press.

Sullivan, B. J. (1979). Diabetes Adjustment Questionnaire. *Psychosomatic Medicine, 41*, 119–137.

Templeton, C. L., Burkhart, M. T., Anderson, B. J., & Bacon, G. E. (1988). A group approach to nutritional problem solving using self-monitoring of blood glucose with diabetic adolescents. *Diabetes Educator, 14*, 189–191.

Travis, L. B., Brouhard, B. H., & Schreiner, B. J. (1987). *Diabetes mellitus in children and adolescents*. Philadelphia: W. B. Saunders.

Viinamaki, H., Niskanen, L., & Tynkkynen, P. (1991). The effect of psychiatric intervention on the metabolic control and mental ability of patients to cope with insulin-dependent diabetes mellitus. *European Journal of Psychiatry, 5*, 37–46.

Warren-Boulton, E., Anderson, B. J., Schwartz, N. L., & Drexler, A. J. (1981). A group approach to the management of diabetes in adolescents and young adults. *Diabetes Care, 4*, 620–623.

Wolanski, R., Sigman, T., & Polychonakos, C. (1996). Assessment of blood glucose monitoring skills in a camp for diabetic children: The effects of individualized feedback counseling. *Patient Education and Counseling, 29*, 5–11.

Wysocki, T., Greco, P., Harris, M., Bubb, J., Elder, C., Harvey, L., & Mcdonnell, K. (1997). Behavior therapy for families of adolescents with IDDM: Maintenance of treatment effects. *Diabetes, 46*(Suppl. 1), 95A.

Wysocki, T., Harris, M. A., Greco, P., Harvey, L. M., McDonell, K., Danda, C. L., Bubb, J., & White, N. H. (1997). Social validity of support group and behavior therapy interventions for families of adolescents with insulin dependent diabetes mellitus. *Journal of Pediatric Psychology, 22*, 635–649.

## Chapter 7

# Management of Urinary Incontinence in Adult Ambulatory Care Populations

JEAN F. WYMAN

### ABSTRACT

During the past decade, research on urinary incontinence and its management has grown significantly. Behavioral therapy is now viewed as an important first line of treatment for stress, urge, and mixed urinary incontinence. This chapter provides a critical review of the intervention studies on lifestyle modifications, bladder training, and pelvic floor muscle training conducted in adult ambulatory care populations that were published in 1988 through 1999. Recommendations for future research are provided.

**Key words: urinary incontinence, stress incontinence, urge incontinence, behavioral therapy, bladder, biofeedback, exercise therapy, pelvic floor, electrical stimulation**

Urinary incontinence is a prevalent and costly health condition that can significantly impair the quality of life in adults. During the past decade, the knowledge base on urinary incontinence and its management has grown tremendously. Behavioral therapies such as bladder training and pelvic floor muscle training are now recommended as the first line of treatment for incontinence (Fantl et al., 1996; Wilson et al., 1999). Practice changes have occurred, with generalist nurses as well as continence nurse specialists assuming a larger role in the initial evaluation and management of incontinent patients. These developments have led to a greater number of individuals seeking and receiving care for their incontinence and to improved health outcomes as a result.

The increased research attention to incontinence has led to several developments that have had or will have a significant influence on clinical practice as well as the conduct of future studies. These include the Agency for Health Care and Policy and Research's (AHCPR; now renamed the Agency for Healthcare Research and Quality) evidence-based practice guidelines on urinary incontinence, which were initially released in 1992 and updated in 1996 (Fantl et al., 1996); publication by the International Continence Society of several reports with recommendations for the standardization of outcome measures for research on lower urinary tract dysfunctions in various populations (Fonda et al., 1998; Lose et al., 1998; Mattiasson et al., 1998; Nordling et al., 1998); the work of the Cochrane Collaboration, which has established a database of clinical trials as well as publishing one systematic review (Roe, Williams, & Palmer, 1999) and several protocols for future reviews on treatments for urinary incontinence; and the recent publication of the *Proceedings of the First International Consultation on Incontinence* (Abrams, Khoury, & Wein, 1999), which provides a comprehensive literature review and consensus opinion of treatment guidelines and research recommendations by international multidisciplinary experts.

This chapter reviews the research on behavioral treatments for urinary incontinence in ambulatory care populations. The focus is on interventions for stress, urge, and mixed incontinence in cognitively intact adults who can independently toilet and adhere to a prescribed treatment. The interventions reviewed include lifestyle modifications, bladder training, and pelvic floor muscle training.

## REVIEW CRITERIA

Reports on the various interventions were obtained by searching MEDLINE, the Cumulative Index for Nursing and Allied Health Literature (CINAHL), and the Cochrane Library from 1988 to April 1999. In addition, reference lists from the *Proceedings of the First International Consultation on Incontinence,* the Agency for Health Care Policy and Research's (AHCPR) clinical practice guideline on urinary incontinence (Fantl et al., 1996), review articles, and published research reports were cross-referenced. Because of the extensive research literature, this review is intended to be representative rather than exhaustive. Criteria used for inclusion in this review were type of participant (e.g., community-dwelling women and men with stress, urge, and mixed incontinence, without mental or physical impairments, who sought treatment in ambulatory care settings); type of treatment (e.g., lifestyle intervention, bladder training, or pelvic floor muscle training) research design (e.g., randomized and nonrandomized controlled trials and prospective cohort studies), with preference given to reviewing randomized controlled trials (RCTs); and publication type (e.g., full published original reports in English). Because of the lack of clinical trials on lifestyle interventions, observational studies were reviewed for the evidence base on these interventions.

## LIFESTYLE INTERVENTIONS

Several modifiable lifestyle factors have been anecdotally or empirically linked to urinary incontinence. These include fluid intake, caffeine consumption, and other dietary factors; constipation; smoking; weight; and physical activity (Fantl et al., 1996). Few studies have investigated the sole effect of modifying these risk factors; those available have examined their effect in women only.

### Fluid and Dietary Modifications

Two studies investigating the effect of fluid and/or caffeine modifications in incontinent women had equivocal results. Dowd, Campbell, and Jones (1996) randomly assigned 58 women (mean age 70.3 years) to one of three groups: (1) increase intake by 500 cc but not to exceed 2,400 cc, (2) decrease intake by 300 cc but not less than a total of 1,000 cc, or (3) maintain baseline intake. Findings were inconclusive partly because of subjects' poor adherence to the fluid intake protocol and partly to the large number of subjects with incomplete diaries (45%). Also, the lack of controlling for baseline fluid intake either at randomization or in the data analysis may have influenced the results. However, on follow-up interviews 3 months postintervention, 20 women reported fewer incontinent episodes and stated that the most significant thing they learned was the need to increase their fluid intake. No relationship was noted between caffeine intake and incontinent episodes.

Tomlinson and her colleagues (1999) reported on the first phase of a behavioral management program in 41 incontinent women (mean age 65.8 years). Women who participated in this phase had to meet at least one inclusion criterion related to a high caffeine intake, inadequate or excessive fluid intake, fluid intake pattern associated with nocturia, infrequent voiding pattern, or constipation. Based on the subjects' patterns, the most common recommendations were to decrease dietary caffeine consumption and increase fluid intake. Other recommendations included altering the timing of fluid intake, reducing excessively long daytime voiding intervals, and changing bowel habits. Linear regression analysis indicated a trend toward a significant relationship between a decrease in caffeine consumption and fewer daytime incontinent episodes. Although a relationship between the increase in fluid intake volume and an increase in voided urine volume was found, there was no relationship to incontinent episodes.

Certain dietary factors that are considered common bladder irritants, such as artificial sweeteners, spicy foods, and citrus fruits, may influence continence status. However, no studies were located that provide evidence to support the recommendation of eliminating these foods from the diet.

## Weight Reduction

Increased body mass index (BMI) has been associated with an increasing risk of urinary incontinence in women (Brown et al., 1996). Two prospective cohort studies evaluating the effect of weight loss on continence status following bariatric surgery in women found significant resolution of stress incontinence (Bump, Sugerman, Fantl, & McClish, 1992; Deitel, Stone, Kassam, Wilk, & Sutherland, 1988) or urge incontinence (Bump et al., 1992). However, no studies were located that reported on incontinence following nonsurgical weight loss programs in mild to moderately overweight individuals.

## Bowel Management

Constipation is cited as a risk factor for incontinence, particularly in the elderly (Fantl et al., 1996). However, no studies were located that specifically examined the effect of bowel management on continence status. In the previously cited study by Tomlinson and her colleagues (1999), recommendations were made to change bowel habits as part of the behavioral self-management program for incontinent women. However, the effect of changes in bowel patterns was not described.

## Smoking Cessation

Smoking has been identified as a risk factor for urinary incontinence (Bump & McClish, 1994; Fantl et al., 1996); however, the evidence is inconclusive. Smoking was not associated with incontinence in a large cross-sectional analysis of women enrolled in a study of osteoporotic fractures (Brown et al., 1996). Although the results are contradictory, two case-control studies in women suggest that smoking is linked to a particular type of incontinence. Bump and McClish (1992) found that smoking was linked to the risk of stress incontinence only, whereas Tampakoudis and his colleagues (Tampakoudis, Tantanassis, Grimbizis, Papaletsos, & Mautelenakis, 1995) found it was linked to motor incontinence (also known as urge incontinence) only. In a large cross-sectional survey of Finnish men, smoking was associated with a greater prevalence of lower urinary tract symptoms, which included urge incontinence (Koskimäki, Hakama, Huhtala, & Tammela, 1998). Risk of symptoms decreased in former smokers the longer the period after smoking cessation. No studies were located that reported on the effect of participation in a smoking cessation program on incontinence.

## Physical Activity

Type and intensity of physical activity is associated with the exacerbation of female incontinence (Bo, Stien, Kulseng-Hanssen, & Kristofferson, 1994;

Davis & Goodman, 1996; Nygaard, Thompson, Svengalis, & Albright, 1994). No studies were located that examined the effects of changes in occupational, recreational, or other daily physical activities on continence status.

Evidence exists that suggests body position during exertional events may help to prevent urine leakage. Norton and Baker (1994) evaluated four postures for reducing urine leakage in 65 women with stress incontinence. Urine loss during coughing was reduced by using a position that involved either crossing the legs or crossing the legs and bending forward. However, these positions, which are not always feasible and/or socially appropriate, have not been tested in an intervention trial.

## BLADDER TRAINING

Bladder training was initially described by Jeffcoate and Francis in 1966 as a treatment for functional disorders of the lower urinary tract in women. It involves a program of patient education that includes urge inhibition strategies, behavioral techniques, and a scheduled voiding regimen. Bladder training has been used to treat detrusor instability, urge incontinence with a stable bladder, genuine stress incontinence, mixed urinary incontinence, and sensory-urgency problems without incontinence.

The mechanism of how bladder training achieves its effects is still poorly understood. Several hypotheses exist, including improved cortical inhibition over detrusor contractions, improved cortical facilitation over urethral closure during bladder filling, improved central modulation of afferent sensory impulses, increased "reserve capability" of the lower urinary tract system, and altered behavior resulting from better individual awareness of circumstances that cause incontinence (Wilson et al., 1999).

Eight studies on bladder training were reviewed: seven RCTs (Columbo, Zanetta, Scalambrino, et al., 1995; Fantl et al., 1991; Lagro-Janssen, Debruyne, Smits, & Van Weel, 1992; O'Brien, Austin, Sethi, P., & O'Boyle, 1991; Szoni, Collas, Ding, & Malone-Lee, 1995; Wiseman, Malone-Lee, & Rai, 1991; Wyman, Fantl, McClish, Bump, & Continence Program, 1998), and one prospective cohort series (Publicover & Bear, 1997). Two trials had an inadequate design, in which subjects within the experimental group received different treatments based on underlying urodynamic diagnosis (O'Brien et al., 1991; Lagro-Janssen et al., 1992). Seven of the eight trials studied women exclusively; two trials also included men (O'Brien et al., 1991; Wiseman et al., 1991). Outcome measures included self-assessment of cure/improvement, voiding diaries, pad tests, condition-specific quality of life, cystometry, and other urodynamic parameters. Follow-up periods were variable, with most RCTs conducting at least one posttreatment evaluation at 3 to 12 weeks postrandomization. Several trials included an additional follow-up at 3 to 12 months posttreatment (Fantl et al., 1991; Lagro-Janssen et al., 1992; Wyman et al., 1998). Although most studies included adherence measures (e.g., diaries or sessions attended), few reported treatment adherence rates. Only one study reported on compliance as a factor affecting treatment outcome (Wyman et al., 1998).

Several variations occurred in the bladder training programs. The initial assigned voiding interval varied from 30 minutes to 2 hours during waking hours only, with 1 hour being the most common interval. The increase in voiding interval ranged from 15 to 60 minutes. Other variations in training programs included the length of the training program (3–12 weeks); use of concomitant treatments such as pelvic floor muscle training (PFMT), bladder pressure biofeedback, and drug therapy; type of urgency inhibition techniques used; and whether fluid modifications were used in the program. Most training programs involved self-monitoring of voiding patterns using a log or diary, with some programs requiring measurement of voided volume. All but one of the studies offered bladder training as an outpatient program with weekly or biweekly visits; one study delivered bladder training via weekly telephone calls for 4 weeks (Publicover & Bear, 1997). Dropout rates from bladder training ranged from 5% to 17%.

There is strong empirical support that bladder training is effective in reducing incontinence severity indices (incontinent episodes, pad test weights, condition-specific quality of life) in women with stress, urge, and mixed incontinence (Fantl et al., 1991; Wyman et al., 1998). Bladder training appears to be equally effective in reducing incontinent episodes in women with detrusor instability, genuine stress incontinence, and both diagnoses. Cure rates reported as no incontinent episodes on a voiding diary were 12%–73% in the RCTs. Improvement rates reported as mean reduction of incontinent episodes ranged from 57% to 87.3% (Fantl et al., 1991; Publicover & Bear, 1997). Because of the small sample of men undergoing bladder training, it is not possible to derive definitive conclusions on its efficacy in men.

Fantl and his associates (1991) studied a 6-week bladder training program in 135 women with sphincteric incompetence (stress incontinence) and detrusor instability with or without sphincteric incompetence. They found that 12% of the treatment group were continent and 76% had reduced their incontinent episodes by at least 50% or more at 6 weeks (mean reduction 57%) as measured by a 7-day voiding diary. Results were maintained 6 months later. There was a 55% improvement in condition-specific quality-of-life scores at 6 weeks, which was also maintained over a 6-month period (Wyman et al., 1997). Significant reductions also were noted with an office pad test and with diurnal and nocturnal frequency. Whereas some women did revert back to normal bladder function following training, no relationship was observed between changes in urodynamic parameters and the number of incontinent episodes (McClish, Fantl, Wyman, Pisani, & Bump, 1991).

Bladder training appears to be as effective as PFMT on immediate and long-term follow-up and as effective as a combination of both therapies on longer-term follow-up in women with stress and/or urge incontinence. In a two-site RCT, Wyman and her colleagues (1998) compared a 12-week program (6 weekly office visits and 6 weeks of mail/telephone contact) of bladder training, biofeedback-assisted pelvic floor muscle (PFM) exercises, and a combination of both therapies in 204 women with genuine stress incontinence or detrusor instability with or without stress incontinence. Treatment adherence rates were assessed by attendance at the weekly office visits, by diaries over the 12-week period, and by self-report at the final follow-up. Cure rates with bladder training determined by a diary were 18% and 16% at 3 and 6 months postrandomization, respectively, versus 13% and 20% in the PFM exercise group and 31% and 27% in the combination therapy group. Improvement rates (i.e., percentage of patients achieving greater than a 50% reduction in incontinent episodes) in the bladder training group was 52% and 46% at 3 and 6 months, 57% and 56% in the PFM exercise group, and 70% and 59% in the combination therapy group. The failure of the combination therapy group to maintain better treatment outcomes at 6 months postrandomization may be related to their slightly lower adherence rate and the greater number of missing diaries at this follow-up, or it may have been an artifact. No differences in cure or improvement rates were noted by women with different urodynamic diagnoses. Improvements in quality of life and symptom distress also were similar between the two groups.

Bladder training appears to have efficacy similar to anticholinergic drug therapy in women and men with detrusor instability. Columbo and his associates (1995) reported that a 6-week course of oxybutynin had a clinical cure rate similar to bladder training (74% vs. 73%, respectively). Although a higher cure rate was noted in women with detrusor instability alone (74% vs. 42%), the relapse rate at 6 months was higher for the drug therapy group, whereas the bladder training group better maintained their treatment outcomes. Symptom improvement in both groups were correlated to changes in bladder stability. Wiseman and her colleagues (1991) found that 34 frail female and male patients who received a placebo and bladder training did equally as well as those patients who received terodiline (recalled from the market) with respect to incontinent episodes, frequency of micturition, and subjective improvement.

## PELVIC FLOOR MUSCLE TRAINING

Pelvic floor muscle training (PFMT), new terminology suggested by the First International Consultation on Incontinence (Wilson et al., 1999), was initially described by Kegel in 1948 as a treatment for urinary incontinence in women. It involves passive or active contractions of the PFM through a variety of training techniques. These techniques include PFM exercises (also referred to as Kegel exercises), biofeedback-assisted PFM exercises, use of intravaginal resistance devices, vaginal weight training, and electrical stimulation. PFMT has been used in the treatment of female stress, urge, and mixed incontinence, as well as in the prevention and treatment of postnatal incontinence and postprostatectomy incontinence.

Several hypotheses exist for how PFMT achieves its effects on continence status. In treatment of stress incontinence, PFMT is thought to increase the speed and force of PFM contraction, which helps to clamp the urethra, increase urethral pressure, and prevent urine loss during abrupt increases in intraabdominal pressure. In women with stress incontinence, PFM contraction may press the urethra against the pubis symphysis, creating a mechanical pressure rise. Strength training also may lead to hypertrophy of the PFMs, which may provide improved structural support to the bladder and urethra. In treatment of urge incontinence, PFM contraction can provide a reflex inhibition of the detrusor muscle, thus reducing bladder contractions that cause leakage to occur (Wilson et al., 1999).

Numerous studies have been conducted on PFMT in women over the past decade. In contrast, research on PFMT in men is quite sparse. Research protocols vary considerably in sample size, training procedures, compliance assessment, outcome measures, and follow-up periods. Compliance measures varied by the training technique: class or office visit attendance, number of biofeedback sessions, number of exercises recorded on a diary or assessed through an electronic meter housed within a home trainer unit, or self-report of overall compliance. Compliance rates tended to be poorly reported except for studies on electrical stimulation, which used electronic home trainer units with built-in adherence monitors. The outcome measures used to evaluate treatment efficacy include self-assessment of improvement, quality-of-life instruments, voiding diaries, pad tests, PFM strength tests, provocative stress tests, and urodynamic parameters. Immediate follow-up periods are variable across studies ranging from 4 weeks to 6 months. Long-term follow-up periods have ranged from 6 months to 4 years.

Efficacy and adherence rates are difficult to compare across studies because of inconsistency in reporting methods and differences in outcome measures. Only recently have PFMT studies reported on quality-of-life changes, using standardized measures. Generally, compliance decreases over time, but it appears to vary depending on the population studied and the amount of daily contractions recommended. For example, in a study of younger Norwegian women, Bo reported that compliance with 36 PFM contractions over 6 months was 93% (Bo, Talseth, & Home, 1999) with no attrition. In contrast, Wells and her colleagues (Wells, Brink, Diokno, Wolfe, & Gillis, 1991) found that older American women were performing

44%–79% of the 90–160 requested contractions at 6 months, with a 34% attrition rate by 6 months.

Seven trials associated greater motivation, higher exercise adherence, and/or attendance at treatment visits or exercise groups with improved outcomes (Bo, Hagen, Kvarstein, Jørgensen, & Larsen, 1990; Glavind, Nøhr, & Walter, 1996; Lagro-Janssen et al., 1992; Laycock & Jerwood, 1993; O'Brien, Austin, Sethi, & O'Boyle, 1991; Sand et al., 1995; Wells, Brink, Diokno, Wolfe, & Gillis, 1991). Attrition rates for PFMT range from 0% to 34% and vary considerably depending on type of treatment, its length, adverse effects, and length of the follow-up period. Although a number of studies have attempted to evaluate predictors of treatment outcomes, findings are often contradictory. No study has had a sufficient sample size to conduct a valid analysis.

Many studies provided insufficient detail on the PFMT protocol to allow study replication. In those reports that did provide details, considerable variation occurred in how PFMT was implemented. In studies using PFM exercises, the strength of the PFM contraction requested ranged from submaximal to maximal, with the majority of studies either employing maximal contractions or not specifying the strength of the contraction. Length of contractions varied from 3 to 40 seconds, and relaxation periods ranged from 5 to 10 seconds.

Some protocols included training for both strength (fast or quick contractions) and endurance (sustained contractions ) of muscle contractions; one study trained for preventive contractions only (Miller, Ashton-Miller, & Delancey, 1998). Other protocols involved a graded exercise program, increasing length of contraction period and/or number of repetitions. The frequency of performing contractions varied from 10 repetitions every hour to sets of contractions performed 3 to 10 times a day; one study used a protocol of exercise every other day (Dougherty, Bishop, Mooney, Gimotty, & Williams, 1993). The total number of contractions per day ranged from 30 to 200, with a majority requesting a total of 45 to 50 daily. Practice audiocassette tapes were provided in some studies. Instruction in PFMT was typically provided as individual teaching and supervision; however, group teaching was used in one study (O'Brien et al., 1991). Some studies used individualized instruction with daily home practice, followed by a weekly group exercise class (Bo et al., 1990). The duration of the training program ranged from 8 weeks to 6 months, with most programs involving a 12-week training protocol.

## Pelvic Floor Muscle Exercises

### STUDIES IN WOMEN

Numerous RCTs have evaluated PFM exercises in women, primarily in those with stress incontinence (Blowman et al., 1991; Bo et al., 1999;

Burns et al., 1993; Dougherty et al., 1993; Ferguson et al., 1990; Henalla, Hutchins, Robinson, & Macvicar, 1989; Lagro-Janssen et al., 1992; Miller, Richardson, et al., 1998; O'Brien et al., 1991; Pieber et al., 1995). Some studies have examined PFM exercises as a preventive intervention during pregnancy or to treat postnatal incontinence (Mørkved & Bo, 1997; Sampselle et al., 1998).

Excellent evidence exists documenting that PFM exercises are effective in strengthening PFM and reducing stress incontinence in women. Cure rates evaluated by diary range from 16% to 30%. Improvement rates by diary range from 60% to 80%. In the studies that evaluated PFM strength, all reported a significant improvement with PFM exercise. However, improvement in PFM strength was not always correlated with improvement in incontinent episodes.

The frequency of daily contractions required to achieve objective improvement appears to be much less than Kegel (1948) reported in his early work. Significant reductions in incontinent episodes as recorded on diary have been found in PFMT programs using as few as 36 to 45 contractions a day (Bo et al., 1990, 1999). Although the majority of protocols require a daily exercise regimen, one study found that exercising every other day resulted in significant reductions in incontinence severity. However, no studies have compared a daily versus every-other-day exercise regimen. Dougherty and her colleagues (1993) used a repeated-measures design and a wait-list control to evaluate a 16-week program of graded PFM exercises performed three times per week by 65 women (mean age 51.3 years) with stress incontinence. There were no significant changes in the urine loss measures (24-hour diary and pad test) and PFM pressure as measured by a water-filled vaginal balloon device following a 4-week control period. Significant reductions in pad test weights and incontinent episodes were noted after 16 weeks of exercise.

Exercise science suggests that use of a resistance device leads to better strength training effects. However, this has not been demonstrated in PFMT studies. Ferguson and her colleagues (1990) evaluated the effectiveness of a 6-week exercise program with and without an intravaginal balloon device in 20 women (mean age 36.5 years) with stress incontinence. There were no differences between subjects who exercised with or without the device in PFM strength or urine loss as measured by a 24-hour home pad test.

The use of an audiocassette practice tape has been recommended to increase adherence. However, studies evaluating the effect of a practice tape on adherence rates for women in PFMT programs have conflicting results, which might be explained by differences in the intensity and frequency of their follow-up. Nygaard and her colleagues (Nygaard, Kreder, Lepic, Fountain, & Rhomberg, 1996) did not find a difference in reduction of incontinent episodes, adherence rates, or dropout rates in 71 women randomized to exercise with and without a practice tape. Subjects were followed with weekly alternating telephone calls and office visits. In contrast, Gallo and Staskin (1997) found that a practice tape did increase adherence rates in 54 women who were seen only once, 4 to 6 weeks after the initial instruction.

The intensity of the exercise program may affect treatment outcomes. Bo and her colleagues (1990) compared a 6-month protocol involving intensive exercise (daily exercises, weekly group exercise session with an enthusiastic instructor, and long-lasting contractions with the supplement of 3–4 fast contractions at the end of each long contraction) versus a standard home exercise program in 52 women (mean age 45.9 years) with stress incontinence. Although both groups increased their muscle strength, the gains were larger in the intensive exercise group, which showed greater reductions on office pad testing and reported an improved leakage index. In this group, 60.1% were continent or almost continent versus 17.3% of the standard exercise group.

Teaching of preventive PFM contraction may help to avoid urine loss with exertional events. Miller and her colleagues (1998) investigated the effect of "Knack," a preventive muscle contraction prior to coughing in 27 women (mean age 68 years). The Knack was effective in reducing urine loss resulting from a medium cough by 98.2% and by 73.3% from a deep cough. Reduction in urine loss was not related to a digital measure of muscle strength.

PFM exercises performed during the prenatal period may help to prevent urinary incontinence symptoms during late pregnancy and the postpartum period. Sampselle and her colleagues (1998) investigated a PFM exercise program (30 contractions per day) taught at 20 weeks gestation in 46 women (mean age 27.2 years) and found that incontinence symptoms measured by a questionnaire were less at 35 weeks gestation and at 6 weeks and 6 months postpartum than in a control group. No significant differences were noted between groups on PFM strength at the two follow-up periods. Initiation of PFM exercises during the postpartum period also appears to reduce incontinence. In a case control study of 99 matched pairs ($N = 198$) of mothers, Mørkved and Bo (1997) tested an 8-week intensive PFM exercise course (36 contractions, three times a week, group exercise class once a week) initiated 8 weeks postpartum and found that the treatment group had significantly less incontinence determined by an office pad test and greater PFM strength than the control group.

## STUDIES IN MEN

Two studies that evaluated PFM exercises in men were located (Chang et al., 1998; O'Brien et al., 1991). In an RCT that included both genders, O'Brien and his colleagues (1991) reported that 77% of the 86 male participants were cured or improved with PFM exercises and/or bladder training. Using a quasi-experimental design, Chang and his colleagues (1998) evaluated a 4-week program of PFM exercises taught in the immediate postoperative period in 50 men (mean age 64–65 years) following transurethral prostatectomy. Significant differences were noted between the treatment and control group in the strength of the PFM contraction and the length between voiding intervals, terminal dribbling, and urinary incontinence which were assessed by questionnaire.

## Biofeedback-Assisted Pelvic Floor Muscle Exercises

Biofeedback is a teaching technique that uses electronic or mechanical monitoring instruments to detect and relay auditory and/or visual display information to the individual about his or her physiologic responses. Biofeedback is used in PFMT to teach muscle awareness and isolation, to help motivate the patient, and to monitor physiologic improvement. It may be provided by single-channel or multichannel feedback (simultaneous measurement of PFM and abdominal or detrusor muscle contraction), using vaginal, anal, and surface electrodes or vaginal or anal balloon devices. Office and home instruments are available for biofeedback training.

### STUDIES IN WOMEN

Six RCTs were located that used biofeedback-assisted PFM exercises; three trials compared biofeedback-assisted PFM exercise to PFM exercise alone (Berghmans et al., 1996; Burns et al., 1993; Glavind et al., 1996), one trial compared biofeedback-assisted PFM exercise with bladder training to PFM exercise (Sherman, Davis, & Wong, 1997), one previously described trial compared biofeedback-assisted PFM exercises to bladder training and a combination of the two therapies (Wyman et al., 1998), and one trial compared biofeedback-assisted PFM exercises taught in the postnatal period to a standard PFM exercise class taught pre- and postpartum (Wilson & Herbison, 1998). The trials vary considerably in sample size, PFM exercise protocols, biofeedback procedures, frequency of contact during treatment phase, outcome measures, and follow-up periods. Although home biofeedback units are available, there is only one prospective cohort study reporting on its use (Hirsch et al., 1999). The majority of studies used vaginal electromyography (EMG) (three studies) or vaginal pressure (one study) for biofeedback. All studies used office biofeedback.

Biofeedback-assisted PFM exercise is efficacious when compared to a no-treatment control group for women with stress incontinence and mixed incontinence (Burns et al., 1993). The empirical support for the superiority of biofeedback-assisted PFM exercise over exercise alone is weak, and further research is needed. Only one study found that biofeedback-assisted PFM exercises were superior to exercises alone; however, there was inadequate control for intensity and frequency of therapist contact between the two groups. Glavind and her colleagues (1996) reported on a 3-month study of 34 women with stress incontinence. Using surface EMG biofeedback administered in four weekly sessions involving four lessons, the cure rate (e.g., less than 1 gm on a pad test) in the biofeedback group was 58% versus 20% in the exercise-alone group, which had weekly sessions involving three lessons.

In the other trials, women in the biofeedback group had results similar to those of the PFM exercise group on subjective improvement, pad tests, and/or voiding diaries (Berghmans et al., 1996; Burns et al., 1993; Sherman et al., 1997). However, women in the biofeedback groups tended to achieve their outcomes sooner (Berghmans et al., 1996), and there may be greater improvements in subjects with more severe incontinence (Burns et al., 1993). Berghmans and his colleagues (1996) reported that women in the biofeedback group achieved significant improvement after 6 sessions of vaginal EMG feedback, whereas it took women in the PFM exercise group 12 sessions to achieve the same level of improvement. In the largest RCT, Burns and her colleagues (1993) evaluated vaginal EMG biofeedback in 123 women with stress and mixed incontinence and found that the biofeedback group achieved higher EMG scores, with quick and sustained muscle contractions, than the PFM exercise group. These scores were correlated with improvement in incontinent episodes. They also noted a trend for the biofeedback group with moderate and severe incontinence to have higher cure/improvement rates than those with mild incontinence.

## STUDIES IN MEN

Three studies using biofeedback-assisted PFM exercise for postprostatectomy incontinence were located (Burgio, Stutzman, & Engel, 1989; Meaglia, Joseph, Chang, & Schmidt, 1990); these vary by the surgical population, the training procedures, the outcome measures, and the follow-up period. Thus, few conclusions can be drawn other than more high-quality research needs to be conducted in this area. Findings are difficult to interpret because of the natural resolution in incontinence that occurs during the first six postoperative months, when many of these studies were conducted.

In one of the first studies conducted, Burgio and her colleagues (1989) used a prospective cohort design to evaluate a biofeedback-assisted training protocol that included 2-hour timed voiding in 20 men with persistent incontinence 6 months postprostatectomy. After one to five biofeedback sessions, patients with urge incontinence had the highest mean reduction of incontinence (80.7%), compared to those with stress incontinence (78.3%) or continual leakage (17%). In the only RCT, Mathewson-Chapman (1997) evaluated a preoperative program using biofeedback-assisted PFM exercise instruction followed by 9 weeks of daily home exercise from postoperative weeks 3–12 in 53 men undergoing radical prostatectomy for localized prostate cancer. The biofeedback group regained continence 51 days after surgery, compared to the control group which became continent at 56 days.

## Pelvic Floor Muscle Exercises versus Drug Therapy

PFMT appears to be equally effective as drug therapy in the treatment of stress and urge incontinence in women. Wells and her colleagues (1991) compared the efficacy of 6-month program of PFM exercises to phenylopropanolamine hydrochloride (50 mg a day, which increased to 50 mg twice a day if leakage continued) in 157 women with urethral incompetency (stress incontinence) or in combination with detrusor hyperactivity when stress incontinence was judged to be the dominant symptom. Subjective improvement was similar in both the PFM exercise and drug therapy groups (77% vs. 84%, respectively), as well as with the number of incontinent episodes recorded on a voiding diary. Cure rates determined by episodes of leakage recorded on a diary were 27% in the PFMT group versus 14% in the drug therapy group. Attrition rate was higher in PFMT (34%) than in the drug therapy group (17%).

In an RCT with 197 women with urge incontinence and urodynamic evidence of detrusor instability, Burgio and her colleagues (1999) compared the efficacy of an 8-week program of a staged, biofeedback-assisted PFMT program, drug therapy (oxybutynin chloride 2.5 mg three times a day, increasing to 5 mg three times a day if needed), and a placebo control condition. PFMT resulted in a greater mean reduction of incontinent episodes (80.7%), compared to drug treatment (68.5%), and both were more effective than the placebo condition (39.4%). Attrition was higher in the control (18.5%) and drug therapy (17.9%) groups than in the behavioral therapy group (6.2%). Compliance rates were not reported. Despite the beneficial effects of drug therapy, only 54.7% said they would continue indefinitely, and 75.5% said they wished to receive another form of treatment. In the behavioral therapy group, only 14.5% said they wished to add drug therapy.

## Vaginal Weight Training

Progressive vaginal weight training was introduced by Plevnik in 1985 as a new method for strengthening and testing PFM in women with stress incontinence, using a set of cone-shaped weights (20–85 gm) (Wilson et al., 1999). The cones provide proprioceptive feedback and prompt a PFM contraction in order to retain the cone. The heaviest weight that can be retained by the patient is worn for a specified period of time while ambulatory, usually 15 minutes twice a day. Protocols vary according to whether PFM exercises are requested in conjunction with cone wearing.

Eight studies were reviewed: four were RCTs (Bo et al., 1999; Cammu & Van Nylen, 1998; Olah, Bridges, Denning, & Farrar, 1990; Pieber et al., 1995), and four were prospective cohort studies (Kondo, Yamada, Morishige, & Niijima, 1996; Peattie, Plevnik, & Stanton, 1988; Wilson & Borland, 1990; Wrigley, 1995). Although the clinical series reported significant improvements with vaginal weight training, the results in RCTs tend to be less impressive. Statistical power is a limitation in most studies because treatment groups are quite small. Thus, it is difficult to derive definitive conclusions about the efficacy of vaginal weight training in comparison to a control group or PFM exercises. Bo and her colleagues (1999) found that women using vaginal cones compared to a no-treatment control group had improved scores on a social activity index and leakage index but had similar outcomes on other subjective measures and pad testing. Cure rate on a pad test was 15%.

Vaginal weight training does not appear to provide additional benefit to PFM exercises alone in either premenopausal and postmenopausal women. Pieber and his colleagues (1995) found similar subjective improvement rates in 46 premenopausal women (mean age 43 years) with mild to moderate stress incontinence undergoing a 3-month program of PFM exercise with (57% improved) and without vaginal cones (53% improved). Similarly, Cammu and Van Nylen (1998) found no differences in treatment outcomes (e.g., subjective improvement, incontinent episodes, pad use, muscle strength) in 60 women (mean age 56.1 years) with stress incontinence undergoing a 3-month program of PFM exercises with and without vaginal cones.

Although vaginal cone instruction and follow-up can be less costly in office practices, there appear to be problems with its acceptability and long-term use. In some studies there was a high attrition rate (42%–47%) (Cammu & Van Nylen, 1998; Kondo et al., 1995; Olah et al., 1990). The adverse effect rate is minimal.

## Electrical Stimulation

Nonimplantable electrical stimulation involves electrical current applied by vaginal, anal, or surface electrodes to produce a contraction of the PFM, along with a reflex inhibition of the detrusor muscle. Great variability exists in the literature regarding the terms used to describe electrical stimulation and the type of current, devices, stimulation parameters, and research protocols that were used. Several types of electrical stimulation, including inferential therapy (two interfering medium-frequency currents) and faradism (low-frequency current with a pulse duration of 1 ms or less), and specifically programmed neuromuscular electrical stimulation has been used. Duration of treatment varied from 15 minutes to 7–8 hours, depending on the type of stimulation; the most common duration was

15 minutes per session. The frequency of stimulation varied from every other day to two or three times a day, typically twice a day. Stimulation was pulsed or continuous, and the lowest pulse duration was 0.1 microseconds. Some studies varied the stimulation protocol according to the type of incontinence, and others used the same protocol for all types (Brubaker, Benson, Bent, Clark, & Schott, 1997). Follow-up periods varied from 4 to 15 weeks. Compliance was assessed in three studies through a built-in compliance meter within the stimulation device (Brubaker et al., 1997; Richardson et al., 1996; Sand et al., 1995).

The ideal research protocol for electrical stimulation is a placebo-controlled, double-blinded study in which electrical stimulation is compared to a sham treatment that uses a similar probe but without the electrical current. Six studies used this protocol to compare active home electrical stimulation provided by a vaginal or anal probe to sham stimulation. Of these, three studies were conducted in women with genuine stress incontinence (Laycock & Jerwood, 1993; Luber & Wolde-Tsadik, 1997; Sand et al., 1995), and one study was conducted in women with detrusor instability, genuine stress incontinence, or a combination of both diagnoses (Brubaker et al., 1997). A fifth study compared electrical stimulation to sham stimulation, with both groups receiving concomitant biofeedback-assisted PFM exercises (Blowman et al., 1991) in women with genuine stress incontinence. A sixth RCT, which compared real versus sham stimulation, included women and men within the same group (Yamanishi et al., 1997); however, because of design problems, no conclusions will be drawn from this trial.

Results are inconsistent among studies that may reflect differences in populations, stimulation devices, stimulation parameters, duration of stimulation, treatment adherence, outcome measures, and follow-up periods. One study suggested that a minimum of 14 weeks of stimulation therapy is necessary to achieve significant objective improvement (Miller & Bavendam, 1996); most of these studies were conducted for 12 weeks or less. Thus, there is insufficient evidence to determine whether electrical stimulation is effective for women with stress, mixed, or urge incontinence. Cure rates evaluated by diary ranged from 0% to 85.7%. Attrition rates were 8%–22%. Adherence rates evaluated by an internal compliance meter ranged from 78.8% to 100%. Adverse effects were inconsistently reported and varied among the studies that reported them; they included 0%–14% for vaginal irritation, 0%–9% for pain, and 0%–3% for urinary tract infection.

Two RCTs did not report improvement on incontinence severity indices. Luber and Wolde-Tsadik (1997) reported no differences in incontinent episodes, leak point pressures, and subjective cure/improvement rates in 54 women with stress incontinence (mean age 53.9 years) who participated in a 12-week program (15 minutes of stimulation twice a day;

50 Hz frequency). Brubaker and her colleagues (1997) found no differences in incontinent episodes or condition-specific quality of life measured by an unstandardized instrument in 157 women with detrusor instability, stress incontinence, or both (mean age 56.9 years) who participated in an 8-week program (20 min of stimulation twice a day, 20 Hz frequency). Compliance rates were similar between groups (78.8% for electrical stimulation vs. 83.7% for sham stimulation). However, 49% of women with detrusor instability had a urodynamic cure (stable on provocative cystometry), whereas none was noted in the sham group. No differences in urodynamic cures were noted between groups for women with stress incontinence.

In contrast, Sand and his colleagues (1995) reported that a 15-week program (15–30 minutes of stimulation twice a day, variable frequency) in 52 women (mean age 53.2 years) was efficacious. Stimulation resulted in significant improvements on weekly incontinent episodes, pad testing, and PFM strength. Cure rates evaluated by diary were 0% in the electrical stimulation group and 6% in the control group, and 20% versus 12%, respectively, as assessed by pad test. Improvement rates (e.g., 50% or more improved) on the diary were 37% in the electrical stimulation group versus 12% in the control group, and 46% versus 18% on the pad test, respectively. Positive outcomes were associated with treatment compliance. No changes were noted in generic quality of life, possibly due to low power.

Limited data are available on the efficacy of surface electrical stimulation, which is becoming more common in clinical practice. Blowman and his colleagues (1991) conducted an RCT that compared surface electrical stimulation using perineal body and buttock electrodes to sham stimulation using a 4-week home stimulation program (60 min per day, 10 Hz frequency) in 14 women (median age 43.5 years) with stress incontinence. Cure rate as reported on a 1-week diary was 85.7% for the treatment group and 16.7% for the control group.

Frequency of home stimulation therapy was evaluated in one study, but results were inconclusive and may have been affected by differential treatment adherence as well as low power. Richardson and his colleagues (1996) found daily and every-other-day stimulation therapy equally effective in reducing incontinent episodes and pad tests in 31 women (mean age 56.9 years) with stress incontinence. However, compliance was significantly higher in the every-other-day stimulation group (100%) than in the daily stimulation group (85%). Subjects who continued device use for 1 year were more likely to maintain a higher cure or improvement rate than were those who discontinued device use.

Electrical stimulation appears to have a similar efficacy to PFM exercise alone (Hahn, Sommar, & Fall, 1991), vaginal weight training alone (Bo et al., 1999; Olah et al., 1990), or the combined use of exercise and vaginal weight training (Laycock & Jerwood, 1993) in treating female stress incontinence. However, in one RCT, PFM exercise was superior to electrical stimulation. Bo and her colleagues (1999) compared a no-treatment control, PFM exercises, vaginal cones, and electrical stimulation (30 min per day, 50 Hz frequency, with variable work/rest cycles) in 107 women with genuine stress incontinence. The greatest improvements in pad test weights and muscle strength were noted in the PFM exercise group in comparison to the other groups.

Only one study was located that compared electrical stimulation to anticholinergic drug therapy (propantheline bromide 7.5 mg–45 mg, two to three times a day) and to bladder training for women with detrusor instability (Smith, 1996). Results were equivocal, which may have been due in part to design flaws.

### Pelvic Floor Muscle Training and Drug Therapy

PFMT may be an excellent adjunct to use with other forms of treatment. Holtedahl, Verelst, and Schiefloe (1998) reported on a population-based RCT of 90 women (mean age 60.6 years) with urinary incontinence and evidence of objective leakage, who were randomized to a 6-month wait-list control or a treatment of estriol, six sessions of physiotherapy (PFM exercises for all subjects; bladder training for urge and mixed incontinence; and graded home electrical stimulation initiated at 20 min a day or every other day for 1–2 months and gradually increased to 7–8 hours during sleeping hours every other day for 4–6 months). Cure/improvement rate at 1 year was 56%.

## SUMMARY AND RESEARCH RECOMMENDATIONS

The quality of the studies on behavioral interventions for urinary incontinence has significantly improved over the past decade. An increasing number of studies are using RCT designs, the gold standard for intervention research, with standardized outcome measurements. In the past 3 years a growing number of incontinence trials have included quality of life in the evaluation of treatment efficacy. However, because of considerable variability in the selection of outcome measures and the reporting of findings, it is difficult to compare results across studies. Future RCTs on incontinence interventions should ideally incorporate a 7-day voiding diary, a home pad test, and a condition-specific quality-of-life instrument as the basic outcome measures.

Several studies had inconclusive results, with no differences noted between treatment groups. In many studies, this may have been due to a small sample size that affected statistical power. These studies could have been improved by performing a power analysis prior to data collection to determine appropriate sample size or by conducting a post hoc power analysis to determine what sample size would have been needed to detect a significant difference between groups.

A surprising number of studies failed to assess or to report treatment adherence rates. Future studies should incorporate standardized measures to evaluate treatment adherence and include analyses that report on the effect of adherence on treatment outcomes.

Research on behavioral treatments to date have been based on theoretical frameworks derived from operant conditioning, empirical data, and/or muscle and exercise physiological principles. Few studies, if any, have incorporated health behavior change theory except for the use of behavioral techniques (e.g., self-monitoring). Although bladder training and PFMT have well-documented short-term efficacy, the long-term maintenance of treatment outcomes tends to be lower. In the few studies that have examined long-term treatment outcomes, most report that adherence rates tend to drop significantly. Future research must reconceptualize these treatment programs using health behavior change theory and design interventions to enhance long-term behavioral change.

Research evidence on the short-term efficacy of bladder training and PFMT as shown on incontinence severity indices (incontinent episodes and pad test weights) is quite strong in women but is virtually lacking in men. Future research with larger sample sizes is needed on both these interventions to document their comparative effectiveness when combined with each other, with lifestyle interventions, antiincontinence devices, and/or drug therapies, as well as their quality-of-life impact, their long-term effectiveness, and their cost-effectiveness, and to determine which subgroups of patients will derive the greatest benefit from their use so that better targeting of patients to particular treatments can occur. The effectiveness of different bladder training and PFMT programs, particularly biofeedback-assisted instruction, should also be compared to determine the parameters of the most effective protocols for different subgroups of patients.

High-quality research is needed on electrical stimulation to better define the parameters of the most effective protocols in different patient subgroups and to determine the advantage of electrical stimulation compared to other forms of PFMT. Research documenting the effectiveness of lifestyle interventions on continence status in the areas of smoking cessation, weight control, fluid and dietary factors, and bowel management also is greatly needed. Finally, future research should address long-term prevention of incontinence in women and men.

## REFERENCES

Abrams, P., Khoury, S., & Wein, A. (Eds.). (1999). *Incontinence: Proceedings of the First International Consultation on Incontinence.* Plymouth, UK: Health Publication.

Berghmans, L. C. M., Frederiks, C. M. A., de Bie, R. A., Weil, E. H. J., Smeets, L. W. H., van Waawijk van Doorn, E. S. C., & Janknegt, R. A. (1996). Efficacy of biofeedback, when included with pelvic floor muscle exercise treatment, for genuine stress incontinence. *Neurourology and Urodynamics, 15,* 37–52.

Blowman, C., Pickles, C., Emery, S., Creates, V., Towell, L., Blackburn, N., Doyle, N., & Walkden, B. (1991). Prospective double blind controlled trial of intensive physiotherapy with and without stimulation of the pelvic floor in treatment of genuine stress incontinence. *Physiotherapy, 77,* 661–664.

Bo, K., Hagen, R. H., Kvarstein, B., Jørgensen, J., & Larsen, S. (1990). Pelvic floor muscle exercise for the treatment of female stress urinary incontinence: 3. Effects of two different degrees of pelvic floor muscle exercises. *Neurourology and Urodynamics, 9,* 489–502.

Bo, K., Stien, R., Kulseng-Hanssen, S., & Kristofferson, M. (1994). Clinical and urodynamic assessment of nulliparous young women with and without stress incontinence symptoms: A case control study. *Obstetrics and Gynecology, 84,* 1028–1032.

Bo, K., Talseth, T., & Holme, I. (1999). Single blind, randomised controlled trial of pelvic floor exercises, electrical stimulation, vaginal cones, and no treatment in management of genuine stress incontinence in women. *British Medical Journal, 318,* 487–493.

Brown, J. S., Seeley, D. G., Fong, J., Black, D. M., Ensrud, K. E., Grady, D., and the Study of Osteoporotic Fractures Research Group. (1996). Urinary incontinence in older women: Who is at risk? *Obstetrics and Gynceology, 87,* 715–721.

Brubaker, L., Benson, J. T., Bent, A., Clark, A., & Shott, S. (1997). Transvaginal electrical stimulation for female urinary incontinence. *American Journal of Obstetrics and Gynecology, 177,* 536–540.

Bump, R. C., & McClish, D. K. (1992). Cigarette smoking and urinary incontinence in women. *American Journal of Obstetrics and Gynecology, 167,* 1213–1218.

Bump, R. C., & McClish, D. M. (1994). Cigarette smoking and pure genuine stress incontinence of urine: A comparison of risk factors and determinants between smokers and nonsmokers. *American Journal of Obstetrics and Gynecology, 170,* 579–582.

Bump, R. C., Sugerman, H. J., Fantl, J. A., & McClish, D. K. (1992). Obesity and lower urinary tract function in women: Effect of surgically induced weight loss. *American Journal of Obstetrics and Gynecology, 167,* 392–399.

Burgio, K. L., Locher, J. L., Goode, P. S., Hardin, J. M., McDowell, B. J., Dombrowski, M., & Candib, D. (1998). Behavioral vs. drug treatment for urge urinary incontinence in older women: A randomized controlled trial. *Journal of the American Medical Association, 280,* 1995–2035.

Burgio, K. L., Stutzman, R. E., & Engel, B. T. (1989). Behavioral training for postprostatectomy urinary incontinence. *Journal of Urology, 141,* 303–306.

Burns, P. A., Pranikoff, K., Nochajski, T. H., Hadley, E. L., Levy, K. J., & Ory, M. G. (1993). A comparison of effectiveness of biofeedback and pelvic muscle exercise treatment of stress incontinence in older community-dwelling women. *Journal of Gerontology: Medical Sciences, 48,* 167–174.

Cammu, H., & Van Nylen, M. (1998). Pelvic floor exercises versus vaginal weight cones in genuine stress incontinence. *European Journal of Obstetrics and Gynecology and Reproductive Biology, 77,* 89–93.

Chang, P. L., Tsai, L. H., Huang, S. T., Wang, T. M., Hsieh, M. L., & Tsui, K. H. (1998). The early effect of pelvic floor muscle exercise after transurethral prostatectomy. *Journal of Urology, 160,* 402–405.

Colombo, M., Zanetta, G., Scalambrino, S., & Milani, R. (1995). Oxybutynin and bladder training in the management of female urinary urge incontinence: A randomized study. *International Urogynecology Journal, 6,* 63–67.

Davis, G. D., & Goodman, M. (1996). Stress urinary incontinence in nulliparous female soldiers in airborne infantry training. *Journal of Pelvic Surgery, 2,* 68–71.

Dietel, M., Stone, E., Kassan, H. A., Wilk, E. J., & Sutherland, D. J. A. (1988). Gynecologic-obstetric changes after loss of massive excess weight following bariatric suregery. *Journal of the American College of Nutrition, 7,* 147–153.

Dougherty, M., Bishop, K., Mooney, R., Gimotty, P., & Williams, B. (1993). Graded pelvic muscle exercise. Effect on stress urinary incontinence. *Journal of Reproductive Medicine, 38,* 684–691.

Dowd, T. T., Campbell, J. M., & Jones, J. A. (1996). Fluid intake and urinary incontinence in older community-dwelling women. *Journal of Community Health Nursing, 13,* 179–186.

Fantl, J. A., Kaschak Newman, D., Colling, J., DeLancey, J. O. L., Keeys, C., Loughery, R., McDowell, B. J., Norton, P., Ouslander, J., Schnelle, J., Staskin, D., Tries, J., Urich, V., Vitousek, S. H., Weiss, B. D., & Whitmore, R. (1996). *Urinary incontinence in adults: Acute and chronic management.* Clinical Practice Guideline, No. 2. Rockville, MD: U.S. Department of Health and Human Services, Public Health Service, Agency for Health Care Policy and Research.

Fantl, J. A., Wyman, J. F., McClish, D. K., Harkins, S. W., Elswick, R. K., Taylor, J. R., & Hadley, E. C. (1991). Efficacy of bladder training in older women with urinary incontinence. *Journal of the American Medical Association, 265,* 609–613.

Ferguson, K. L., McKey, P. L., Bishop, K. R., Kloen, P., Verheul, J. B., & Dougherty, M. C. (1990). Stress urinary incontinence: Effect of pelvic muscle exercise. *Obstetrics and Gynecology, 75,* 671–675.

Fonda, D., Resnick, N. M., Colling, J., Burgio, K., Ouslander, J. G., Norton, C., Ekelund, P., Versi, E., & Mattiasson, A. (1998). Outcome measures for research of lower urinary tract dysfunction in frail older people. *Neurourology and Urodynamics, 17,* 273–282.

Gallo, M. L., & Staskin, D. R. (1997). Cues to action: Pelvic floor muscle exercise compliance in women with stress urinary incontinence. *Neurourology and Urodynamics, 16,* 167–177.

Glavind, K., Nøhr, S. B., & Walter, S. (1996). Biofeedback and physiotherapy versus physiotherapy alone in treatment of genuine stress urinary incontinence. *International Urogynecology Journal and Pelvic Floor Dysfunction, 7,* 339–343.

Hahn, I., Sommar, S., & Fall, M. (1991). A comparative study of pelvic floor training and electrical stimulation for the treatment of genuine female stress urinary incontinence. *Neurourology and Urodynamics, 10,* 545–554.

Henalla, S. M., Hutchins, C. J., Robinson, P., & Macvicar, J. (1989). Nonoperative methods in the treatment of female genuine stress incontinence of urine. *Journal of Obstetrics and Gynecology, 9,* 222–225.

Hirsh, A., Weirauch, G., Steimer, B., Bihler, K., Peschers, U., Bergauer, F., Leib, B., & Dimpfl, T. (1999). Treatment of female urinary incontinence with EMG-controlled biofeedback home training. *International Urogynecology Journal and Pelvic Floor Dysfunction, 10,* 7–10.

Holtedahl, K., Verelst, M., & Schiefloe, A. (1998). A population based, randomized, controlled trial of conservative treatment for urinary incontinence in women. *Acta Obstetrica et Gynecologica Scandinavica, 77,* 671–677.

Jeffcoate, T. N. A., & Francis, W. J. (1966). Urgency incontinence in the female. *American Journal of Obstetrics and Gynecology, 94,* 604–618.

Kegel, A. H. (1948). Progressive resistance exercise in the functional restoration of the perineal muscles. *American Journal of Obstetrics and Gynecology, 56,* 238–248.

Kondo, A., Yamada, Y., Morishige, R., & Niijima, R. (1996). An intensive programme for pelvic floor muscle exercises: Short and long-term effects on those with stress urinary incontinence. *Acta Urologica Japan, 42,* 853–859.

Koskimäki, J., Hakama, M., Huhtala, H., & Tammela, T. L. J. (1998). Association of smoking with lower urinary tract symptoms. *Journal of Urology, 159,* 1580–1582.

Lagro-Janssen, A. L. M., Debruyne, F. M. J., Smits, A. J. A., & Van Weel, C. (1992). The effects of treatment of urinary incontinence in general practice. *Family Practice, 9,* 284–289.

Laycock, J., & Jerwood, D. (1993). Does pre-modulated interferential therapy cure genuine stress incontinence? *Physiotherapy, 79,* 553–560.

Lose, G., Fantl, J. A., Victor, A., Walter, S., Wells, T. L., Wyman, J., & Mattiasson, A. (1998). Outcome measures for research in adult women with symptoms of lower urinary tract dysfunction. *Neurourology and Urodynamics, 17,* 255–262.

Luber, K. M., & Wolde-Tsadik, G. (1997). Efficacy of functional electrical stimulation in treating genuine stress incontinence: A randomized clinical trial. *Neurourology and Urodynamics, 16,* 543–551.

Mathewson-Chapman, M. (1997). Pelvic muscle exercise/biofeedback for urinary incontinence after prostatectomy. *Journal of Cancer Education, 12,* 218–223.

Mattiasson, A., Djurhuus, J. C., Fonda, D., Lose, G., Nordling, J., & Stöherer, M. (1998). Standardization of outcome studies in patients with lower urinary tract dysfunction: A report on general principles from the Standardization Committee of the International Continence Society. *Neurourology and Urodynamics, 17,* 249–254.

McClish, D. K., Fantl, J. A., Wyman, J. F., Pisani, G., & Bump, R. C. (1991). Bladder training in older women with urinary incontinence: Relationship between outcome and changes in urodynamic observations. *Obstetrics and Gynecology, 77,* 281–286.

Meaglia, J. P., Joseph, A. C., Chang, M., & Schmidt, J. D. (1990). Post-prostatectomy urinary incontinence: Response to behavioral training. *Journal of Urology, 144,* 674–676.

Miller, J. L., & Bavendam, T. (1996). Treatment with the Reliance urinary control insert: One-year experience. *Journal of Endourology, 10,* 287–292.

Miller, J. M., Ashton-Miller, J. A., & DeLancey, J. O. L. (1998). A pelvic muscle pre-contraction can reduce cough-related urine loss in selected women with mild stress urinary incontinence. *Journal of the American Geriatrics Society, 46,* 870–874.

Miller, K., Richardson, D. A., Siegel, S. W., Karram, M. M., Blackwood, N. B., & Sand, P. K. (1998). Pelvic floor electrical stimulation for genuine stress incontinence: Who will benefit and when? *International Urogynecology Journal and Pelvic Floor Dysfunction, 9,* 265–270.

Mørkved, S., & Bo, K. (1997). The effect of postpartum pelvic floor muscle exercise in the prevention and treatment of urinary incontinence. *International Urogynecology Journal and Pelvic Floor Dysfunction, 8,* 217–222.

Nordling, J., Abrams, P., Ameda, K., Andersen, J. T., Donovan, J., Griffiths, D., Kobayshi, S., Koyanagi, T., Schäfer, Yalla, S., & Mattiasson, A. (1998). Outcomes measures for research in treatment of adult males with symptoms of lower urinary tract dysfunction. *Neurourology and Urodynamics, 17,* 263–262.

Norton, P. A., & Baker, J. W. (1994). Postural changes can reduce leakage in women with stress urinary incontinence. *Obstetrics and Gynecology, 84,* 770–774.

Nygaard, I. E., Kreder, K. J., Lepic, M. M., Fountain, K. A., & Rhomberg, A. T. (1996). Efficacy of pelvic floor muscle exercises in women with stress, urge, and mixed urinary incontinence. *American Journal of Obstetrics and Gynecology, 174,* 120–125.

Nygaard, I. E., Thompson, F. L., Svengalis, S. L., & Albright, J. P. (1994). Urinary incontinence in elite nulliparous athletes. *Obstetrics and Gynecology, 84,* 183–187.

O'Brien, J., Austin, M., Sethi, P., & O'Boyle, P. (1991). Urinary incontinence: Prevalence, need for treatment, and effectiveness of intervention by nurse. *British Medical Journal, 303,* 1308–1312.

Olah, K. S., Bridges, N., Denning, J., & Farrar, D. J. (1990). The conservative management of patients with symptoms of stress incontinence: A randomized, prospective study comparing weighted vaginal cones and interferential therapy. *American Journal of Obstetrics and Gynecology, 162,* 87–92.

Peattie, A. B., Plevnik, S., & Stanton, S. L. (1988). Vaginal cones: A conservative method of treating genuine stress incontinence. *British Journal of Obstetrics and Gynecology, 95,* 1049–1053.

Pieber, D., Zivkovic, F., Tamussino, K., Ralph, G., Lippit, G., & Fauland, B. (1995). Pelvic floor exercise alone or with vaginal cones for the treatment of mild to moderate stress urinary incontinence in premenopausal women. *International Urogynecology Journal and Pelvic Floor Dysfunction, 6,* 14–17.

Plevnik, S. (1985). New method for testing and strengthening of pelvic floor muscles. *Neurourology and Urodynamics, 4,* 267–268.

Publicover, C., & Bear, M. (1997). The effect of bladder training on urinary incontinence in community-dwelling older women. *Journal of Wound, Ostomy, and Continence Nurses, 24,* 319–324.

Richardson, D. A., Miller, K. L., Siegel, S. W., Karram, M. M., Blackwood, N. B., & Staskin, D. R. (1996). Pelvic floor electrical stimulation: A comparison of daily and every-other-day therapy for genuine stress incontinence. *Urology, 48,* 110–118.

Roe, B., Williams, K., & Palmer, M. (1999). Bladder training for urinary incontinence (Cochrane Review). In *The Cochrane Library,* Issue 1, Oxford: Update Software.

Sampselle, C. M., Miller, J. M., Mims, B. L., Delancey, J. O. L., Ashton-Miller, J. A., & Antonakos, C. L. (1998). Effect of pelvic muscle exercise on transient incontinence during pregnancy and after birth. *Obstetrics and Gynecology, 91,* 406–412.

Sand, P. K., Richardson, D. A., Staskin, D. R., Swift, S. E., Appell, R. A., Whitmore, K. E., & Ostergard, D. R. (1995). Pelvic floor electrical stimulation in the treatment of genuine stress incontinence: A multicenter, placebo-controlled trial. *American Journal of Obstetrics and Gynecology, 173*, 72–79.

Sherman, R. A., Davis, G. D., & Wong, M. F. (1997). Behavioral treatment of exercise-induced incontinence among female soldiers. *Military Medicine, 162*, 690–694.

Smith, J. J. (1996). Intravaginal stimulation randomized trial. *Journal of Urology, 155*, 127–130.

Szonyi, G., Collas, D. M., Ding, Y. Y., & Malone-Lee, J. G. (1995). Oxybutynin with bladder training for detrusor instability in elderly people: A randomized controlled trial. *Age and Ageing, 24*, 287–291.

Tampakoudis, P., Tantanassis, T., Grimbizis, G., Papaletsos, M., & Mantalenakis, S. (1995). Cigarette smoking and urinary incontinence in women: A new calculative method of estimating the exposure to smoke. *European Journal of Obstetrics and Gynecology and Reproductive Biology, 63*, 27–30.

Tomlinson, B. U., Dougherty, M. C., Pendergast, J. F., Boyington, A. R., Coffman, M. A., & Pickers, S. M. (1999). Dietary caffeine, fluid intake and urinary incontinence in older rural women. *International Urogynecology Journal and Pelvic Floor Dysfunction, 10*, 22–28.

Wells, T. J., Brink, C. A., Diokno, A. C., Wolfe, R., & Gillis, G. L. (1991). Pelvic muscle exercise for stress urinary incontinence in elderly women. *Journal of the American Geriatrics Society, 39*, 785–791.

Wilson, P. D., Bo, K., Bourcier, A., Hay-Smith, J., Staskin, D., Nygaard, I., Wyman, J., & Shepherd, A. (1999). Conservative management in women. In P. Abrams, S. Khoury, & A. Wien (Eds.), *Incontinence: Proceedings from the First International Consultation on Incontinence* (pp. 579–636). Plymouth, UK: Health Publication.

Wilson, P. D., & Borland, M. (1990). Vaginal cones for the treatment of genuine stress incontinence. *Australian and New Zealand Journal of Obstetrics and Gynecology, 30*, 157–160.

Wilson, P. D., & Herbison, G. P. (1998). A randomized controlled trial of pelvic floor muscle exercises to treat postnatal urinary incontinence. *International Urogynecology Journal and Pelvic Floor Dysfunction, 9*, 257–264.

Wiseman, P. A., Malone-Lee, J., & Rai, G. S. (1991). Terodiline with bladder retraining for detrusor instability in elderly people. *British Medical Journal, 302*, 994–996.

Wrigley, T. (1995). The effect of training with vaginal weighted cones and pelvic floor exercises on the strength of the pelvic floor muscles: A pilot study. *International Urogynecology Journal and Pelvic Floor Dysfunction, 6*, 4–9.

Wyman, J. F., Fantl, J. A., McClish, D. K., Bump, R. C., and the Continence Program for Women Research Group. (1998). Comparative efficacy of behavioral interventions in the management of female urinary incontinence. *American Journal of Obstetrics and Gynecology, 179*, 999–1007.

Wyman, J. F., Fantl, J. A., McClish, D. K., Harkins, S. W., Taylor, J. R., & Ory, M. G. (1997). Effect of bladder training on quality of life of older women with urinary incontinence. *International Urogynecology Journal and Pelvic Floor Dysfunction, 8*, 223–229.

Yamanishi, T., Yashuda, K., Sakakibara, R., Hattori, T., Ito, H., & Murakami, S. (1997). Pelvic floor electrical stimulation in the treatment of stress incontinence: An investigational study and a placebo controlled double-blind trial. *Journal of Urology, 158*, 2127–2131.

# Chapter 8

# Family Interventions to Prevent Substance Abuse: Children and Adolescents

CAROL J. LOVELAND-CHERRY

## ABSTRACT

Substance abuse often begins in adolescence and is a major factor determining health outcomes for adolescents and adults; thus, it is an important focus for prevention strategies. The use of drugs, especially alcohol, can lead to chronic addiction to substances as well as contribute to a number of common chronic conditions. These conditions include cancer, cardiovascular disease, disability from accidents or violence, and unplanned pregnancy and are major causes of morbidity and mortality among adolescents and adults. As the major social unit responsible for socialization of children and stabilization of adult personalities, the family has been the target of prevention efforts. In this chapter the empirical literature on family interventions to prevent substance use in adolescents is critically reviewed, generalizations and implications for practice identified, and directions for future research projected.

**Key words: adolescence, family, interventions, substance use, prevention, community-based**

The empirical literature describing family-based interventions directed at prevention of substance use and abuse among adolescents is critiqued to identify major generalizations, implications for nursing practice, and directions for future research. The review focuses on prevention programs and does not include interventions directed at the treatment of substance abuse. Family prevention strategies, the significance of substance abuse for the health of adolescents, a summary of family protective and risk factors, and an overview of the proposed mechanisms underlying the family influence are presented as background for the critique of relevant published studies.

A comprehensive on-line search using MEDLINE and Mirlyn was conducted with the search keywords *children, adolescents, substance abuse, substance use, prevention, family, nursing, alcohol, marijuana, smoking,* and *drugs.* Inclusion criteria comprised manuscripts (1) published in refereed journals, (2) published in English, (3) reporting the results of research, (4) with a stated focus of prevention of substance abuse in adolescents, (5) indicating the family as the target of the intervention, and (6) published between January 1990 and June 1999. Manuscripts were excluded if they were descriptions of programs and their implementation but were not systematic evaluations of the programs within a research framework. Two major categories of family interventions are included: (1) interventions that contained a family-focused component embedded within a broader program and (2) interventions that focused exclusively on the family as the target of intervention. Although identification of 92 relevant references resulted from the literature search, only 13 intervention programs that met the inclusion criteria were identified. Of those 13, only 1 was authored by a nurse researcher.

For each study, the following components were evaluated: (1) category of family intervention (embedded vs. exclusive), (2) adequacy of design and study methods, (3) conceptual framework or approach, (4) format of the intervention, (5) content of the intervention, (6) the population, including diversity and sampling plan, (7) level (universal, selective, indicated) of intervention, and (8) magnitude and duration of effects.

## EXTENT AND SIGNIFICANCE OF ADOLESCENT SUBSTANCE USE

Substance use and abuse, especially the use of alcohol, is a major factor in morbidity and mortality in the United States, with "nearly one third of premature deaths . . . attributable to the abuse of addictive substances, most prominently tobacco and alcohol." Further, cigarette smoking has been identified as the "single most preventable behavioral factor in illness, disability, and death" (Pentz, MacKinnon, et al., 1989, p. 713). The full consequences of alcohol misuse in the United States are difficult to estimate because, although alcohol misuse contributes to various health and social problems, the direct involvement of alcohol misuse in these problems can be inferred only from health and social statistics. This misuse of alcohol has been identified as responsible for over 100,000 premature deaths per year, including approximately 44% of the more than 45,000 traffic crash fatalities, and costing over $148 billion in 1992 in health care, premature death, lowered productivity, and crime (National Institute on Drug Abuse, 1997). For many adolescents, alcohol experimentation is limited to a brief period, but even for youthful experimenters, especially those who overindulge, negative consequences can ensue in the form of illness;

death due to adverse drug reactions or overconsumption; unwanted pregnancy and diseases due to risky sexual behavior; injury or death from accidents or violence; and problems with parents, school personnel, or law enforcement (Abbey, Ross, & McDuffie, 1994; Biglan, Duncan, Ary, & Smolkowski, 1990; Lowry et al., 1994; Orpinas, Basen-Enquist, Grunbaum, & Parcel, 1995).

Persistent substance use is a factor in the development of chronic conditions such as cardiovascular disease, cancer, and disabilities from accidents and violent incidents. A smaller percentage of adolescents will develop substance dependence, leading to progressive increases in psychological, interpersonal, financial, and physical problems (Arria, Dohey, Mezzich, Bukstein, & Van Thiel, 1995; Botvin, Baker, Dusenbury, Tortu, & Botvin, 1990; Clapper, Buka, Goldfield, Lipsitt, & Tsuang, 1995; Eggert, Thompson, Herting, & Nicholas, 1994; C. A. Johnson et al., 1990; Kandel, Yamaguchi, & Chen, 1992). Unfortunately, addictive disorders often become chronic conditions and persist into adulthood. Further, prolonged persistent use of drugs, especially alcohol, contributes to the development of other chronic conditions. Thus, adolescent substance use contributes to a number of chronic conditions and can, in the instance of addiction, itself become a chronic condition.

Substance abuse among adolescents steadily declined from the beginning of the 1980s until 1992. In 1992 an upswing in reported substance use among adolescents, particularly younger adolescents, was noted. The increase continued until a leveling off appeared in 1998 (Johnston, O'Malley, & Bachman, 1998b). Most recent data on the proportion of 12th-graders reporting use of major substances in their lifetime, based on the Monitoring the Future Study, are marijuana 49%, alcohol 87%, cigarettes 65.3%, hallucinogens 14%, and cocaine 9.3%. Alcohol continues to be the most commonly used substance among adolescents (Johnston, O'Malley, & Bachman, 1998a). The greatest increases have been in marijuana and cocaine use and in use among eighth-grade students.

## UNDERLYING DYNAMICS OF FAMILY INFLUENCE

Two major pathways of family influence in substance abuse have been identified. The first, based on an increasing number of twin studies, is the role of genetic factors in substance use and abuse (Merikangas, Dierker, & Fenton, 1998). Convincing evidence exists for both general substance use and associated conduct disorder (e.g., Grove, Eckert, Heston, Bouchard, Segal, & Lykken, 1990) and specific drugs (Claridge, Ross, & Hume, 1978; Gurling, Grant, & Dangl, 1985; Jang, Lively, & Vernon, 1995; Pedersen, 1981).

The second pathway of influence is through the effects of the family environment. The family continues to be the major unit for the socialization of children, including the development of attitudes and behaviors (Kumpfer, 1998; Loveland-Cherry, Ross, & Kaufman, 1999). Parents and siblings are powerful role models for children and adolescents.

Genetic risk often can be moderated by environments. Thus, both pathways of influence are important to consider in the prevention of adolescent substance abuse. Clearly, a large number of individuals with significant biological or inherited risk for substance abuse avoid becoming involved in abusive or addictive behaviors. Some of the amelioration of risk is accomplished through the enhancement of protective factors, often through interventions with the family unit.

## FAMILY PROTECTIVE AND RISK FACTORS

A number of factors that either place adolescents at higher risk or protect adolescents from substance use have been identified. These protective and risk factors can be classified as inherited biological risk, environmental risk, behavioral risk, and age-related risk. The family is an important conduit for several of the classifications of risk and protective factors. Clearly, inherited biological risk is transmitted within the intergenerational structure of families. The family is a critical environment for the development of children; it is the locus of daily living, meeting basic needs such as shelter, nourishment, and health care. Beliefs, norms, expectancies, and behaviors largely are developed and maintained within the family. One hypothesis regarding peer influences on adolescents' beliefs and behaviors proposes that peers are selected on the basis of salient values. The competing hypothesis is that peers directly influence the development of substance use among adolescents. The important role that families play in the prevention of adolescent substance use is well established in terms of risk and protective factors.

The factors specific to families that are associated with increased risk of adolescent substance use include parental and sibling substance use (Hawkins, Catalano, & Miller, 1992), permissive or inconsistent parental discipline (Brook, Whiteman, Balka, & Hamburg, 1992; Dielman, Butchart, & Shope, 1993), parental approval of adolescent substance use (Johnson & Pamdina, 1991; Dielman, Butchart, Shope, & Miller, 1990–1991), and poor parent–child relationships (Baumrind, 1991; Brook, Brook, Gordon, Whiteman, & Cohen, 1990).

Family factors that protect adolescents from alcohol use include a cohesive, supportive family environment (Barnes & Windle, 1987; Brook et al., 1992; Cohen & Rice, 1995; Loveland-Cherry, Leech, Laetz, & Dielman, 1996); clear rules for expected behavior (Andrews, Hops, Ary, Tildeslye, & Harris, 1993; Oetting & Beauvais, 1987); and consistent, high levels of parental monitoring (Biglan et al., 1995; Dishion, Patterson, Stoolmiller,

& Skinner, 1991; Steinberg, Fletcher, & Darling, 1994). Protective factors have been demonstrated to positively influence adolescents' behavior and also to mediate the effects of risk factors (Brook et al., 1990). The presence of protective factors is consistent with the concept of family resiliency (Johnson, Bryant, Strader, Bucholtz, Berbaum, Collins, & Noe, 1996).

Family risk and protective factors provide direction for developing strategies for prevention; therefore, interventions have been developed to target and be implemented with families. Often the intervention activities are done with parents or are structured to be done interactively by parents and the adolescents. Some of the interventions promote the involvement of the entire family unit. In addition to targeting either select members of the family or the entire family unit, the interventions are targeted to address adolescents and families at different levels of risk.

## LEVEL OF INTERVENTION

Family prevention strategies can be structured at several levels, commonly identified in the substance abuse field as universal, selective, or indicated. Universal prevention programs are directed at the general population; selective programs are designed for individuals or families who have identified risk factors, such as a family history of alcohol addiction; and indicated programs are focused on individuals or families who evidence problem behaviors such as, for adolescents, school problems, destructive behavior, or problems involving school, family, and/or police. Family prevention interventions have been developed that focus on one or more of the three levels.

## TARGETS FOR PREVENTION OF ADOLESCENT SUBSTANCE ABUSE

Initially, family interventions were not common in prevention of adolescent alcohol use. By far, the largest number of programs for preventing adolescent substance use are school-based. Access to large numbers of adolescents is most easily achieved by sampling groups or sites where they congregate, and schools are the most convenient of these settings. Growing recognition of the multiple contexts that influence adolescent substance abuse motivated consideration of alternative targets for intervention. The cumulative evidence supporting the importance of family protective and risk factors directed attention to targeting families for intervention. Interventions targeted at families have been developed both as components of broader programs and as single-component programs. The former interventions are discussed as embedded family interventions and the latter as exclusive family interventions.

## Embedded Family Interventions

Broad-based programs delivered within schools and communities often include a family component. The very nature of these programs, the integrated format, makes it difficult to tease out the effects of each of the specific components, including those targeted at families. These broad-based programs are usually directed at the universal level of prevention, that is, at the general population. Integrated community prevention programs have demonstrated significant reductions in adolescent substance use (Pentz, Dwyer, et al., 1989; Perry et al., 1996). Embedded family interventions generally are components of either a community-based or a school-based intervention. Reports of six embedded family interventions were identified. Although there may be similarities in the embedded family interventions in community- and school-based programs, the differences are significant enough that they are reviewed separately.

### COMMUNITY-BASED EMBEDDED FAMILY INTERVENTIONS

Reports of three programs (Midwestern Prevention Project, Project Northland, Creating Lasting Connections) that met the previously stated criteria for community-based embedded family interventions were found. All of the reported programs are examples of community-based trials using a multicomponent, multilevel approach. Two of the programs, the Midwestern Prevention Project (Pentz et al., 1989; Rohrbach et al., 1995) and the Project Northland (Perry et al., 1993, 1996; Williams et al., 1999), were reported in multiple publications.

*Conceptual Approach.*    Conceptual approaches for community-based adolescent substance abuse prevention programs are primarily integrated models that incorporate appropriate components from a variety of theories focused at various system levels. Wagenaar and Perry (1995), in their review of theories related to alcohol behaviors (e.g., problem behavior theory, social learning theory), cogently illustrate the need to consider multiple levels of factors, and they propose an integrated theory of drinking. The Creating Lasting Connections program is based on a model that includes community engagement, parent resiliency, and youth resiliency as predictors of adolescent outcomes. The Midwestern Prevention Project and Project Northland are conceptualized within comprehensive ecological models that include influences from multiple levels of the social environment, including individual, family, peer group, school, and community.

*Format and Content.*    The Midwestern Prevention Project and Project Northland incorporate a school-based component, a community involvement or organization component, and a parent education and organization component. A mass media program also is included within the Midwestern

Prevention Project. The Creating Lasting Connections project focused intervention on church communities, families, and individual youth.

The Midwestern Prevention Project consisted of a 10-session youth educational program on skills training for resistance of drug use, 10 homework sessions involving active interviews and role plays with parents and family members, and mass media coverage (Pentz, Dwyer, et al., 1989, p. 3260). The program component was titled Indiana Students Taught Awareness and Resistance (STAR). The family component included parent-child homework assignments, parent organization at school sites, parenting skills training workshops, and parent participation in community organization activities. Homework assignments were made as part of the youth educational sessions in science or health education classes and completed with parents and family members. Follow-up on the homework was part of the classroom component. At each of participating schools, a program implementation committee, consisting of the school principal, a school staff member, student peer leaders, and parents who were active in school activities, was established. These committees coordinated both the parenting skills workshops and other school-based activities for parents. Parents and children participated in the two-session parenting skills workshops focused on increasing parent-child communication, the establishment of family rules and expectations, and parental support of drug-free behaviors. At the community level, parents were encouraged to participate in a community coalition and on subcommittees that targeted parent-child program issues.

Each year of the Northland Project interventions was developed around a theme: Slick Tracy Home Team Program, Amazing Alternatives! and Power Lines. Within each of these themes, complementary components—behavioral curricula, peer leadership, parental involvement, and community changes—were developed and implemented. For the behavioral curricula, teachers were trained to implement classroom sessions. Selected and volunteer peer leaders were involved in training sessions and coordinating alcohol-free events, producing a regional newsletter. At the community level, task forces were established to support the adolescent groups and other alcohol-free activities, and press releases were distributed for publication in local newspapers and school newsletters. The parental component included parent-child activities using a comic book format, a newsletter with alcohol-related parenting suggestions, events at the schools, facilitators for local teen groups, and membership on community task forces.

The Creating Lasting Connections takes a different approach from the broad community one used in the Midwestern Prevention Project and Northland projects. The goal of the intervention was to build community, family, and youth resiliency through church communities. Church Advocacy Team (CAT) members were recruited from the church communities and trained in the study purposes and protocols. CATs then recruited high-risk families to participate in the parent/guardian and youth component of the program. Activities included participation in training modules and follow-up case management services.

All of the community-based embedded family interventions attended to the developmental level of the participating adolescents and their families in designing program components. Consideration of developmental issues is especially well illustrated in the program components at each grade level in Project Northland. Since the intervention was conducted over 3 years, it was important to vary the activities according to current issues that adolescents and their families are facing. In the first year, grade 6, the parent intervention component used a comic book format and related activities around an appealing character, Slick Tracy. In the second year, grade 7 parents are involved with Amazing Alternatives! and working with the student groups. By year 3, grade 8 parents are invited to attend a play that models parent-child communication and to plan an alcohol-free party. Activities at each year address the age-appropriate issues for adolescents.

*Population.*    Adolescents and their families were recruited through schools in the Midwestern Prevention Project and Project Northland. For the Midwestern Prevention Project, 22,500 students were enrolled from sixth or seventh grades in 15 communities in the Kansas City metropolitan area and from three cohorts of students from 57 middle or junior high schools in 12 school districts in the Indianapolis area. Study participants at both sites were primarily White, 75% and 72%, respectively, reflecting the racial distribution of the communities. In Project Northland, 2,351 primarily White adolescents were recruited from 24 school districts in rural and small towns in Minnesota. For the Creating Lasting Connections project, a total of 486 families were recruited from 14 African American urban (four) and White suburban (three) and rural (seven) church communities, but analyses were based on 97 parents/guardians and 120 youth ages 12–14 who had complete data from three waves of data collection. The characteristics of the subset of participants used for the analyses could not be determined from the information presented. No analyses comparing the effects of the intervention by racial or ethnic group were evident.

*Level of Intervention.*    Both the Midwestern Prevention Project and Project Northland interventions were developed at the universal level, for the general population. In the Creating Lasting Connections project, the CATs were trained to recruit families with characteristics that would place them at highest risk for substance use. The characteristics were not specified in the publication. Consequently, specific classification of the level of the intervention was not possible but was inferred to be at the selective level—those families and individuals with identified risk factors for substance use.

*Adequacy of Design.*    All of the community-based embedded programs used controlled designs to evaluate outcomes of the interventions. The Midwestern Prevention Project used a quasi-experimental design in Kansas City and a randomized experimental design in Indianapolis. In Project Northland, schools or school districts were randomized either to the intervention condition or to a reference or delayed program control condition; repeated measures with four waves of data collection were used. A randomized block design with repeated measures (three waves) was used in the family and youth components of the Creating Lasting Connections.

*Magnitude and Duration of Effects.*    As would be expected from a developmental perspective, overall substance use increased in the samples for all three projects. Short-term and long-term effects were measured for all three programs but for different variables and at different time points. No direct effects on alcohol and other drug (AOD) use were proposed in the Creating Lasting Connections program because the literature consistently supports no direct effects for programs lasting 1 year or less. However, indirect effects on adolescent AOD through the moderator of family resiliency were proposed and supported. Parents in the intervention group demonstrated an increase in AOD resiliency. Short-term effects (measured at 6–7 months) were noted for AOD use. As parents increased their AOD knowledge and beliefs, decreased their quantity of smoking tobacco products, and decreased their likelihood of punishing adolescents for misconduct, adolescents experienced delayed onset of alcohol use. Delay in other drug use was found as parents increased adolescents' involvement in setting non-AOD family rules and positive family communication and self-image and decreased their frequency of alcohol use and family conflict, and family pathology. Long-term effects (measured at 1 year) on AOD use were found as a number of the direct effects on parents' resiliency were sustained. Short-term effects were measured at 6–7 months and long-term effects at 1 year.

In Project Northland, effects were measured each spring following the initial intervention year. Results support significant effects of the intervention in reducing the onset and prevalence of alcohol use, tobacco use, and changes in specific predictive factors.

In the Midwestern Prevention Project, short-term effects (at 1 year postintervention) on decreasing alcohol, tobacco, and marijuana use were evident for adolescents receiving the intervention. Long-term effects (3 years) were found for reducing tobacco and marijuana use but not for alcohol use.

## SCHOOL-BASED EMBEDDED FAMILY INTERVENTIONS

The four identified embedded family interventions were components of school-based programs: Metropolitan Area Child Study, Keep a Clear Mind,

Adolescent Transitions Program, and Start Taking Alcohol Risks Seriously (STARS). This set of intervention programs differed from many of the more traditional school-based programs in that they had an embedded family intervention and may or may not have had a classroom intervention. The Metropolitan Area Child Study, Keep a Clear Mind, and Adolescent Transitions Program each has a classroom component. STARS for Families Program does not have a classroom component but provides standardized health consultations by nurses in the school setting.

***Conceptual Approach.*** All of the school-based embedded programs were based on an identified conceptual model. The Metropolitan Area Child Study program builds on a family systems perspective that integrates components of functional, sequential, structural-strategic, and psychoeducational approaches (Tolan & McKay, 1996).

The STARS project is based on the Multi-component Motivational Stages prevention model (Werch, 1997; Werch, Pappas, Carlson, & DiClemente, 1999). The model builds on the stages of change in habits from the transtheoretical model (Prochaska & DiClemente, 1983). Keep a Clear Mind is based on a social skills model; the description of the theoretical model for Keep a Clear Mind is limited to a general statement (Werch, Young, Clark, Garrett, Hooks, & Kersten, 1991).

The Adolescent Transitions Program is based on a social interactional framework and uses a multiple gating model approach to parent intervention. The latter "can best be described as a tiered strategy, with each level of intervention building on the previous one" (Dishion, Kavanagh, & Kiesner, 1998).

***Format and Content.*** Metropolitan Area Child Study consists of three increasingly intensive levels of intervention "designed to increase prosocial behavior and problem-solving skills and decrease use of aggression" (Tolan & McKay). The first level is focused on enhancing the classroom programs; the second level adds peer relationship training, and the third level combines the peer relationship training and a family intervention. The family intervention has 20 sessions organized in five phases; the first five sessions include preengagement, joining and assessment, and problem identification. The remaining sessions allocate two sessions each to monitoring, family rules, reframing, accenting the positive, and listening skills. The program incorporates four modes of intervention: family groups, individual meeting with families, weekly telephone calls, and homework assignments.

The multiple gating approach (interventions at multiple levels—universal, selective, indicated) used in Adolescent Transitions Program directs the three components that build on each other: Family Resource Room includes the use of self-check exercises, books, videotapes, media on effective parenting and norms, classroom-based parent-child exercises that support family management practices, dissemination of specific information, and screening and assessment. The next level of the intervention, Family Check-Up, consists of an assessment of strengths and needs of the adolescent and family and a family feedback session. Motivational interviewing is used to complete the assessment, and the FRAMES model (Miller & Rollnick, 1991) guides the family feedback session. The acronym FRAMES stands for feedback, responsibility, advice, menu of intervention options, empathy, and self-efficacy. The third level of the intervention, Family Intervention, involves the use of "several protocols by behavioral, structural, and eclectic family therapists working with problematic adolescents" (Dishion et al., 1998, p. 218).

The STARS program combines two strategies: a standardized health consultation by a nurse and mailed prevention postcards to parents. The nurse completes the health consultation, using a standardized checklist of 12 risk factors for substance use, and incorporates preintervention data to target the intervention. The mailed postcards contain key facts that were tailored to address a risk factor specific to the parent's adolescent child, based on preintervention data. Parents received up to 10 postcards (Werch et al., 1999).

In the Keep a Clear Mind program, adolescents received four weekly lessons: alcohol, tobacco, marijuana, and tool for avoiding drugs. The weekly topic was introduced by either a project assistant or the classroom teacher, and then the lesson was distributed to the children to take home and complete with their parents. Assignments were to be returned by the end of the week (Werch et al., 1991).

*Population.*    The school-based embedded family interventions were implemented with diverse populations. The Metropolitan Area Child Study recruited children identified as being "at risk for developing serious antisocial behavior due to elevated aggression compared to classmate" from four schools randomly assigned to the family interventions component. The children were from grades 2, 3, and 5 and were selected on the basis of ratings by teachers on the Teacher's Report Form and rated by peers as being disruptive or socially rejected. Just over half of the children (54%) were from a suburban low-income community and the remainder (46%) from an inner-city community. The sample included 327 African American (40.9%), Latino (37.6%), White (21%), and other (0.5%) families.

In the Keep a Clear Mind project, the participants were 511 students from 23 fourth-, fifth-, and sixth-grade classes from six elementary school in two adjacent school districts in northwest Arkansas. The students were mostly (93%) White and had a mean age of 10.4 years. Parents ($n = 1,022$) of the students also were participants.

Participants in the STARS program were 650 sixth-grade students recruited from a neighborhood and a bused middle school in the economically disadvantaged inner city of Jacksonville, Florida. Children had to be enrolled in school and have less than 50% absenteeism to be eligible for the study. The sample consisted of African American (85%), Caucasian (12%), and other (3%) students.

In the Adolescent Transitions Program, 119 families of high-risk adolescents participated in the multilevel intervention. Participants were recruited from schools in Oregon, screened for risk status, and randomly assigned to one of four conditions. A second sample, of 39 families, was recruited as a quasi-experimental control.

*Level of Intervention.*    The interventions for the school-based embedded family programs were structured across all three levels: universal, selective, and indicated. The Metropolitan Area Child Study intervention focused on high-risk children and would be considered selective. Both the STARS and Keep a Clear Mind programs were universal interventions directed at lower risk children. The Adolescent Transitions Program was unique in its use of a multiple gating approach that included universal, selective, and indicated components with at-risk families.

*Adequacy of Design.*    The Metropolitan Area Child Study, Keep a Clear Mind, STAR, and Adolescent Transitions Program all used a randomized, controlled, repeated-measures design. Measures of study variables were completed prior to the intervention, with postintervention measures at varying times—immediately, 6 months, and 1 year postintervention.

*Magnitude and Duration of Effects.*    Outcome variables and effects of the interventions varied. Some programs measured recent (7-day and 30-day) alcohol use (STARS, Adolescent Transitions Program ), heavy drinking (STARS), and intention to use alcohol in the future (STARS, Keep a Clear Mind). Some measured parent variables in addition to adolescent variables (Adolescent Transitions Program, Keep a Clear Mind, Metropolitan Area Child Study). The results of two pilot studies of the STARS program support a reduction in adolescents' alcohol use, as well as positive changes in adolescents' perceptions of adult drinking, susceptibility to alcohol problems, and intention to stop or reduce drinking (Werch, 1997).

Results of the Adolescent Transitions Program intervention provide interesting insights into possible untoward effects from specific components. For participants assigned to the parent focus and 10 focus conditions, there were immediate reductions in observed and reported family conflict. Additionally, participants in the parent focus showed improvements in problem behaviors at school and in tobacco use. The foci that brought high-risk adolescents together, however, resulted in increases in problem behaviors at school and in tobacco use (Dishion & Andrews, 1995).

## Exclusive Family Interventions

A third group of prevention programs is focused on and limited to intervention directly with the family. In contrast to family interventions that are embedded within a broader program, these interventions are developed specifically for and are implemented with families. Reports of seven exclusive family interventions were reviewed: Strengthening Families Program/ Iowa Strengthening Families Program (Kumpfer, 1998; Kumpfer, Molgaard, & Spoth, 1996; Spoth, Redmond, & Lepper, 1999); Preparing for the Drug Free Years (Catalano, Kosterman, Hagerty, Hawkins, & Spoth, 1998; Spoth, Redmond, Haggerty, & Ward, 1995); Family Effectiveness Training (Szapocznik, Santisteban, Rio, Perez-Vidal, Santisteban, & Kurines, 1989); Michigan State University Multiple Risk Child Outreach Program (Maguin, Zucker, & Fitzgerald, 1994; Nye, Zucker, & Fitzgerald, 1999); Parent-Based Intervention Strategies to Reduce Adolescent Alcohol-Impaired Driving (Jaccard & Turrisi, 1999); Child and Parent Relations (Loveland-Cherry et al., 1999); and SUPER STARS (Emshoff, Avery, Raduka, Anderson, & Calvert, 1996). Two of the interventions, Strengthening Families Program and Preparing for the Drug Free Years, have been implemented in more than one study, and the intervention by Jaccard is in the process of being implemented.

CONCEPTUAL APPROACH

A variety of theoretical models provide the direction for the exclusive family interventions. Several, but not all, of the theoretical approaches included a focus on risk and protective factors from different perspectives. The Strengthening Families Program has been guided by three models: originally, the Values-Attitudes-Stressors-Coping Skills and Resources Model, then the Resiliency Model and the Social Ecology Model of Adolescent Substance Use (Kumpfer, 1998; Kumpfer et al., 1996). Preparing for the Drug Free Years is guided by the social development model, an integration of social control, social learning, and differential association theories (Catalano et al., 1998). Family Effectiveness Training is focused on family patterns of interaction and intergenerational conflict conceptualized as constituting the high-risk syndrome (Szapocznik et al., 1989). A intergenerational risk model that "incorporates a broadly based, systemic model that includes a focus on family factors as well as individual child factors" underlies the work of Zucker and colleagues (Maguin et al., 1994, p. 106). The program for Adolescent Drunk Driving is based on Jaccard's behavioral alternative model, a specific case of the more general decision theoretical frameworks (Jaccard & Turisi, 1999). The Child and Parent Relations program is guided by a conceptual model that integrates social-cognitive skills, problem behavior, and family systems theories (Loveland-Cherry et al., 1999). SUPER STARS incorporates protective and risk factors from both individual and family perspectives as a basis for the intervention (Emshoff et al., 1996).

## FORMAT AND CONTENT

In contrast to the embedded family interventions, the exclusive family interventions all involved direct contact with either groups of families or individual families. The programs were implemented in schools (Dishion, 1998), churches, and family homes in rural and urban communities (Loveland-Cherry et al., 1999; Nye, Zucker, & Fitzgerald, 1999).

The Strengthening Families Program is "a highly structured, 14-week, comprehensive family-focused curriculum" (Kumpfer, 1998, p. 168). The program is lengthened by 2 weeks if baseline and follow-up measures of families are done. There are three components to the Strengthening Families Program, which are implemented concurrently: (1) parent training, (2) children's skills training, and (3) family skills training. Each of the components is led by trained staff in sessions that last 2½ to 3 hours each. For each session, parents and children attend separate classes for the first hour, work together in family sessions during the second hour, and spend the third hour in meals and family fun activities. The basic approach is to have children and parents learn skills separately and then practice them together in a family group. A 7-week universal modification of the Strengthening Families Program was developed for use with junior high children and their families in Iowa (ISFP).

Preparing for the Drug Free Years is implemented in groups through a series of five 2-hour workshop sessions, with a recently revised format of 10 1-hour sessions for use in workplace settings (Catalano et al., 1998). Trained leaders recruited from the community conduct the workshops. The sessions are supplemented by a family activity book, family meetings, and videotapes. The major topics for the intervention include preventing drug abuse in the family, setting family norms on drugs and alcohol, resisting peer influence through refusal skills, managing family conflict, and strengthening family bonds.

Zucker and colleagues (Nye et al., 1999) designed a program consisting of approximately 28 sessions implemented in two phases over a 10-month period. In the first phase, child management skills were emphasized in weekly sessions and two between-sessions telephone contacts. When families successfully acquired the parenting skills, biweekly sessions and weekly telephone contacts were provided in the second phase "to support and reinforce the child management techniques" and address significant marital and other family problems.

The Family Effectiveness Training program was designed for Hispanic families of preadolescents who are at risk for future drug abuse. The intervention consists of 13 weekly sessions of 1.5 to 2 hours, which are conducted by a facilitator. The Family Effectiveness Training program is operationalized within the Strategic Structural Systems approach developed by Szapocznik, Santisteban, Rio, Perez-Vidal, Santisteban, and Kurtines (1989), which evolved from Minuchin's (1974) structural family systems work, and Haley's (1973) and Madanes's (1981) strategic concepts. The 13 sessions cover three components: family development, bicultural effectiveness training, and strategic structural family systems therapy.

The goal of the Child and Parent Relations program is to develop parent and family assets that are proposed to maximize protective factors and minimize parent and family risk factors, with the ultimate goal of reducing adolescent alcohol use and misuse. Parents participated in three hour-long in-home sessions, with family meetings afterward, and follow-up telephone calls. The intervention was implemented when the child was in the last year of elementary school, with a booster intervention in seventh grade. The sessions focused on general parenting skills and family functioning as well as on factors specific to alcohol use and misuse.

The SUPER STARS consisted of nine 2-hour sessions for children ages 6–11 years and their parents or surrogate parents held at a local agency, such as a boys' or girls' club. Participants completed seven core sessions within 2 weeks and two booster or family reunion sessions at 1 and 3 months after the core sessions. Two versions of the program were created, one primarily African American families and one for families from diverse ethnic groups. The intervention focused on enhancing individual and family protective factors and minimizing risk factors within a framework of prosocial bonding. The program is organized around the importance of family and culture. Sessions were implemented with groups of families, usually with 8 to 10 families.

## POPULATION

The exclusive family interventions were evaluated with a variety of families of both elementary school age children and adolescents in rural and urban areas. The selective level interventions (Strengthening Families Program, Family Effectiveness Training, Nye, Zucker, & Fitzgerald, 1999) were implemented with families with a family member with identified substance abuse problems. The universal interventions were implemented with diverse families from the general population. Two interventions, Strengthening Families Program and Preparing for the Drug Free Years, have been implemented in multiple settings with diverse populations.

The Strengthening Families Program has been implemented with a variety of populations in urban and rural areas. The elementary age (6–12 years old) intervention was developed with a sample of 71 intervention families, 47 no-treatment matched families, and 90 families from the general population in Salt Lake City. The program was modified and evaluated with African American families in Alabama and Detroit, with multiethnic families in Utah, with Asian and Pacific Islander families in Hawaii, and with Hispanic families in Denver. The modified universal intervention for junior high students and their families was implemented with 446 families of sixth graders in rural Iowa as part of Project Family (Spoth, Redmond, Hockaday, & Shin, 1996).

Preparing for the Drug Free Years has been implemented in seven studies with primarily white families (84%–90%), with one exception: a sample of Hispanic, African American, Samoan, and Native American families in the Seattle area. The samples ranged from 24 families of pediatric patients in HMO clinics to 759 families from the general population. One sample consisted of families who viewed a TV special and subsequently attended workshops. Most recently, the intervention has been implemented and evaluated with rural Iowa families as part of Project Family (Spoth et al., 1996).

The Zucker intervention was implemented with families with at least one parent with an alcohol abuse problem and a target male child between the ages of 3 and 5 years recruited from local district court records of men convicted of driving while impaired or driving under the influence of liquor. All of the men met the diagnostic criteria for probable or definite alcoholism. The 52 eligible families were assigned to studies with both parents participating or only the mother participating.

The Family Effectiveness Training program was specifically designed for Hispanic families with high-risk preadolescents. The sample for the study consisted of 79 such families who had come to a treatment center seeking assistance for a behavioral or psychological problem in a child 6 to 12 years of age and had maladaptive interactions . The greatest proportion of the sample was Cuban (76%).

Participants in the Child and Parents Relations study were two cohorts of 428 adolescents and their parents recruited from three midwestern school districts. One cohort was primarily White (86%), and the other had approximately equal proportions of African American and White participants.

Participants in the African American version of the SUPER STARS program consisted of 290 parents or parent surrogates and 382 children from low-income neighborhoods in Atlanta. Nearly all of the participants (96.9%) described themselves as African American, most (79.9%) were female, and 81.4% of the adults were partners of the parent of the study child.

## LEVEL OF INTERVENTION

Exclusive family interventions included both universal- and selective-level foci. The Strengthening Families Program is a selective-level intervention with two versions that target different high-risk populations: elementary school–age children of drug abusers and their families and high-risk junior high school students and their families. Other selective-level interventions included the Family Effectiveness Training, SUPER STARS, and the very early intervention by Nye, Zucker, and Fitzgerald (1999). Preparing for the Drug Free Years, Child and Parent Relations, and the Parent Intervention to Reduce Adolescent Alcohol-Impaired Driving are all universal-level interventions.

## ADEQUACY OF DESIGN

Generally, the exclusive family interventions have been evaluated in clinical trials using randomized repeated-measures design. For those programs, such as the Strengthening Families Program and Preparing for the Drug Free Years, that have been implemented as demonstration projects, a noncontrolled pretest-posttest design was used to evaluate both process and outcomes; this same design was used to evaluate the SUPER STARS program. The use of a Solomon Four Group design in two studies (Loveland-Cherry et al., 1999; Szapocznik et al., 1989) had a number of drawbacks, including reducing the power of tests of significance by reducing the subsample size and resulting in a number of families without pretest data, which complicated data analyses. The trade-off of evaluating the effects of testing did not compensate for these negative consequences, as no significant testing effect was found. In fact, a randomized, controlled repeated-measures design was selected for the second phase of the Child and Parent Relations study rather than the Solomon Four Group design.

## MAGNITUDE AND DURATION OF EFFECTS

As with the embedded family interventions, the outcome variables were not consistent across studies. In some instances, adolescent substance use was considered an outcome variable. In other studies, the effects of the intervention on parent behaviors and attitudes; family functioning; and adolescents' self-concept, self-efficacy, self-esteem, and/or problem behaviors were measured.

Effects for the Strengthening Families Program were most evident when all three components of the intervention were implemented as a package. For the integrated intervention, children's risk and protective factors for drug use improved, and tobacco and alcohol use decreased in older children who had already reported use of these substances. Parents reported reduced drug use and increased parenting efficacy (Kumpfer, 1998). Results of a 5-year follow-up from a quasi-experimental evaluation of implementation of the Strengthening Families Program support the maintenance of positive changes in parenting skills and family functioning. With some exceptions, positive results have been documented in the replications with diverse populations. Preliminary results from an experimental design study support positive effects on parent-child affective quality, intervention-targeted behaviors, and general child management from pretest to posttest (Kumpfer, 1998) and effects of moderate magnitude in reduction in alcohol initiation at 1- and 2-year follow-up of the Iowa Strengthening Families Program (Spoth, Redmond, & Lepper, 1999).

Across the experimental studies of the Preparing for the Drug Free Years effectiveness, there is evidence of improvement in targeted parenting behaviors, general child management, and parent-child affective quality (Catalano et al., 1998). The effects are evident at 1-year follow-up. Other evaluation has focused on recruitment and participation in the intervention.

In the Family Effectiveness Training program, measures of current dysfunction in the identified child and in family structure and functioning were examined at 13 weeks following interventions and at 6 months following the clinical extension. Findings for children indicate positive effects on behavior, personality, inadequacy problems, and feelings about themselves and, for families, improvements in family structure, resonance, and developmental stage. Effects on measures of family environment were evident only on the fathers' perception of expressiveness.

Findings through a 4-year follow-up for one cohort of participants and through a 3-year follow-up for the second cohort indicate that adolescents in the Child and Parent Relations program condition had decreased alcohol use and misuse compared to those in the control condition. Further, the effects seem to be evident for adolescents who reported no prior drinking at pretest. No effects of the intervention on parenting and family measures were evident.

Both process and outcomes were evaluated for the SUPER STARS program. Results of the process evaluation indicated that the leaders were well trained; there was high implementation fidelity and positive reactions from participants. Significant pretest-posttest changes were observed for children's feeling good about their family, themselves, and their looks; pride in family history; how they feel; the importance of learning about Africa; and their choosing not to fight. For parents, there were significant positive differences in family cohesion, parental behavior, racial pride, family communication, and conflict resolution. No significant differences in children's drug use were observed, but the numbers of children reporting drug use were small, ranging form one to three individuals.

## CONCLUSIONS

The interventions and studies reviewed were impressive both in the scope of the variables that were targeted for intervention, the use of theory-based strategies, the strengths of the designs, the diversity of the populations, and the demonstrated effects of the interventions. Demonstrating the effectiveness of prevention interventions is difficult and can be costly. Studies have been more successful in demonstrating short-term effectiveness than long-term outcomes. A related issue is that of costs and benefits. Few studies evaluate the cost of interventions or the feasibility of implementing the interventions outside the context of a research project.

The notion that it is more effective to target interventions to specific at-risk groups has received increased support. Universal interventions can be directed toward the general population (primary prevention, health promotion) or targeted to specific groups: subgroups that are identified as being at high risk and in the early stages of problem behaviors (secondary prevention, early intervention) or specific groups or individuals who evidence problem behaviors (tertiary prevention, treatment and rehabilitation). Debate continues on where the emphasis for interventions is most effective in this continuum. Botvin, Baker, Dusenbury, Tortu, and Botvin (1990) argue for the effectiveness and efficiency of a focus on groups identified as high risk. A counterargument is that all adolescents are at risk for the major factors that potentially affect their health and that intervening at the universal level is most cost-effective. The evidence for the level of choice for intervention is equivocal and will require multiple controlled studies to determine adequately which approach is most effective.

## Implications for Nursing Practice

Nursing, as a practice discipline, has numerous opportunities to intervene in the prevention of adolescent substance abuse and thereby reduce the incidence of chronic conditions associated with substance use. Families have long been an identified client group for nursing intervention. The empirical evidence for the effectiveness of family interventions to reduce adolescent substance use is sufficiently established to provide direction for nursing intervention in this area.

Traditionally, the majority of nurses practice in settings and within reimbursement structures that are more conducive to a focus on individuals. However, recent shifts in health care emphasize the need to focus on population-based interventions implemented by collaborative, multidisciplinary teams. Nursing has expertise in the areas of family, health behavior change, and health promotion that can make valuable contributions to reducing adolescent substance use.

## Directions for Future Research

Recommendations for future research in the area of use of family interventions to decrease adolescent substance use are clearly and concisely summarized by Etz, Robertson, and Ashery (1998) within six categories: (1) etiology, (2) prevention intervention content, (3) research methodology, (4) prevention methodology, (5) dissemination, and (6) prevention services research. Considerable evidence exists regarding the factors that influence adolescent substance use. How these factors interact and the degree of impact for subgroups (e.g., racial/ethnic groups, males vs. females) is less well understood. The studies reviewed employed a number of different strategies with families. The relative impact of various approaches with diverse populations should be evaluated through replication studies. Additional research, focused on determining the most appropriate timing and dosage levels for interventions, is needed.

Major issues related to recruitment and retention of families must be addressed in future research. Although some efforts have been made to tailor interventions to meet specific needs of certain families, much remains to be done to identify the dimensions that are most critical for consideration in targeting families to maximize effects. Additional research also is needed in the areas of costs of interventions and the feasibility of implementing interventions in nonresearch contexts.

Targeting families for prevention of adolescent substance use is an area of research with considerable potential for decreasing chronic conditions. Nursing has much to contribute to building the knowledge basic to prevention intervention with families and yet has played a limited role in this important field of study.

## REFERENCES

Abbey, A., Ross, L. T., & McDuffie, D. (1994). Alcohol's role in sexual assault. In R. R. Watson (Ed.), *Drug and alcohol abuse reviews: Vol. 5. Addictive behaviors in women* (pp. 97–123). Totowa, NJ: Humana Press.

Andrews, J. A., Hops, H., Ary, D., Tildesley, E., & Harris, J. (1993). Parental influence in early adolescent substance use: Specific and nonspecific effects. *Journal of Early Adolescence, 13*, 285–310.

Arria, A. M., Dohey, M. A., Mezzich, A. C., Bukstein, O. G., & Van Thiel, D. H. (1995). Self-reported health problems and physical symptomatology in adolescent alcohol abusers. *Journal of Adolescent Health, 16*, 226–231.

Barnes, G. M., & Windle, M. (1987). Family factors in adolescent alcohol and drug abuse. *Pediatrician, 14*, 13–18.

Baumrind, D. (1991). The influence of parenting style on adolescent competence and substance use. *Journal of Early Adolescence, 11*(1), 56–95.

Biglan, A., Duncan, T. E., Ary, D. V., & Smolkowski, K. (1995). Peer and parental influences on adolescent tobacco use. *Journal of Behavioral Medicine, 18*(4), 315–330.

Botvin, G. J., Baker, E., Dusenbury, L., Tortu, S., & Botvin, E. M. (1990). Preventing adolescent drug abuse through a multimodal cognitive-behavioral approach: Results of a 3-year study. *Journal of Consulting and Clinical Psychology, 58*(4), 437–446.

Brook, J. S., Brook, D. W., Gordon, A. S., Whiteman, M., & Cohen, P. (1990). The psychosocial etiology of adolescent drug use: A family interactional approach. *Genetic, Social and General Psychology Monographs, 116*(2), 111–267.

Brook, J. S., Whiteman, M., Balka, E. B., & Hamburg, B. A. (1992). African-American and Puerto Rican drug use: Personality, familial, and other environmental risk factors. *Genetic, Social, and General Psychology Monographs, 118*(4), 417–438.

Catalano, R. F., Kosterman, R., Hagerty, K., Hawkins, J. D., & Spoth, R. L. (1998). A universal intervention for the prevention of substance abuse: Preparing for the Drug-Free Years. *National Institute on Drug Abuse Research Monograph, 177,* 130–159.

Clapper, R. L., Buka, S. L., Goldfield, E. C., Lipsitt, L. P., & Tsuang, M. T. (1995). Adolescent problem behaviors as predictors of adult alcohol diagnoses. *International Journal of the Addictions, 30*(5), 507–523.

Claridge, G., Ross, E., & Hume, W. I. (1978). *Personality differences and biological variations.* Oxford: Pergamon Press.

Cohen, D. A., & Rice, J. C. (1995). A parent-targeted intervention for adolescent substance use prevention: Lessons learned. *Evaluation Review, 19*(2), 159–180.

Dielman, T. E., Butchart, A. T., & Shope, J. T. (1993). Structural equation model tests of patterns of family interaction, peer alcohol use, and intrapersonal predictors of adolescent alcohol use and misuse. *Journal of Drug Education, 23,* 273–316.

Dielman, T. E., Butchart, A. T., Shope, J. T., & Miller, M. (1990–1991). Environmental correlates of adolescent substance use and misuse: Implications for prevention programs. *International Journal of the Addictions, 25*(7A & 8A), 855–880.

Dishion, T. J., Kavanagh, K., & Kiesner, J. (1998). Prevention of early adolescent substance abuse among high-risk youth: A multiple gating approach to parent intervention. *National Institute on Drug Abuse Research Monograph, 177,* 208–228.

Dishion, T. J., Patterson, G. R., Stoolmiller, M., & Skinner, M. L. (1991). Family, school, and behavioral antecedents to early adolescents' involvement with antisocial peers. *Developmental Psychology, 27,* 172–180.

Eggert, L. L., Thompson, E. A., Herting, J. R., & Nicholas, L. J. (1995). Reducing suicide potential among high-risk youth: Tests of a school-based prevention program. *Suicide and Life-Threatening Behavior, 25,* 276–296.

Emshoff, J., Avery, E., Raduka, G., Anderson, D. J., & Calvert, C. (1996). Findings from SUPER STARS: A health promotion program for families to enhance multiple protective factors. *Journal of Adolescent Research, 11,* 68–96.

Etz, K. E., Robertson, E. B., & Ashery, R. S. (1998). Drug abuse prevention through family-based interventions: Future research. *National Institute on Drug Abuse Research Monograph, 177,* 1–11.

Grove, W. M., Eckert, E. D., Heston, L., Bouchard, T. J., Segal, N., & Lykken, D. T. (1990). Heritability of substance abuse and antisocial behavior: A study of monozygotic twins reared apart. *Biological Psychology, 27,* 1293–1304.

Gurling, H. M., Grant, S., & Dangl, J. (1985). The genetic and cultural transmission of alcohol use, alcoholism, cigarette smoking and coffee drinking: A review and an example using a log linear cultural transmission model. *British Journal of the Addictions, 80*(3), 269–279.

Haley, J. (1973). *Uncommon therapy.* New York: W. W. Norton.

Hawkins, J. D., Catalano, R. F., & Miller, J. Y. (1992). Risk and protective factors for alcohol and other drug problems in adolescence and early adulthood: Implications for substance abuse prevention. *Psychological Bulletin, 112*(1), 64–105.

Jaccard, J., & Turrisi, R. (1999). Parent-based intervention strategies to reduce adolescent alcohol-impaired driving. *Journal of Studies on Alcohol,* (Suppl. 13), 84–93.

Jang, K. L., Livesly, W. J., & Vernon, P. A. (1995). Alcohol and drug problems: A multivariate behavioral genetic analysis of co-morbidity. *Addiction, 90,* 1213–1221.

Johnson, C. A., Pentz, M. A., Weber, M. D., Dwyer, J. H., Baer, N., MacKinnon, D. P., & Hansen, W. B. (1990). Relative effectiveness of comprehensive community programming for drug abuse prevention with high-risk and low-risk adolescents. *Journal of Consulting and Clinical Psychology, 58*(4), 447–456.

Johnson, K., Bryant, D., Strader, T., Bucholtz, G., Berbaum, M., Collins, D., & Noe, T. (1996). Reducing alcohol and other drug use by strengthening community, family, and youth resiliency: An evaluation of the Creating Lasting Connections program. *Journal of Adolescent Research, 11,* 36–67.

Johnson, V., & Pandina, R. J. (1991). Effects of the family environment on adolescent substance use, delinquency, and coping styles. *American Journal of Drug and Alcohol Abuse, 17*(1), 71–88.

Johnston, L. D., O'Malley, P. M., & Bachman, J. G. (1998a). Drug use by American young people begins to turn downward [On-line].

Johnston, L. D., O'Malley, P. M., & Bachman, J. G. (1998b). *National survey results on drug use from Monitoring the Future study, 1975–1997.* Washington, DC: U.S. Government Printing Office.

Johnston, L. D., O'Malley, P. M., & Bachman, J. G. (1999). *National survey results on drug use from the Monitoring the Future study, 1975–1998. Vol. 1: Secondary school students.* Rockville, MD: National Institute on Drug Abuse. [Web page]. Manuscript in preparation.

Kandel, D. B., Yamaguchi, K., & Chen, K. (1992). Stages of progression in drug involvement from adolescence to adulthood: Further evidence for the gateway theory. *Journal of Studies on Alcohol, 53,* 447–457.

Kumpfer, K. L. (1998). Selective prevention interventions: The Strengthening Families program. *National Institute on Drug Abuse Research Monograph, 177,* 160–207.

Kumpfer, K. L., Molgaard, V., & Spoth, R. (1996). The strengthening families program for the prevention of delinquency and drug use. In R. D. Peters & R. J. McMahon (Eds.), *Preventing childhood disorders, substance abuse, and delinquency* (pp. 241–267). Thousand Oaks, CA: Sage.

Loveland-Cherry, C. J., Leech, S. L., Laetz, V. B., & Dielman, T. E. (1996). Correlates of alcohol use and misuse in 4th grade children: Psychosocial, peer, parental and family factors. *Health Education Quarterly, 23*(4), 497–511.

Loveland-Cherry, C. J., Ross, L. T., & Kaufman, S. R. (1999). Effects of a home-based family intervention on adolescent alcohol use and misuse. *Journal of Studies on Alcohol,* (Suppl. 13), 94–102.

Lowry, R., Holtzman, D., Truman, B. I., Kann, L., Collins, J. L., & Kolbe, L. J. (1994). Substance use and HIV-related sexual behaviors among U.S. high school students: Are they related? *American Journal of Public Health, 84,* 1116–1120.

Madanes, C. (1981). *Strategic family therapy.* San Francisco: Jossey-Bass.

Maguin, E., Zucker, R. A., & Fitzgerald, H. E. (1994). The path to alcohol problems through conduct problems: A family-based approach to very early intervention with risk. *Journal of Research on Adolescence, 4,* 249–269.

Merikangas, K. R., Dierker, L., & Fenton, B. (1998). Familial factors and substance abuse: Implications for prevention. *National Institute on Drug Abuse Research Monograph, 177,* 12–41.

Miller, W. R., & Rollnick, S. (1991). *Motivational interviewing: Preparing people to change addictive behavior.* New York: Guilford Press.

Minuchin, S. (1974). *Families and family therapy.* Cambridge, MA: Harvard University Press.

National Institute on Drug Abuse. (1997). *Ninth special report to the U.S. Congress on alcohol and health.* (National Institute of Health Publication No. 97-4017). Bethesda, MD: Author.

Nye, C. L., Zucker, R. A., & Fitzgerald, H. E. (1999). Early family-based intervention in the path to alcohol problems: Rationale and relationship between treatment process characteristics and child and parenting outcomes. *Journal of Studies on Alcohol,* (Suppl. 13), 10–21.

Oetting, E. R., & Beauvais, F. (1987). Common elements in youth drug abuse: Peer clusters and other psychosocial factors. *Journal of Drug Issues,* 133–151.

Orpinas, P. K., Basen-Engquist, K., Grunbaum, J. A., & Parcel, G. S. (1995). The co-morbidity of violence-related behaviors with health-risk behaviors in a population of high school students. *Journal of Adolescent Health, 16,* 216–225.

Pedersen, N. (1981). Twin similarity for usage of common drugs. In L. Gedda (Ed.), *Twin Research 3, Part C: Epidemiological and Clinical Studies* (pp. 53–59). New York: Wiley-Liss.

Pentz, M. A., Dwyer, J. H., MacKinnon, D. P., Flay, B. R., Hansen, W. B., Wang, E. Y., & Johnson, C. A. (1989). A multi-community trial for primary prevention of adolescent drug abuse: Effects on drug use prevalence. *Journal of the American Medical Association, 261,* 3259–3266.

Pentz, M. A. MacKinnon, D. P., Flay, B. R., Hansen, W. B., Johnson, C. A., & Dwyer, J. H. (1989). Primary prevention of chronic diseases in adolescence: Effects of the Midwestern Prevention Project on tobacco use. *American Journal of Epidemiology, 130*(4), 713–724.

Perry, C. L., Williams, C. L., Forster, J. L., Wolfson, M., Wagenaar, A. C., Finnegan, J. R., McGovern, P. G., Veblen-Mortenson, S., Komro, K. A., & Anstine, P. S. (1993). Background, conceptualization, and design of a community-wide research program on adolescent alcohol use: Project Northland. *Health Education Research, 8,* 125–136.

Perry, C. L., Williams, C. L., Veblen-Mortenson, S., Toomey, T. L., Komro, K. A., Anstine, P. S., McGovern, P. G., Finnegan, J. R., Forster, J. L., Wagenaar, A. C., & Wolfson, M. (1996). Project Northland: Outcomes of a community-wide alcohol use prevention program during early adolescence. *American Journal of Public Health, 86,* 956–965.

Prochaska, J., & DiClemente, C. D. (1983). Stages and processes of self-change of smoking: Toward an integrative model of self-change. *Journal of Consulting Clinical Psychology, 51,* 390–395.

Rohrbach, L. A., Hodgson, C. S., Broder, B. I., Montgomery, S. B., Flay, B. R., Hansen, W. B., & Pentz, M. A. (1995). Parental participation in drug abuse prevention: Results from the Midwestern Prevention Project. In G. M. Boyd, J. Howard, & R. A. Zucker (Eds.), *Alcohol problems among adolescents: Current directions in prevention research* (pp. 173–195). Hillsdale, NJ: Erlbaum.

Spoth, R., Redmond, C., Haggerty, K., & Ward, T. (1995). A controlled parenting skills outcome study examining individual difference and attendance effects. *Journal of Marriage and the Family, 57,* 449–464.

Spoth, R., Redmond, C., Hockaday, C., & Shin, C. (1996). Barriers to participation in family skills preventive interventions and their evaluations. *Family Relations, 15,* 247–254.

Spoth, R., Redmond, C., & Lepper, H. (1999). Alcohol initiation outcomes of universal family-focused preventive interventions: One- and two-year follow-ups of a controlled study. *Journal of Studies on Alcohol,* (Suppl. 13), 103–111.

Steinberg, L., Fletcher, A., & Darling, N. (1994). Parental monitoring and peer influences on adolescent substance use. *Pediatrics, 93*(6), 1060–1064.

Szapocznik, J., Santisteban, D., Rio, A., Perez-Vidal, A., Santisteban, D., & Kurtines, W. M. (1989). Family effectiveness training: An intervention to prevent drug abuse and problem behaviors in Hispanic adolescents. *Hispanic Journal of Behavioral Sciences, 11*(1), 4–27.

Tolan, P. H., & McKay, M. M. (1996). Preventing serious antisocial behavior in inner-city children: An empirically based family intervention program. *Family Relations, 45,* 148–155.

Wagenaar, A. C., & Perry, C. L. (1995). Community strategies for the reduction of youth drinking: Theory and application. In G. M. Boyd, J. Howard, & R. A. Zucker (Eds.), *Alcohol problems among adolescents: Current directions in prevention research* (pp. 197–223). Hillsdale, NJ: Erlbaum.

Werch, C. E. (1997). Expanding the stages of change: A program matched to the stages of alcohol acquisition. *American Journal of Health Promotion, 12,* 34–37.

Werch, C. E., Pappas, D. M., Carlson, J. M., & DiClemente, C. C. (1999). Six-month outcomes of an alcohol prevention program for inner-city youth. *American Journal of Health Promotion, 13*(4), 237–240.

Werch, C. E., Young, M., Clark, M., Garett, C., Hooks, S., & Kesten, C. (1991). Effects of a take-home drug prevention program on drug-related communication and beliefs of parents and children. *Journal of School Health, 61,* 346–350.

Williams, C. L., Perry, C. L., Farbakhsh, K., & Veblen-Mortenson, S. (1999). Project Northland: Comprehensive alcohol use prevention for young adolescents, their parents, schools, peers and communities. *Journal of Studies on Alcohol,* (Suppl. 13), 112–124.

Chapter 9

# School-Based Interventions for Primary Prevention of Cardiovascular Disease: Evidence of Effects for Minority Populations

JANET C. MEININGER

## ABSTRACT

The purposes of this review were to analyze and evaluate the results of school-based studies that have used population-wide approaches for primary prevention of cardiovascular diseases and to assess the extent to which strategies tested to date have been effective for minority populations in the United States. The literature included in the review was restricted to studies published between 1986 and August 1999; they sampled elementary, middle, or high school students and incorporated a control or comparison group. There were no consistent effects of school-based interventions on blood pressure, lipid profiles, or measures of body mass and obesity. There was evidence that changes in knowledge and health behaviors occurred. Findings are interpreted within the context of population-wide approaches to prevention, and recommendations for future research directions are discussed.

**Key words: adolescents, cardiovascular risk factors, children, primary prevention, school-based interventions**

Atherosclerotic processes begin in childhood, although the clinical consequences may not become apparent until middle or old age (Sternby, Fernandez-Britlo, & Nordet, 1999; Strong et al., 1999). Atherosclerosis not only begins in childhood, but its rate of progression in young adults is linked to elevated risk factors (McGill, McMahan, Malcom, Oalmann, & Strong, 1997; McGill et al., 1998). Recent findings from the Bogalusa autopsy study document a prospective relationship between multiple risk factors and the severity of asymptomatic coronary and aortic atherosclerosis in young persons (Berenson et al., 1998).

Approximately half of all children in the United States exhibit one or more cardiovascular risk factors, with one-fourth to one-third having at least one elevated risk factor at entry to elementary school (Williams & Wynder, 1993). Alarming trends in the United States include an increase between 1986 and 1996 in the prevalence of obesity among 11- to 14-year-olds that is accompanied by an increase in systolic blood pressure (Luepker, Jacobs, Prineas, & Sinaiko, 1999) and a decline in physical activity among youth (Department of Health and Human Services, 1996). Significant ethnic differences in cardiovascular disease risk factors have been documented as early as 6 to 9 years of age and widen with increasing age. Specifically, body mass index was higher for African American and Mexican American girls than for Anglo girls, and blood pressure levels were higher for African American girls than for Anglo girls in every age group. Smoking prevalence was highest for Anglo girls and boys, especially among those from low socioeconomic circumstances (Winkleby, Robinson, Sundquist, & Kraemer, 1999).

The rationale for intervening early in life to prevent cardiovascular diseases is further documented by reports over the past two decades that risk factors and health behaviors in children and adolescents track over time and are predictive of adult profiles (Kelder, Perry, Klepp, & Lytle, 1994; Sinaiko, Donahue, Jacobs, & Prineas, 1998). Because risk factors become established early in life, track from childhood into adulthood, and are linked to the development of atherosclerosis, interventions that begin early in life are essential for primary prevention of cardiovascular diseases.

Preventive interventions are classified as population-wide or high-risk approaches (Rose, 1980). In the population-wide approach, interventions are directed to the entire population or subpopulation and are designed to shift the risk factor distribution of the population downward. In the high-risk approach the aim is to identify particular individuals with elevated risk-factor levels and direct specific programs to those individuals to lower their risk. Any substantial impact on the incidence of disease can be achieved only by shifting the risk-factor distribution of the entire population to a lower level. This is because a relatively small proportion of total cases occurs at the high end of the distribution of any risk factor; the vast majority of cases occur in the middle of the distribution, where large numbers of individuals are exposed to moderate levels of risk. Thus, interventions directed only toward those in the highest risk groups will not effectively reduce cardiovascular disease for the population as a whole.

School-based studies have been instituted to test population-wide interventions to improve cardiovascular health. The vast majority of children and adolescents in the United States can be reached through schools. In addition to providing cognitive learning opportunities in the classroom, health behaviors can be influenced through physical education programs and food service modifications. These interventions have the potential to prevent or reduce obesity and smoking, decrease levels of total and low-density lipoprotein cholesterol, increase high-density lipoprotein cholesterol, decrease blood pressure, and increase physical activity and cardiovascular fitness. The purposes of this review were to analyze and evaluate results of school-based studies that have used population-wide approaches for primary prevention of cardiovascular diseases and to assess the extent to which strategies tested to date have been effective for minority populations in the United States.

## SCOPE OF REVIEW

This review focused on intervention studies published in English between 1986 and August 1999. Studies were identified through MEDLINE and the Cumulative Index to Nursing and Allied Health Literature (CINAHL) databases and reference lists of published articles. The following groups of key words were searched: those describing risk factors (blood pressure, lipids, obesity, physical inactivity), the age groups of interest (school-age children and adolescents), and the type of program (school-based program, cardiovascular health promotion/disease prevention, primary prevention, population-wide approaches). Criteria for inclusion were as follows: (1) the intervention was population-wide or "universal" (i.e., subjects were not selected on the basis of a high-risk status on one or more variables; (2) the study was conducted in the United States; (3) the target population for the intervention was in elementary, middle, and/or high school, and the sample was selected from one or more schools; (4) the design incorporated a control or comparison group (randomized or nonrandomized); and (5) outcomes included one or more anthropometric or physiological cardiovascular disease risk factors, including measurement of blood pressure, the lipid profile, and/or obesity.

There have been several recent reviews related to cardiovascular health in children and adolescents, but they encompass a different scope of studies. Resnicow and Robinson (1997) used a semiquantitative approach to review and summarize outcomes of school-based cardiovascular disease prevention studies conducted in the United States and abroad. Meininger (1997) reviewed school-based studies and discussed implications for nursing practice. Several reviewers have focused on physical activity (Baranowski, Anderson, & Carmack, 1998; Miller, Balady, & Fletcher, 1997; Pender, 1998; Stone, McKenzie, Welk, & Booth, 1998). Others have focused on dietary interventions, highlighting the prevention and treatment of obesity and cardiovascular health promotion (Kennedy, 1998; Story, 1999; Van Horn & Kavey, 1997). This review is distinguished by its biobehavioral focus; studies that link cognitive and behavioral interventions with physiological outcomes are reviewed. It extends previous studies by assessing potential impact of designs and methods on study outcomes and focusing on evidence that strategies for primary prevention of cardiovascular disease are effective in minority populations. Following a critical review and synthesis, trends and directions for future research are discussed.

## REVIEW OF STUDIES

Ten projects met the inclusion criteria for this review and are summarized in Table 9.1. They are presented in chronological order, from the earliest to the most recently published. The size and description of the sample, design, the intervention and its theoretical basis, the outcome variables, and the results are presented. In the following sections, designs and methods are critically analyzed, and findings across all studies are synthesized.

### Samples

Most studies focused on school-age children in the third through sixth grades. One recent study targeted middle school children (Gortmaker et al., 1999). Two studies included only adolescent participants (Ellison, Capper, Stephenson, et al., 1989; Killen et al., 1988). In addition to the fact that school-age children may be more amenable than adolescents to changes in behaviors that influence the cardiovascular risk profile (Kelder et al., 1994), differential maturation of subjects during puberty could bias the estimates of intervention effects. These effects cannot be detected or controlled in the absence of individual measurements of growth and development. The studies by Killen and colleagues (1988, 1989) illustrates the problem of capturing changes in cardiovascular risk factors over time in the midst of rapid physical and psychosocial changes that take place during adolescence.

A wide range of ethnic groups is represented among the studies reviewed. Nevertheless, we have very little information on differential effects of interventions by ethnicity. An exception is the San Diego Family Health Project (Atkins et al., 1990; Nader et al., 1989) in which Anglo Americans and Mexican Americans were compared. Although significant reduction in diastolic blood pressure was observed, there was, overall, a greater observable effect of the intervention for Anglo families. This may have been due to (1) confounding of ethnicity and socioeconomic status, resulting in less ability to detect change among the less advantaged Mexican American participants, and (2) the methods of measurement presented barriers for the less educated Mexican American participants.

Differential selection and attrition of participants is a concern both for internal and external validity of these studies. Internal validity is of prime importance because of the potential for interaction between selection

**TABLE 9.1   Overview of School-Based Cardiovascular Risk Reduction Studies: Know Your Body, New York**

| Project | Sample | Study design | Intervention | Outcome variables | Results |
|---|---|---|---|---|---|
| **First Author (year)** Walter et al. (1988) | **Age group/grade** (at baseline) 4th grade (9.1 yr) | **Design** Randomization within districts matched demographically | **Target (provider)** Child behavior (Classroom teacher) | Knowledge | Increased ($p<.05$) We Br |
| **Project name** Know Your Body | **Size** 37 schools $n = 3388$ | **Unit of randomization/ analysis** Schools/schools | **Program components** **Content** Nutrition Physical fitness Smoking **Methods** Curriculum Information Motivation Behavioral skills | Total fat Total cholesterol HDL cholesterol Systolic BP Diastolic BP Pulse rate recovery index Ponderosity index | Decreased ($p<.05$) We Decreased ($p<.05$) We n. s. n. s. n. s. n. s. n. s. |
| **Location** Bronx, NY (Br) Westchester, NY (We) | **Ethnic group %** Bronx  Westchester 49 B  10 B 25 W  84 W 23 H  2 H 3 O  4 O | **Duration of follow-up** (from baseline) 1, 2, 3, and 5 years | **Duration/intensity of intervention** 5 yr/2 hr/wk | | |
| | **Indicators of SES** Mean annual income Bronx $22,126 Westchester $55,904 | **Long-term follow-up** (in absence of intervention) None | **Theoretical framework(s)** Health belief model Cognitive development theory | | |
| | **Response rate** (as % of baseline participants) Bronx 66% Westchester 80% | | | | |

**TABLE 9.1    Overview of School-Based Cardiovascular Risk Reduction Studies: Know Your Body, New York (Continued)**

| Project | Sample | Study design | Intervention | Outcome variables | Results |
|---|---|---|---|---|---|
| **First author (year)** Bush, Zuckerman, Taggart, et al. (1989); Bush, Zuckerman, Theiss, et al. (1989) | **Age group/grade** 4th–6th grade/ 10.5 years **Size** 9 schools $n = 1041$ **Ethnic group %** 100 B | **Design** Randomized blocks design (by SES) **Unit of randomization/ analysis** School/subject **Duration of initial follow-up** (from baseline) 2 years (Intended as a 5-yr study) | **Target (provider)** Child behavior (Classroom teacher) **Program components Content** Nutrition Physical fitness Smoking **Methods** Curriculum Information Motivation Behavioral skills Information for parents Community advisory board | Knowledge Total fat Saturated fat Cholesterol Systolic BP Diastolic BP Total cholesterol HDL-Cholesterol Total/HDL ratio Ponderosity index Triceps skinfold Fitness | Increased ($p < .05$) n. s. n. s. n. s. Decreased ($p = .001$) Decreased ($p < .0001$) n. s. Increased ($p < .0001$) Decreased ($p < .0001$) n. s. n. s. Increased ($p = .01$) |
| **Project name** Know Your Body in Washington, DC **Location** Washington, DC | **Indicators of SES** 3 SES levels Low, 36% Middle, 29% High, 35% **Response rate** 41.4% (at 2 yr) | **Long-term follow-up** (After withdrawal of intervention) None reported | **Duration/intensity of intervention** 1.5 hr/week for 2 yr **Theoretical framework(s)** Social cognitive theory PRECEDE framework | | |

| First author (year) | Killen et al. (1988, 1989) |
|---|---|
| **Project name** | Stanford Adolescent Heart Health Program |
| **Location** | Northern California |
| **Age group/grade** | 10th grade / 14–16 years |
| **Size** | 1130 — 4 schools |
| **Ethnic group %** | 2 B   13 A   69 W   10 O   6 H |
| **Indicators of SES** | 50% college educated fathers |
| **Response rate** (as % of baseline participants) | 78% |
| **Design** | Randomized blocks design (by school size and ethnic distribution) |
| **Unit of randomization/analysis** | School/subject — Behavioral skills |
| **Duration of initial follow-up** (from baseline) | 4 months (2 mo after completion of intervention) |
| **Long-term follow-up** (in absence of intervention) | None after initial follow up |
| **Target (provider)** | Adolescent behavior (Project teacher) |
| **Program components** Content | Physical activity; Nutrition; Smoking prevention |
| **Methods** | Information; Resistance skills |
| **Duration/intensity of intervention** | 7 wk/20–50 min/session; 20 sessions |
| **Theoretical framework(s)** | Social cognitive theory; Social inoculation theory |

|  |  |
|---|---|
| Knowledge | Increased ($p < .0001$) |
| Exercise | Increased ($p < .0003$) |
| Diet | Improved ($p < .0001$) |
| Smoking | Decreased ($p = .009$) |
| Heart rate | Decreased ($p < .0001$) |
| Body mass | Smaller increase ($p = .05$) |
| Tripceps skinfold | Decreased ($p = .004$) |
| Subscapular skinfold | Decreased ($p = .01$) |
| Systolic BP | n. s. |
| Diastolic BP | n. s. |

**TABLE 9.1 Overview of School-Based Cardiovascular Risk Reduction Studies: Know Your Body, New York (Continued)**

| Project | Sample | Study design | Intervention | Outcome variables | Results |
|---|---|---|---|---|---|
| **First author (year)** Ellison et al. (1989) | **Age group/grade** 15 years (mean) **Size** 2 schools | **Design** Nonrandomized, concurrently controlled study with crossover | **Target (provider)** Food service personnel (Project nutritionist) | Sodium intake Systolic BP Diastolic BP | Decreased ($p = .001$) Decreased ($p = .01$) Decreased ($p = .001$) |
| **Project name** Exeter-Andover | $n = 309$ intervention $n = 341$ control | **Unit of randomization/ analysis** Not randomized | **Program components Content** Food purchasing and preparation to reduce sodium | | |
| **Location** New England | **Ethnic group %** 77 W | **Duration of initial follow-up** (from baseline) 2 academic years (1 intervention, 1 control) | **Duration/intensity of intervention** 24 wk during 7-mo interval | | |
| | **Indicators of SES** Private boarding schools | **Long-term follow-up** (in absence of intervention) None after initial follow-up | **Theoretical framework(s)** None specified | | |
| | **Response rate** 77% intervention 82% control | | | | |

|  |  |
|---|---|
| **First author (year)** | Nader et al. (1989) Atkins et al. (1990) |
| **Project name** | San Diego Family Health Project |
| **Location** | San Diego, CA |
| **Age group/grade** | 5th–6th graders |
| **Size** | 206 families recruited from 12 schools; 163 children |
| **Ethnic group %** | 46 AA 54 MA |
| **Indicators of SES** | Primarily low SES |
| **Response rate** | 91% of baseline families remained at 12 months |
| **Design** | Randomized blocks design (by SES) |
| **Unit of randomization/ analysis** | Schools/individuals |
| **Duration of initial follow-up** (from baseline) | 2 years |
| **Long-term follow-up** (in the absence of intervention) | None after initial follow-up |
| **Target (provider)** | Child and parent behavior (Trained graduate students) |
| **Program components** | |
| **Content** | Diet Exercise |
| **Methods** | Family evening sessions Information Exercise Behavioral skills Healthy snacks |
| **Duration/intensity of intervention** | 1 yr (3 mo intensive; 9 mo maintenance) |
| **Theoretical framework(s)** | Social cognitive theory |
| Knowledge | Increased ($p = .0001$) |
| Fat | Decreased AA ($p = .0005$) MA n. s. |
| Salt | Decreased AA ($p = .0001$) MA n. s. |
| Exercise | n. s. AA and MA |
| Body mass | n. s. AA and MA |
| Systolic BP | n. s. AA and MA |
| Diastolic BP | Decreased AA ($p = .02$) MA ($p = .02$) |
| Heart rate | n. s. AA and MA |
| Cholesterol | n. s. AA and MA |
| LDL cholesterol | n. s. AA and MA |

**TABLE 9.1  Overview of School-Based Cardiovascular Risk Reduction Studies: Know Your Body, New York (*Continued*)**

| Project | Sample | Study design | Intervention | Outcome variables | Results |
|---|---|---|---|---|---|
| **First author (year)** Berenson et al. (1991) | **Age group/grade** 4th–5th grade | **Design** Randomization of schools | **Target (provider)** Child and parent behavior (Classroom and PE teachers) | Knowledge | Not reported |
| Arbeit et al. (1992) | **Size** 4 schools n = 556 | **Unit of randomization/ analysis** Schools/students | School environment (lunch, PE) | Fitness | Increased, 5th grade boys ($p < .01$) |
| **Project name** Heart Smart Program | **Ethnic group %** 58 W 32 B 10 O | **Duration of initial follow-up** (from baseline) 1 school year | **Program components** **Content** Nutrition Physical fitness Smoking prevention | Body mass Total cholesterol Triglyceride HDL cholesterol | Not reported Not reported Not reported Increased ($p < .05$) |
| **Location** Jefferson Parish, Louisiana | **Indicators of SES** Lower middle income | **Long-term follow-up** (in the absence of intervention) None reported | **Methods** School lunch alternatives Information Behavioral skills Parent education Teacher education | LDL cholesterol VLDL cholesterol Systolic BP Diastolic BP | Not reported Not reported Not reported Not reported |
| | **Response rate** (as % of baseline) 26%–52% (varied by outcome variable) | | **Duration/intensity of intervention** Curriculum: 15–35 hr/yr PE: 12 lessons Lunch modification: 1 yr | | |
| | | | **Theoretical framework(s)** Social cognitive theory PRECEDE model | | |

**First author (year)**
Howard et al. (1996)

**Age group/grade** (at baseline)
4th–6th grade

**Project name**
Cardiovascular Risk Reduction for the Classroom

**Size**
1 school
$n = 98$

**Ethnic group %**
Not specified

**Location**
Parochial school

**Indicators of SES**
Not specified

**Response rate** (as % of baseline participants)
87%

**Design**
Randomized blocks design (by grade)

**Unit of randomization/analysis**
Class/student

**Duration of follow-up** (from baseline)
1 year after the program
Knowledge at 1 month and 1 year

**Long-term follow-up** (in absence of intervention)
None after initial follow up

**Target (provider)**
Child behavior (provider not specified)

**Program components**

**Content**
Smoking
Hypertension
Diet
Physical activity

**Methods**
Classroom curriculum

**Duration/intensity of intervention**
5 weeks
40 min/wk

**Theoretical framework(s)**
Not specified

|  |  |
| --- | --- |
| Knowledge | Increased 1 mo $p = .007$ |
|  | n. s. 1 year |
| Self-report |  |
| Diet | n. s. |
| Physical activity | Increased ($p < .02$) |
| Body mass | n. s. |
| Triceps skinfold | n. s. |
| Systolic BP | n. s. |
| Diastolic BP | n. s. |
| Total cholesterol | n. s. |
| LDL cholesterol | n. s. |

**TABLE 9.1  Overview of School-Based Cardiovascular Risk Reduction Studies: Know Your Body, New York (Continued)**

| Project | Sample | Study design | Intervention | Outcome variables | Results |
|---|---|---|---|---|---|
| **First author (year)** Harrell et al. (1996) | **Age group/grade** (at baseline) 3rd–4th grade 8–11 years old | **Design** Randomized blocks design (by region and urban/rural) | **Target (provider)** Child behavior (Classroom and PE teachers) | **School-level analysis** Self-report Knowledge Physical activity | Increased $p < .05$ Increased $p < .05$ |
| **Project name** Cardiovascular Health in Children (CHIC) | **Size** 12 schools $n = 1274$ | **Unit of randomization/ analysis** School/school and individual | **Program components Content** Nutrition Smoking prevention Physical fitness | Cholesterol Systolic BP Diastolic BP Skinfolds | n. s. n. s. n. s. n. s. |
| **Location** North Carolina, 3 regions Urban/rural in each region | **Ethnic group %** 74 W 20 B 6 O | **Duration of follow-up** (from baseline) 8–10 weeks | **Methods** Classroom curriculum PE classes | Body mass index Aerobic power | n. s. n. s. |
| | **Indicators of SES** Parental education <12 years, 17.6% | **Long-term follow-up** (in absence of intervention) None reported | **Duration/intensity of intervention** 8 weeks 2–3 times/week | **Individual level analysis** Self-report Knowledge Physical activity | Increased $p < .05$ n. s. |
| | **Response rate** (as % of baseline participants) 95% | | **Theoretical framework(s)** Development of positive health behavior model | Cholesterol Systolic BP Diastolic BP Skinfolds Body mass index Aerobic power | Decreased $p < .05$ n. s. n. s. Decreased $p < .05$ n. s. Increased $p < .05$ |

**First author (year)**
Leupker et al. (1996)

**Project name**
Child and Adolescent Trial for Cardiovascular Health (CATCH)

**Location (sites)**
California
Louisiana
Minnesota
Texas

**Age group/grade**
3rd–4th grade (mean 8 yr at baseline)

**Size**
96 schools
$n = 4019$

**Ethnic group %**
69 W    14 H
13 B     4 O

**Indicators of SES**
Not reported

**Response rate** (as % of baseline)
100% schools
79% students

**Design**
Randomization by schools

**Unit of randomization/analysis**
School/school; individual controlling for site and random effects of school within site

**Duration of initial follow-up** (from baseline)
3 school years

**Long-term follow-up** (in absence of intervention)
yes—see below

**Target (provider)**
Individual and family
Behavior and school environment (Food service, classroom, & PE teachers)

**Program components**
**Program content**
Nutrition
Diet
Smoking
Physical fitness

**Program methods**
Information
Behavioral skills
Physical education
Food service changes
Home curriculum

**Duration/intensity of intervention**
5–12 wk/yr, 15–24 sessions; environmental interventions over 3 years

|  |  |
|---|---|
| **School level** | |
| Lunch | |
| Total fat | Decreased ($p < .001$) |
| Saturated fat | Decreased ($p < .01$) |
| Sodium | n. s. |
| Potassium | Increased ($p < .01$) |
| Physical education | |
| Moderate–vigorous | Increased ($p < .02$) |
| Vigorous activity | Increased ($p < .04$) |
| **Student level** | |
| Diet knowledge | Increased ($p < .001$) |
| Total fat intake | Decreased ($p < .01$) |
| Saturated fat intake | Decreased ($p < .01$) |
| Cholesterol intake | Decreased ($p < .05$) |
| Total activity | n. s. |
| Vigorous activity | Increased ($p < .003$) |
| Body mass | n. s. |
| Skinfolds | n. s. |
| Systolic BP | n. s. |
| Diastolic BP | n. s. |
| Cholesterol | n. s. |
| Heart rate | n. s. |
| HDL cholesterol | n. s. |
| Apolipoprotein B | n. s. |

**Theoretical framework(s)**
Social cognitive theory

**TABLE 9.1   Overview of School-Based Cardiovascular Risk Reduction Studies: Know Your Body, New York** (*Continued*)

| Project | Sample | Study design | Intervention | Outcome variables | Results |
|---|---|---|---|---|---|
| **First author (year)** Nader et al. (1999) | **Age group/grade** 8th grade  Size $n = 3714$ | **Long-term follow-up** (the absence of intervention)  3 years | None | **Student level** | |
| | | | | Diet knowledge | Maintained ($p = .001$) |
| | | | | Total fat | Maintained ($p = .002$) |
| | | | | Saturated fat | Maintained ($p = .008$) |
| | | | | Cholesterol | n. s. |
| | | | | Total activity | n. s. |
| **Project name** Child and Adolescent Trial for Cardiovascular Health (CATCH) 3-year maintenance study | **Response rate** (as % of baseline cohort)  73% | | | Vigorous activity | Maintained ($p = .001$) |
| | | | | Body mass | n. s. |
| | | | | Skinfolds | n. s. |
| | | | | Systolic BP | n. s. |
| | | | | Diastolic BP | n. s. |
| | | | | Total cholesterol | n. s. |
| | | | | HDL cholesterol | n. s. |
| | | | | Apolipoprotein B | n. s. |

| **First author (year)** | Gortmaker et al. (1999) |
|---|---|
| **Project name** | Planet Health |
| **Location** | Massachusetts |
| **Ethnic group %** | 66 W    14 H<br>13 B    7 O |
| **Indicators of SES** | Median annual income of areas studied, $35,000 |
| **Response rate** (as % of baseline participants) | 83% |
| **Age group/grade** (at baseline) | 6th–8th grade |
| **Size** | 10 schools<br>$n = 1560$ |
| **Design** | Randomized schools matched by town and ethnic composition |
| **Unit of randomization/ analysis** | Schools/cluster randomization adjusting for individual covariates |
| **Duration of follow-up** (from baseline) | End of 2nd school year after baseline |
| **Long-term follow-up** (in absence of intervention) | None beyond initial follow-up |
| **Target (provider)** | Child behavior (Classroom teachers of major subjects and PE) |
| **Program components** **Content** | Reduce TV<br>Physical activity<br>Reduce fat<br>Increase fruit and vegetable consumption |
| **Methods** | Information<br>Cognitive and behavioral skills<br>Behavioral supports<br>Funding of teacher-initiated proposals |
| **Duration/intensity of intervention** | 2 school years (16 sessions/yr) |
| **Theoretical framework(s)** | Behavioral choice theory<br>Social cognitive theory |

| Outcome measure | Result |
|---|---|
| Index based on body mass and triceps skinfold | Decreased girls ($p = .05$)<br>boys n. s. |
| **Self-report** | |
| TV viewing | Decreased ($p < .05$) |
| Physical activity | n. s. |
| Fat | n. s. |
| Saturated fat | n. s. |
| Fruits and vegetables | Increased, girls ($p = .05$) |
| Total intake | Less increase, girls ($p = .05$) |

A = Asian; AA = Anglo American; B = Black; BP = blood pressure; Br = Bronx; H = Hispanic; MA = Mexican American; n.s. = not significant; O = other; We = Westchester; W = White.

factors and the intervention, leading to biased estimates of the intervention effect. In most reports, the response rates are reported and participants are compared with nonparticipants on available relevant data, such as sociodemographic characteristics and knowledge of cardiovascular disease risk factors.

Attrition was a major problem in some of the studies. Loss to follow-up is an issue in studies of longer duration and in lower socioeconomic groups that may be more mobile. For instance, the Know Your Body program in Washington, DC (Bush, Zuckerman, Taggart, et al., 1989; Bush, Zuckerman, Theiss, et al., 1989), was designed as a 5-year study. However, only 41.4% of the baseline participants were available for remeasurement after 2 years, and 17.5 % were available after 4 years. These difficulties in studying cohorts of children longitudinally are recognized by investigators. Investigators involved in the CATCH (Child and Adolescent Trial for Cardiovascular Health) study and the CHIC (Cardiovascular Health in Children) study have published articles on strategies for recruiting and maintaining study cohorts (Frauman, Criswell, & Harrell, 1998; Lytle, 1998).

## Study Designs

Although individuals cannot be randomized in school-based prevention studies, schools within districts or regions provide natural groupings that can be randomized. The most common design was randomization of schools within districts after matching on characteristics such as socioeconomic status. Many authors acknowledged the difficulty in having enough schools to consider this the unit of randomization and analysis. Further, an appropriate method of analysis must be employed to correspond to the cluster randomization procedure (Donner & Klar, 1994; Zucker et al., 1995). Because students within a school are more similar to each other than to students in other schools, the probability of making a Type I error is increased unless this lack of independence of observations is considered in the analysis. A multilevel analysis is recommended so that Type I error can be controlled while allowing for the analysis of covariates or interaction terms that are measured at the student level (Basen-Engquist et al., 1997). As noted in Table 9.1, the method of analysis was appropriate for the method of randomization in many instances.

## Theoretical Frameworks and Methods

A recent study (Howard, Bindler, Synoground, & Van Gemert, 1996) relied on cognitive interventions to increase knowledge of cardiovascular health and risk factors and their modification; in most studies attempts to increase knowledge were combined with development of specific skills. These approaches were based in social cognitive theory (Bandura, 1986). One group of investigators pointed out the lack of fit between the values inherent in social learning theory and the cultural values of minority populations in the United States, in this case, Mexican Americans (Nader et al., 1989).

Recognizing the profound influence of media and peers, many intervention studies are enhanced with social pressure resistance training derived from McGuire's (1964) social inoculation theory. Implementation of other programs, such as the Know Your Body project in Washington, DC, were guided by PRECEDE (Predisposing, Reinforcing, and Enabling Constructs in Educational Diagnosis and Evaluation), a framework that incorporates influences of the wider community on children's behavior (Green, Kreuter, Deeds, & Partridge, 1980). Stage of development was considered in the design of cognitive (Piaget & Inhelder, 1969) as well as behavioral interventions (Bruhn & Parcel, 1982).

Although some projects altered the environment of the schools by changing the school lunch options and enhancing the physical education curriculum, all the studies but one placed a major emphasis on changing the behavior of individuals. The exception was a study by Ellison and colleagues (Ellison, Capper, Goldberg, Witschi, & Stare, 1989; Ellison, Capper, Stephenson, et al., 1989), who directed the intervention to the food service personnel of a boarding school. Thus, the environment of the school was altered through changes in the food, but no attempt was made to change the health behaviors of the students. Recent studies (Harrell et al., 1996; Luepker et al., 1996) combined behavioral approaches with substantial changes to the school environment. A few studies have reached beyond the school and involved the families of students and/or the community (Berenson, Arbeit, Hunter, Johnson, & Nicklas, 1991; Bush, Zuckerman, Taggart, et al., 1989; Leupker et al., 1996; Nader et al., 1989)

The CATCH study explicitly incorporated interventions directed at the individual, family, and school levels, acknowledging the importance of modifying the environments that direct and support behaviors. Family participation was added as an arm of the study, with extensive process evaluation measures to document the dose effect of family involvement. The level of adult participation (dose) was related to the students' attitudes, knowledge, and beliefs about diet and physical activity, but not behavior (Nader et al., 1996).

For the most part, programs have been developed and implemented using theoretical frameworks, but empirical results have not been used to explicitly test and revise the theoretical bases of interventions. In recent reviews, Baranowski and colleagues (1998) and Pender (1998) have discussed the need for rigorous theory testing in relation to physical activity interventions.

## Providers, Duration, and Intensity of Interventions

In the vast majority of the interventions, classroom and physical education teachers have been trained to deliver the individual interventions. Planet

Health (Gortmaker et al., 1999) varied the providers of an intervention for middle school students by incorporating sessions within the existing school curriculum; classroom teachers in four major subjects (language arts, math, science, and social studies) and physical education delivered the intervention. The importance of training and support of teachers was emphasized by many authors, and lack of consistent or intensive delivery of the intervention by school personnel was cited as a possible source of weak or null effects. In the CATCH study there was an extensive process evaluation to monitor the participation of school staff in training, the dose of the intervention that was actually delivered, the fidelity to the protocol, and the compatibility of the program with the schools' needs (Lytle, Davidann, et al., 1994). Projects in which study personnel were involved directly in delivering the intervention include a recent study by a nurse researcher (Howard et al., 1996), the Stanford Adolescent Heart Health Program (Killen et al., 1988), and the San Diego Family Health Project (Nader et al., 1989).

The duration of interventions ranged from 5 weeks to 5 years. Intensity of programs varied considerably across studies. Increasing the length of intervention was offset by the difficulties of maintaining study cohorts and programs of sufficient intensity over long periods of time. Overall, there appeared to be no relationship between program duration/intensity and program outcomes.

## Outcome Variables and Results

None of the early studies that used primarily cognitive strategies made a significant impact on reducing body fat or body mass. Furthermore, it was noted in one project that obese children were less likely to participate in follow-up measurements (Bush, Zuckerman, Taggart, et al., 1989; Bush, Zuckerman, Theiss, et al., 1989). Overall, three of nine studies that measured body mass or skinfolds had significant effects; two of these studies had differential effects by gender. The CHIC study, which included an 8-week exercise program as well as 8 weeks of classes on nutrition and smoking, resulted in a decrease in skinfold thickness but had no effect on body mass index (Harrell, McMurray, Bangdiwala, et al., 1996). In middle school students participating in Planet Health, an index based on body mass and triceps skinfold thickness was significantly reduced in females but not males (Gortmaker et al., 1999). A more consistent effect of intervention on body mass and skinfold thickness was observed for 10th grade females than for males in the Stanford Adolescent Health Study (Killen et al., 1988).

Although the interventions in these three studies differed in methods, providers, and length of intervention, each specifically addressed physical activity and/or reduction of obesity. The CHIC study incorporated an exercise intervention in the physical education curriculum. The Stanford Adolescent Health intervention covered a number of topics in addition to physical activity but was delivered by project staff as part of the physical education curriculum. Planet Health was designed to reduce obesity by intervening to reduce TV time, increase intake of fruits and vegetables, reduce fat intake, and increase physical activity.

Three of nine studies that included blood pressure as an outcome variable reported a significant decrease in blood pressure; each of the studies had a restricted sample and thus cannot be considered representative of the general population of children and adolescents. These studies were (1) the Know Your Body study in Washington, DC, an investigation focused on African American children (Bush, Zuckerman, Taggart, et al., 1989; Bush, Zuckerman, Theiss, et al., 1989); (2) the Exeter-Andover study, which was conducted in two private boarding schools (Ellison, Capper, Stephenson, et al., 1989); and (3) the San Diego Family Health Project, which decreased diastolic blood pressure of Anglo American but not Mexican American participants (Atkins et al., 1990; Nader et al., 1989).

These three studies used vastly different interventions to produce a decrease in blood pressure. The Washington DC Know Your Body study of African American children was cognitively based and reported outcomes after 2 years of intervention. Ellison and colleagues (1989) intervened for a period of 1 academic year by changing the school food preparation without attempting to change the behavior of individual students. In the San Diego study, the intervention entailed extensive involvement of family members for 3 months and was followed by a 9-month maintenance intervention. Features shared by the three studies are (1) interventions that took place over long periods of time, and (2) study groups consisting of highly selected participants, not representative of broad, diverse populations. Selection may have affected the internal as well as external validity of the Know Your Body in Washington DC study and the San Diego Family Health Projects; this source of bias was discussed by the authors. These studies provided limited evidence that school-based studies can have an impact on blood pressure.

Four of seven studies that measured at least one lipid profile variable reported an improvement in total cholesterol or HDL-cholesterol. Two of these studies reported an increase in HDL-cholesterol: the Washington, DC Know Your Body Study (Bush, Zuckerman, Taggart, et al., 1989) and the Heart Smart Program (Arbeit et al., 1992; Berenson et al., 1991). In both studies the intervention took place over a long period of time (1–2 years), but both had extremely low response rates. There may have been selective attrition or interaction between the intervention and selection factors. A decrease in total cholesterol was observed in the Westchester sample of the Know Your Body study (Walter, Hofman, Vaughan, & Wynder, 1988) and at the individual level of analysis in the CHIC study (Harrell, McMurray, Bangdiwala, et al., 1996). In neither of these analyses was the cluster randomization aspect of the study taken into account, increasing the possibility of a Type I error. Across all studies, effects on physiological and anthropometric risk factors were minimal.

There was more consistent evidence that changes in knowledge and behavior occurred. Most studies incorporated a knowledge component and demonstrated a significant increase in knowledge among intervention participants compared with control participants. Four of six studies that measured fitness level or heart rate reported significant improvements for the intervention group compared with controls. Four of five studies had an increase in reports of exercise associated with the intervention. Importantly, in the CATCH study, the intervention group maintained a significantly higher level of vigorous activity 3 years after completion of the intervention (Nader et al., 1999).

Six of eight studies that assessed dietary intake, often by self-report, produced significant improvements in one or more dietary components. A pattern that emerges with inspection of the dietary outcomes in Table 9.1 is that the significant results were not consistent across gender and ethnic groups. In the Know Your Body studies, improvements were achieved for dietary intake for Westchester students but not for those in the Bronx or for African Americans in the Washington, DC study. Likewise, Anglo Americans but not Mexican Americans in the San Diego Family Health Project improved. Gortmaker and colleagues (1999) reported an increase in fruit and vegetable intake for females but not for males. Studies of long-term effects on dietary patterns are needed to justify interventions beginning in youth. Results of the CATCH maintenance study provide encouraging results; 3 years after intervention, maintenance of a significant reduction in total fat and saturated fat was observed among eighth-graders (Nader et al., 1999).

## RECENT TRENDS

Recent trends identified during the process of conducting this review are (1) initiation of interventions directed to preschool children, (2) increased emphasis on long-term outcomes of school-based interventions, and (3) development of culturally sensitive interventions.

Williams, one of the developers of the early Know Your Body studies in elementary schools, described a demonstration and education research project designed to evaluate effectiveness of a cardiovascular risk reduction program in preschool centers (Williams et al., 1998). This effort is based on the rationale that risk factors linked to diet (i.e., hypercholesterolemia and obesity) are prevalent by 3 years of age and track over time. Outcomes not yet published include cholesterol, nutrition knowledge, changes in dietary intake at home and at school, growth, and body fatness.

Only one of the studies reviewed, CATCH, published data on long-term maintenance of intervention effects. As noted previously, the results were positive for maintenance of diet knowledge, reduction in fat and saturated fat intake, and vigorous physical activity 3 years after completion of the intervention (Nader et al., 1999). Currently, a nurse-led study, CHIC II, is following students in rural schools in North Carolina until high school graduation. The difficulties and expense of following large cohorts over long periods of time may limit the number of studies with long-term outcomes.

With few exceptions, the studies in this review included participants from multiple ethnic groups. However, there was no evidence that any of the interventions were designed to be culturally sensitive. In striking contrast is the recent development of the Pathways study to prevent obesity in Native American children (Gittelsohn et al., 1998). Formative research was used to design culturally sensitive interventions; to respond to parent, teacher, and community needs, and to develop culturally appropriate instruments. Another example is a study in which focus group responses were used to develop heart disease education and prevention programs for adult, immigrant Latinos in the Washington, DC area (Moreno et al., 1997). Recognizing the need for a framework for developing culturally sensitive health promotion and disease prevention interventions, Resnicow, Baranowski, Ahluwalla, and Braitwaite (1999) not only delineated the dimensions of such a framework but also proposed research that is needed to test culturally sensitive programs.

In spite of the advantages of school-based studies, this approach does not address the needs of some vulnerable groups such as homeless youths and school dropouts (Ensign & Santelli, 1998). These groups may have high-risk cardiovascular profiles in conjunction with major social, psychological, and physical problems but lack access to primary care services. It is not likely that risk factors would be addressed for these groups until target organ damage begins to occur in young and middle adulthood. Innovative approaches will be required to reach high-risk, vulnerable groups.

## SUMMARY AND FUTURE DIRECTIONS

In summary, there were no consistent effects of school-based interventions on the risk factor profiles of children and adolescents. More significant effects on blood pressure and lipids were observed for earlier compared with later studies. Later studies incorporated behavioral as well as cognitive strategies and were combined with interventions to address the school environment, the families of student participants, or total community interventions. In spite of these enhancements, measurable changes in physiological risk factor profiles were rare. The CATCH study, one of the most rigorous in design and methods, with ethnically and geographically diverse samples, was not able to demonstrate an impact on physiological or anthropometric outcomes (Luepker et al., 1996). There was evidence, however, that changes in knowledge and health behaviors occurred with multifaceted school-based interventions. Changes in risk factors were not consistent across gender and ethnic groups. This pattern of differential results leads to the conclusion that gender-specific and culturally sensitive interventions will be required. Further, assumptions and values of theoretical models must be evaluated for their cultural relevance.

Even when there were statistically significant results, the effects were small. The impact of these programs should be interpreted within the context of population-wide strategies. Using this approach to achieve a very small reduction of the mean value of a risk factor for an entire population may lower disease rates more than much larger changes in the segment of the population that is at high risk. For instance, it has been estimated by Kottke, Puska, Salonen, Tuomilehto, and Nissinen (1985), that a 4% reduction in cholesterol, a 15% reduction in smoking, and a 3% reduction in diastolic blood pressure would reduce deaths due to coronary artery disease by 18%. In contrast, a high-risk approach, focusing on the subset of the population in the highest quartile on all three risk factors and lowering the average cholesterol of this group by 34%, smoking by 20%, and diastolic blood pressure to below 90 mm Hg, would result in a 2% to 9% reduction of deaths due to coronary disease in the same population. These estimates were based on heart disease mortality rates in North America and Finland, populations that have a relatively high incidence of heart disease.

In the CHIC study, Harrell and colleagues (Harrell, McMurray, Gansky, Bangdiwalla, & Bradley, 1999) compared the outcomes of population-wide and high-risk approaches. Analyses of the impact on population mean values indicated that the high-risk approach achieved a lower level of improvement in the cardiovascular health of the target population. Furthermore, they found that a school-based, population-wide approach was as effective in reducing risk-factor levels of high-risk children (defined as those with two or more risk factors) as a small group approach that specifically targeted the high-risk segment of the population (Harrell et al., 1998). The population-wide approach has other advantages. High-risk children are not singled out or labeled, and the costs of broad-based screening programs are eliminated.

Multiple levels of interventions that go beyond targeting changes in behaviors of individuals and school environments may be required. Family involvement in interventions has produced very disappointing results. Broader public health interventions are recommended with school and community linkages, combined with mass media messages and policy changes, to reinforce interventions at the individual, family, school, and community levels. There is very little research to substantiate this recommendation, with the exception of the Class of 1989 study, which was a school-based intervention embedded in a larger effort, the Minnesota Heart Health

Program, a project designed to reduce cardiovascular risk in whole communities. Although physiological risk factors of the students in this study were not measured as outcomes (and thus not included in this review), sustained changes in physical activity and food choices were reported (Kelder, Perry, & Klepp, 1993; Kelder et al., 1994). Further work on school-based studies embedded within interventions at the community level, such as mass media campaigns and education and screening programs for adults, should be pursued.

## REFERENCES

Arbeit, M. L., Johnson, C. C., Mott, D. S., Harsha, D. W., Nicklas, T. A., Webber, L. S., & Berenson, G. S. (1992). The Heart Smart cardiovascular school health promotion: Behavior correlates of risk factor change. *Preventive Medicine, 21,* 18–32.

Atkins, C. J., Senn, K., Rupp, J., Kaplan, R. M., Patterson, T. L., Sallis, J. F. J., & Nader, P. R. (1990). Attendance at health promotion programs: Baseline predictors and program outcomes. *Health Education Quarterly, 17*(4), 417–428.

Bandura, A. (1986). *Social foundations of thought and action.* Englewood Cliffs, NJ: Prentice-Hall.

Baranowski, T., Anderson, C., & Carmack, C. (1998). Mediating variable framework in physical activity interventions. *American Journal of Preventive Medicine, 15*(4), 266–297.

Basen-Engquist, K., Parcel, G. S., Harrist, R., Kirby, D., Coyle, K., Banspach, S., & Rugg, D. (1997). The Safer Choices Project: Methodological issues in school-based health promotion intervention research. *Journal of School Health, 67*(9), 365–371.

Berenson, G. S., Arbeit, M. L., Hunter, S. M., Johnson, C. C., & Nicklas, T. A. (1991). Heart Smart cardiovascular health promotion for elementary school children. *Annals of the New York Academy of Sciences, 623,* 299–313.

Berenson, G. S., Srinivasan, S. R., Bao, W., Newman, W. P. I., Tracy, R. E., & Wattigney, W. A. (1998). Association between multiple cardiovascular risk factors and atherosclerosis in children and young adults. *New England Journal of Medicine, 338,* 1650–1656.

Bruhn, J., & Parcel, G. (1982). Current knowledge about the health behavior of young children: A conference summary. *Health Education Quarterly, 9,* 142–166.

Bush, P. J., Zuckerman, A. E., Taggart, V. S., Theiss, P. K., Peleg, E. O., & Smith, S. A. (1989). Cardiovascular risk factor prevention in Black schoolchildren: The "Know Your Body" evaluation project. *Health Education Quarterly, 16,* 215–227.

Bush, P. J., Zuckerman, A. E., Theiss, P. K., Taggart, V. S., Horowitz, C., Sheridan, M. J., & Walter, H. J. (1989). Cardiovascular risk factor prevention in Black schoolchildren: Two-year results of the "Know Your Body" program. *American Journal of Epidemiology, 129*(3), 466–482.

Department of Health and Human Services. (1996). *Physical activity and health: A report of the surgeon general.* Atlanta: Centers for Disease Control and Prevention.

Donner, A., & Klar, N. (1994). Methods for comparing event rates in intervention studies when the unit of allocation is a cluster. *American Journal of Epidemiology, 140*(3), 279–289.

Ellison, R. C., Capper, A. L., Goldberg, R. J., Witschi, J. C., & Stare, F. J. (1989). The environmental component: Changing school food service to promote cardiovascular health. *Health Education Quarterly, 16(2),* 285–297.

Ellison, R. C., Capper, A. L., Stephenson, W. P., Goldberg, R. J., Hosmer, D. W. J., Humphrey, K. F., Ockene, J. K., Gamble, W. J., Witschi, J. C., & Stare, F. J. (1989). Effects on blood pressure of a decrease in sodium use in institutional food preparation: The Exeter-Andover Project. *Journal of Clinical Epidemiology, 42(3),* 201–208.

Ensign, J., & Santelli, J. (1998). Comparison of adolescents at a school-based health clinic with homeless adolescents. *Archives of Pediatric and Adolescent Medicine, 152,* 20–24.

Frauman, A. C., Criswell, E. S., & Harrell, J. S. (1998). Strategies for conducting intervention research in schools. *Western Journal of Nursing Research, 20(2),* 243–250.

Gittelsohn, J., Evans, M., Helitzer, D., Anliker, J., Story, M., Metcalfe, L., Davis, S., & Cloud, P. I. (1998). Formative research in a school-based obesity prevention program for Native American school children (Pathways). *Health Education Research, 13(2),* 251–265.

Gortmaker, S. L., Peterson, K., Wiecha, J., Sobol, A. M., Dixit, S., Fox, M. K., & Laird, N. (1999). Reducing obesity via a school-based interdisciplinary intervention among youth. *Archives of Pediatric and Adolescent Medicine, 153,* 409–418.

Green, L. W., Kreuter, M. W., Deeds, S. G., & Partridge, K. B. (1980). *Health education planning: A diagnostic approach.* Palo Alto, CA: Mayfield.

Harrell, J. S., Gansky, S. A., McMurray, R. G., Bangdiwala, S. I., Frauman, A. C., & Bradley, C. B. (1998). School-based interventions improve heart health in children with multiple cardiovascular disease risk factors. *Pediatrics, 102(2),* 371–380.

Harrell, J. S., McMurray, R. G., Bangdiwala, S. I., Frauman, A. C., Gansky, S. A., & Bradley, C. B. (1996). Effects of a school-based intervention to reduce cardiovascular disease risk factors in elementary-school children: The Cardiovascular Health In Children (CHIC) study. *Journal of Pediatrics, 128(6),* 797–805.

Harrell, J. S., McMurray, R. G., Gansky, S. A., Bangdiwala, S. I., & Bradley, C. B. (1999). A public health vs. a risk-based intervention to improve cardiovascular health in elementary school children: The Cardiovascular Health In Children Study. *American Journal of Public Health, 89(10),* 1529–1535.

Howard, J. K. H., Bindler, R. M., Synoground, G., & Van Gemert, F. C. (1996). A cardiovascular risk reduction program for the classroom. *Journal of School Nursing, 12(4),* 4–11.

Kelder, S. H., Perry, C. L., Klepp, K. I. (1993). Community-wide youth exercise promotion: Long-term outcomes of the Minnesota Heart Health Program and the Class of 1989 Study. *Journal of School Health, 63(5),* 218–223.

Kelder, S. H., Perry, C. L., Klepp, K. I., & Lytle, L. (1994). Longitudinal tracking of adolescent smoking, physical activity, and food choice behaviors. *American Journal of Public Health, 84(7),* 1121–1126.

Kennedy, C. M. (1998). Childhood nutrition. In J. J. Fitzpatrick (Ed.), *Annual Review of Nursing Research, 16,* 3–38.

Killen, J. D., Robinson, T. N., Telch, M. J., Saylor, K. E., Maron, D. J., Rich, T., & Bryson, S. (1989). The Stanford Adolescent Heart Health Program. *Health Education Quarterly, 16(2),* 263–283.

Killen, J. D., Telch, M. J., Robinson, T. N., Maccoby, N., Taylor, B., & Farquhar, J. W. (1988). Cardiovascular disease risk reduction for tenth graders. *Journal of the American Medical Association, 260*(12), 1728–1733.

Kottke, T. E., Puska, P., Salonen, J. T., Tuomilehto, J., & Nissinen, A. (1985). Projected effects of high-risk versus population-based prevention strategies in coronary heart disease. *American Journal of Epidemiology, 121,* 697–704.

Luepker, R., Jacobs, D. R., Prineas, R. J., & Sinaiko, A. R. (1999). Secular trends of blood pressure and body size in a multi-ethnic adolescent population: 1986–1996. *Journal of Pediatrics, 134*(6), 668–674.

Luepker, R. V., Perry, C. L., McKinlay, S. M., Nader, P. R., Parcel, G. S., Stone, E. J., Webber, L. S., Elder, J. P., Feldman, H. A., Johnson, C. C., Kelder, S. H., & Wu, M. (1996). Outcomes of a field trial to improve children's dietary patterns and physical activity. *Journal of the American Medical Association, 275*(10), 768–776.

Lytle, L. A. (1998). Lessons from the Child and Adolescent Trial for Cardiovascular Health (CATCH): Interventions with children. *Current Opinion Lipidology, 9,* 29–33.

Lytle, L. A., Johnson, C. C., Bachman, K., Wambsgans, K., Perry, C. L., Stone, E. J., & Budman, S. (1994). Successful recruitment strategies for school-based health promotion: Experiences from CATCH. *Journal of School Health, 64*(10), 405–409.

McGill, H. C. J., McMahan, C. A., Malcom, G. T., Oalmann, M. C., & Strong, J. P. (1997). Effects of serum lipoproteins and smoking on atheroscleroisis in young men and women. *Arteriosclerosis, Thrombosis and Vascular Biology, 17*(1), 95–106.

McGill, H. C. J., McMahan, C. A., Tracy, R. E., Oalmann, M. C., Cornhill, J. F., Herderick, E. E., & Strong, J. P. (1998). Relation of postmortem renal index of hypertension to atherosclerosis and coronary artery size in young men and women. *Arteriosclerosis, Thrombosis and Vascular Biology, 18*(7), 1108–1118.

McGuire, W. (1964). Inducing resistance to persuasion. In L. Berkowitz (Ed.), *Advances in experimental social psychology* (pp. 191–229). New York: Academic Press.

Meininger, J. C. (1997). Primary prevention of cardiovascular disease risk factors: Review and implications for population-based practice. *Advanced Practice Nursing Quarterly, 3*(2), 70–79.

Miller, T. D., Balady, G. J., & Fletcher, G. F. (1997). Exercise and its role in the prevention and rehabilitation of cardiovascular disease. *Annals of Behavioral Medicine, 19*(3), 220–229.

Moreno, C., Alvarado, M., Balcazar, H., Lane, C., Newman, E., Ortiz, G., & Forrest, M. (1997). Heart disease education and prevention program targeting immigrant Latinos: Using focus group responses to develop effective interventions. *Journal of Community Health, 22*(6), 435–450.

Nader, P. R., Sallis, J. F., Patterson, T. L., Abramson, I. S., Rupp, J. W., Senn, K. L., Atkins, C. J., Roppe, B. E., Morris, J. A., Wallace, J. P., & Vega, W. A. (1989). A family approach to cardiovascular risk reduction: Results from the San Diego Family Health Project. *Health Education Quarterly, 16*(2), 229–244.

Nader, P. R., Sellers, D. E., Johnson, C. C., Perry, C. L., Stone, E. J., Cook, K. C., Bebchuk, J., & Luepker, R. V. (1996). The effect of adult participation in a school-based family intervention to improve children's diet and physical activity: The Child and Adolescent Trial for Cardiovascular Health. *Preventive Medicine, 25,* 455–464.

Nader, P. R., Stone, E. J., Lytle, L. A., Perry, C. L., Osganian, S. K., Kelder, S.,

Webber, L. S., Elder, J. P., Montgomery, D., Feldman, H. A., Wu, M., Johnson, C., Parcel, G. S., & Leupker, R. V. (1999). Three-year maintenance of improved diet and physical activity: The CATCH Cohort. *Archives of Pediatric and Adolescent Medicine, 153,* 695–704.

Pender, N. J. (1998). Motivation for physical activity among children and adolescents. In J. J. Fitzpatrick (Ed.) *Annual Review of Nursing Research, 16,* 139–172.

Piaget, J. & Inhelder, B. (1969). *The Psychology of the Child.* New York: Basic Books.

Resnicow, K., Baranowski, T., Ahluwalla, J. S., & Braithwaite, R. L. (1999). Cultural sensitivity in public health: Defined and demystified. *Ethnicity and Disease, 9,* 10–21.

Resnicow, K., & Robinson, T. (1997). School-based cardiovascular disease prevention studies: Review and synthesis. *Annals of Epidemiology, 7*(S7), S14–S31.

Rose, G. (1980). Relative merits of intervening on whole populations versus high-risk individuals only. In R. M. Lauer & R. B. Shekelle (Eds.), *Childhood prevention of atherosclerosis and hypertension* (pp. 351–566). New York: Raven Press.

Sinaiko, A. R., Donahue, R. P., Jacobs, D. R. J., & Prineas, R. J. (1998). Relation of weight and rate of increase in weight during childhood and adolescence to body size, blood pressure, fasting insulin, and lipids in young adults. *Circulation, 99,* 1471–1476.

Sternby, N. H., Fernandez-Britlo, J. E., & Nordet, P. (1999). Pathobiological Determinants of Atherosclerosis in Youth (PBDAY Study) 1986–96. *Bulletin of the World Health Organization, 77*(3), 250–257.

Stone, E., McKenzie, T. L., Welk, G. J., & Booth, M. L. (1998). Effects of physical activity interventions in youth. *American Journal of Preventive Medicine, 15*(4), 298–315.

Story, M. (1999). School-based approaches for preventing and treating obesity. *International Journal of Obesity, 23*(2), S43–S51.

Strong, J. P., Malcom, G. T., McMahan, C. A., Tracy, R. E., Newman, W. P., Herderick, E. E., & Cornhill, J. F. (1999). Prevalence and extent of atherosclerosis in adolescents and young adults: Implications for prevention from the Pathobiological Determinants of Atherosclerosis in Youth Study. *Journal of the American Medical Association, 281*(8), 727–735.

Van Horn, L., & Kavey, R. E. (1997). Diet and cardiovascular disease prevention: What works? *Annals of Behavioral Medicine, 19*(3), 197–212.

Walter, H. J., Hofman, A., Vaughan, R. D., & Wynder, E. L. (1988). Modification of risk factors for coronary heart disease: Five-year results of a school-based intervention trial. *New England Journal of Medicine, 318*(17), 1093–1100.

Williams, C., & Wynder, E. (1993) A child health report card 1992. *Preventive Medicine, 22*(4), 604–628.

Williams, C. L., Squillace, M. M., Bollella, M. C., Brotanek, J., Campanaro, L., D'Agostino, C., Pfau, J., Sprance, L., Strobino, B. A., Spark, A., & Boccio, L. (1998). Healthy Start: A comprehensive health education program for preschool children. *Preventive Medicine, 27,* 216–223.

Winkleby, M. A., Robinson, T. N., Sundquist, J., & Kraemer, H. C. (1999). Ethnic variation in cardiovascular disease risk factors among children and young adults. *Journal of the American Medical Association, 281,* 1006–1013.

Zucker, D. M., Lakatos, E., Webber, L. S., Murray, D. M., McKinlay, S. M., Feldman, H. A., Kelder, S. H., & Nader, P. R. (1995). Statistical design of the Child and Adolescent Trial for Cardiovascular Health (CATCH): Implications of cluster randomization. *Controlled Clinical Trials, 16,* 96–118.

## PART II

# Milestones in Nursing Research

Chapter 10

# Breakthroughs in Scientific Research: The Discipline of Nursing, 1960–1999

SUE K. DONALDSON

### ABSTRACT

The period of 1960 to 1999 was an era of evolution and rapid growth of scientific research in the discipline of nursing during which specific knowledge realms, or subfields of the discipline, emerged and scientific breakthroughs occurred. This review presents the milestones or scientific breakthroughs of the era in the context of the prevailing thinking within and beyond the discipline of nursing. The nature of each scientific breakthrough in nursing is characterized as to the transdisciplinary change in thinking brought about by the work. The pathfinders for each scientific breakthrough are identified as well as their pathfinding modes. Opportunities for future scientific breakthroughs in nursing are presented.

**Key words: nursing science, nursing research, nursing research realms, research pathfinders, nurse researchers, scientific breakthroughs, discipline of nursing, research opportunities, evolution of nursing science**

This review offers three views of nursing science for the period 1960 to 1999: first, breakthroughs in nursing research that were selected by using a set of criteria for scientific work that has changed thinking about human health within and beyond the discipline of nursing; second, the pathfinders and the nature of the breakthrough; third, opportunities for future breakthroughs as fields of contemporary research and approaches for stimulating development of new scientific disciplinary realms. Each scientific research breakthrough is presented: (a) as the emergence of a new or reconceptualized realm of nursing knowledge, (b) in the context of predominant thinking in nursing at that time, and (c) in the context of prevailing scientific knowledge and practice in other disciplines. Whenever possible, the name stated for the breakthrough realm is that used by the pathfinder; in other cases, an appropriate name for the new scientific research realm was selected to capture the collective of work that constitutes the critical mass in terms of the selection criteria. The intent of presenting each scientific research breakthrough in its historical and contemporary context is to elucidate the significant change in scientific thinking represented by each. Emerging and future breakthroughs also are discussed in terms of their potential for changing scientific thinking and extending nursing knowledge to other disciplines.

## Definition of Scientific Breakthrough

The term *breakthrough* was defined as knowledge that transcends its discipline of origin, in this case nursing. The rationale for focusing on scientific research is that this form of nursing knowledge is the most likely to be adopted by other disciplines, especially by health professional disciplines that seek scientific evidence as the basis for clinical practice.

## Nursing Science and Disciplinary Realms

The definition of nursing research used in this paper is empirical scientific inquiry that generates knowledge from the perspective of the discipline of nursing (S. K. Donaldson & Crowley, 1978). The focus on science in this review thus excludes nonscientific scholarly inquiry in the discipline, even though this type of work also has been significant in shaping the discipline and professional practice of nursing.

The nursing perspective was identified as that focusing on phenomena of humans, as individuals or personal social groups, and their health, including health status, health-related processes and behaviors, health determinants, and dynamics of health. In the broadest terms, this perspective yields a view of the ecology of personal human health for individuals and families. This is distinct from the medical perspective of human disease and the public health perspective of the ecology of population health; the discipline of public health addresses the health of large aggregates of humans who do not necessarily have a personal relationship.

The health phenomena for the nursing breakthroughs are those that relate to the experience, health status, or behavior of intact humans as opposed to function or status of their cells, organs, or organ system per se. Animal research was included only if the overall objective was to explain health phenomena of intact humans. The intent was to select research in which the contribution was primarily to the discipline of nursing; this excluded research focused on pathology; pathophysiology and disease mechanisms; and nonintegrated, isolated body systems per se, which are the primary focus of biomedical disciplines. Research considered core to other nonnursing human and behavioral science disciplines, such as sociology and anthropology, also was not included even though the researcher may have been a nurse. Within the eligible nursing disciplinary scientific body of work, there was no intent to select breakthroughs with regard to a particular theoretical formation, conceptual model, scientific design, subject or unit of analysis, or specific human health phenomenon addressed by the work.

## Breakthrough Criteria

The criteria used to select the breakthroughs for purposes of this review are those that identify scientific nursing knowledge that changed the prevailing thinking about a human health phenomenon. As a result, all of the research breakthroughs identified in this review represent a new realm of scientific knowledge in the discipline of nursing, achieved either per se solum or through reconceptualization of former realms. In addition and most important, the new nursing knowledge transcended the discipline of nursing and changed thinking about the health phenomenon in other disciplines. Thus, acknowledgment by other disciplinary scientists that the nursing research is the source of the new view or paradigm was essential to its classification as a breakthrough. The evidence used was publication of the nursing research in scientific journals of other fields and incorporation of the nursing knowledge in scientific studies of nonnurse researchers. Meeting the criterion of acceptance of the nursing disciplinary knowledge by other disciplines was the major characteristic distinguishing the scientific research identified as breakthroughs in this review from other significant research and scholarly work in nursing.

## Identification of Pathfinders

The pathfinders were those nurse scientists who were identified by their peers as the originating thought leaders for their field or scientific realm. The second criterion for identifying pathfinders for each breakthrough realm was principal authorship of the first published peer-reviewed reports of data-based research in the field. Researchers who followed the pathfinder at a later time in the identified realm are not addressed, even though the excellence of their work may have greatly refined or expanded the knowledge in the field. Contemporary pathfinders for a given field or research realm are listed together even though they may not have worked or published together. Nonnurse collaborators and coauthors of the seminal scientific work are not included as pathfinders but can be identified in the citations of the reference list.

The majority of the pathfinders for each breakthrough realm in this review were interviewed by the author. These interviews were essential to gain an understanding of their views as to how they conceptualized the new field in the context of prevailing ideas in nursing and related fields.

The published literature contains very little of the information gleaned from the interviews because, according to the pathfinders, their scientific publications do not contain the full historical context of their work nor the fit of the new knowledge with the emerging discipline of nursing. Unpublished quotations in the text that follows were derived from personal written remarks sent to the author by the pathfinders after the interviews.

## REALMS OF BREAKTHROUGHS IN NURSING SCIENTIFIC RESEARCH

### Breakthrough in Person and Family Health

Nursing is the only health science discipline to focus its research on health phenomena of humans in three contexts: (a) as autonomous individuals; (b) as members of intimate social groups, such as a family; and (c) as family units (Haber, 1998). Earliest conceptualizations of the discipline of nursing emphasized the individual human as the unit of analysis and as the recipient of nursing care (S. K. Donaldson & Crowley, 1978). In both clinical practice and nursing research, family members and the family were usually addressed only as they influenced the health status of the individual patient. However, pathfinder Jeanne Quint Benoliel explored, in the early 1960s, the subjective experiences of patients and of their families during transitions in health following diagnosis of a life-threatening illness. Benoliel is the first nurse researcher to study a health phenomenon of humans in all three contexts relevant to the discipline of nursing and is the pathfinder who established the disciplinary realm of person and family health through her program of scientific research. Benoliel (née Quint) studied the subjective experience of humans; as persons, family members, and families over time periods in which they adapted to the realization of a life-threatening illness (Quint, 1963).

At the time that Benoliel initiated her first longitudinal clinical research—using qualitative methods (Quint, 1962) to study the personal experiences of women following mastectomy for breast cancer and the related experience of their families—nurses in general were focused on the physical tasks of physical care for patients. Fairman (1997) notes that, from the 1930s through the 1950s, Isabel Stewart's formulation of nursing science was dominant. Stewart's formulation was an efficiency model of work, and it was the prevailing paradigm for nursing research and nursing education. Stewart's paradigm fit well with the nature of nurses' training in hospital schools of the era, which was based on procedure and method and relied heavily on skilled task performance rather than on problem solving. Although Virginia Henderson offered a different view of nursing science, beginning in the mid-1940s—a focus on patients with research grounded in physical and behavioral sciences—Henderson's view was not supported by the nursing leadership of the 1950s (Fairman, 1997). Research in nursing in the 1950s focused on methodologic issues, student problems, and educational curricula (Fairman, 1997).

In terms of families, Brodie (1997) points out that in the 1950s and early 1960s the emphasis on physical care, directed exclusively toward individual patients, was so prevalent that even mothers of sick children were excluded from hospitals where their children were patients. Infrequently, mothers of hospitalized children were viewed as contributing to the well-being of the child, but these mothers were not seen as objects of nursing care in their own right (Brodie, 1997). When placed in this context and at the forefront of scientific research in nursing, the revolutionary nature of Benoliel's work becomes apparent. She is the scientific pathfinder for the disciplinary perspective of patient and family health and was the first researcher to launch a major sustained program of scientific research in the discipline of nursing.

The breakthrough nature of Benoliel's research is attributable to its impact on medicine and the field of medical sociology. In the early 1960s it was not common practice for physicians to inform women, even after mastectomy, that they had breast cancer. At times, family members were informed and they decided whether the woman should be told. This withholding of information by physicians emanated in part from the anticipated reaction of the woman to the diagnosis of cancer and the stigmatization of persons diagnosed with cancer. Nurses in the early 1960s generally followed the mode of communication established by the physician, and the nursing care was primarily physical tasks performed following mastectomy. But the pattern of communication with women with breast cancer also reflected the fears, anxieties, and comfort level with the diagnosis of cancer that the physicians and nurses themselves held, their association of cancer with a death sentence, and the dearth of effective therapies for cancer (Quint, 1965).

In this context, Benoliel partnered with physicians and surgeons and included, as a major focus of her exploratory research, documentation of the rationale and consequences of information control by physicians and nurses. Benoliel demonstrated the benefits, to the patient and the family, of direct and full communication of the diagnosis of cancer and the prognosis of the disease by the physicians and nurses (Quint, 1963, 1965, 1972b). The results of her research had a profound impact not only on the practice of nursing but also on the practice of medicine and on the field of medical sociology (Quint, 1963, 1965, 1966, 1972b; Quint, Strauss, & Glaser, 1964).

In addition to the revolutionary nature of Benoliel's research in the discipline of nursing and the analysis of informational control in medicine, her work established the study of stages of the dynamic process and time stages of adaptation of humans to life-threatening illness. The nature of the life-threatening event varied in her research from diagnosis of cancer in women (Quint, 1963) and diabetes in adolescents (Quint, 1970, 1977) to persons with terminal illness regardless of the precipitating health problem (Quint et al., 1964). Pathfinder Ruth McCorkle joined Benoliel in establishing the field of adaptive stage transitional care. They established the transition services model of practice, which became the basis of graduate education for many leaders in hospice and palliative care (Benoliel, personal communication, Sept. 29, 1998). Benoliel and McCorkle (1978) are well known for their holistic approach to terminal illness, which emanates from their nursing research in adaptive stage transitional care. They established the methodological and content foundation of this realm of nursing research, including development of widely used tools, such as the social dependence scale and the patient symptom distress scale, that are specific to human experience rather than to disease (Benoliel & McCorkle, 1983; McCorkle, Quint-Benoliel, & Young, 1980). They extended the knowledge they generated to behavioral science in general (G. Donaldson, McCorkle, Georgialou, & Benoliel, 1986).

## Breakthroughs in Pain Management

The disciplinary scientific realm of pain management has a three-phase breakthrough. The first phase originates with the research of pathfinder Jean E. Johnson, published in 1973. Her work was subsequently refined and embellished by her own studies and those of a large cadre of nurse scientists in the field of pain management. Johnson is the pathfinder of this important field because she was the first to challenge the prevailing thinking of the 1960s about the "measurement of pain and the cognitive processes involved in the pain experience" (personal communication, J. Johnson, Sept. 1998).

Johnson's research (1973) challenged the use of attribution theory in the conceptualization of human emotional response to painful physical stimuli. The favored hypothesis in the 1960s was that when human subjects attribute their pain sensations to a neutral source (i.e., neutral source attribution) they have less of an emotional response than when they attribute the same sensations to the threatening, actual source (Nisbett & Schachter, 1966; Schachter & Singer, 1962). In her laboratory study of humans, Johnson forewarned the subjects as to the exact physical source of the painful sensations they would experience from a threatening stimulus and showed that this forewarning accounted for a reduction in emotional response. This research led to the discarding of the neutral source attribution theory for pain across all fields and thus is a scientific breakthrough in nursing.

Prior to Johnson's (1973) research, the prevailing thought in medicine and science derived from a biological paradigm in which pain tolerance was measured as reflex withdrawal from a painful stimulus of varying intensity. Pain threshold was defined as the intensity of stimulation at which pain is first noticed or perceived. The debate in the late 1950s and early 1960s was the relationship of this type of pain measurement to cognitive processes associated with the human experience of pain. There were disagreements as to the relationship of the sensory-discriminative (i.e., physiological) mechanisms versus the emotional-reactive (i.e., psychological) mechanisms underlying pain tolerance versus pain threshold responses (Beecher, 1959; Casey & Melzack, 1967; Melzack & Wall, 1965).

Johnson settled the debate with a laboratory study of male subjects in which she demonstrated that people are able to rate the physical intensity of the painful stimulus and the degree of distress experienced from it on separate scales and that these scales provide reliable and valid measures of the components of pain. Her work also makes obsolete the notion of pain threshold as an indicator of "psychological response" to pain (Johnson, 1973). This research changed the thinking in the multidisciplinary field of pain and also influenced the clinical assessment of pain in that the research provided validated tools, such as the patient subjective experience rating scales (Johnson & Rice, 1974; Johnson, Fuller, & Endress, 1978). The subjective aspects of Johnson's work were breakthroughs in the scientific field of pain management, but in nursing they follow the pathfinding research of Benoliel in the focus on the human experience and anticipatory information sharing with the patient (Quint, 1962).

A second breakthrough in nursing research emanates from the work of pathfinder Gayle G. Page, whose seminal work changed the primary rationale for clinical pain management from that of humanitarian relief of unbearable misery to that of disease control and survival. Page has demonstrated, through her animal laboratory research, that pain can kill (Page & Ben-Eliyahu, 1998). Page's research on rats focuses on surgical pain managed with morphine as an adjunct to anesthesia, both pre- and postoperatively (Page, Ben-Eliyahu, & Liebeskind, 1994; Page, Ben-Eliyahu & McDonald, 1997; Page, Ben-Eliyahu, Yirmiya, & Liebeskind, 1993).

The multidisciplinary science context of Page's pathfinding demonstrates that her work was based on a substantial existing knowledge base; however, she and her collaborators offered new evidence that altered the clinical perspective of pain. Prior research of others had demonstrated that, in laboratory animals, stress and pain result in inhibition of immune function and enhancement of tumor growth (Keller, Weiss, Schleifer, Miller, & Stein, 1981; Laudenslager, Ryan, Drugan, Hyson, & Maier, 1983; Lewis, Shavit, Terman, Gale, & Liebeskind, 1983/84; Sklar & Anisman, 1979; Visintainer, Volpicelli, & Seligman, 1982). Corollary clinical studies of humans had demonstrated that acute pain associated with surgery and trauma could increase morbidity and mortality (Cousins, 1991; Tønnesen, 1989). It also was known that surgery decreases human immune function

(Page, McDonald, & Ben-Eliyahu, 1998). What Page and collaborators demonstrated was that, in rats, management of acute surgical pain (morphine with anesthesia) reversed the immune-suppressant and tumor-enhancing effects of surgery (Page et al., 1993, 1997). This research introduced acute pain of surgery as the factor responsible for the surgery-induced suppression of immune function and enhancement of metastatic tumor growth. It is interesting to note that pathfinder Gayle Page integrated psychoneuroimmunology, the major conceptualization of another realm of nursing research (Kiecolt-Glaser, Page, Marucha, MacCallum, & Glaser, 1998; Page & Ben-Eliyahu, 1998), Psychobiological health, discussed later. Page's research also crosses over into the clinical practice field of oncology nursing.

A third breakthrough in nursing research in the realm of pain management is attributable to pathfinder Christine Miaskowski. Prior to her work and that of co-workers, researchers had already shown sex differences in human responses to nociceptive stimuli and painful conditions: women reported lower pain tolerance and higher distress for a given stimulus intensity (Fillingim & Maixner, 1995). Clinical research also showed sex variations in the pain experience (Unruh, 1996). However, no one had demonstrated corollary sex differences in analgesic responses, making it unclear whether the basis of the sex difference in pain experience was in cognitive or in pain-modulating mechanisms. The human clinical study conducted by Miaskowski and collaborators (Gear, Gordon, et al., 1996; Gear, Miaskowski, et al., 1996) demonstrated that kappa-opioids produce significantly greater analgesia in women than in men and strongly suggests a sex difference in kappa-opioid-activated endogenous pain-modulating mechanisms. The link to another nursing realm, that of women's health, was made by Miaskowski and co-workers in the recommendation that future studies include women in luteal and follicular phases of their cycle (Gear, Gordon, et al., 1996; Miaskowski, 1997).

## Breakthroughs in Neonatal and Young Child Development

Kathryn E. Barnard began her research in the 1960s (Hammer & Barnard, 1966) with her study of mentally retarded adolescents. She shifted her emphasis in the 1970s to prevention of developmental health problems and became the nursing research pathfinder in neonatal and young child development. Her research focused on the identification and assessment of children at risk of developmental and health problems, such as infants who were seriously ill, abused, or neglected or who failed to thrive (Barnard, 1973; Barnard & Collar, 1973). The significance of Barnard's research as the basis for health care in early intervention with infants and children with disabilities was recognized in her being asked to share her research findings with the 1974 President's Committee on Mental Retardation (Barnard, 1976).

From the beginning, Barnard's research emphasized the family, following the path of Benoliel, as discussed above, and she explicated the family perspective in publications within and beyond nursing (Barnard, 1979; Barnard & Bee, 1983; Barnard, Bee, & Hammond, 1984; Barnard, Wenner, et al., 1977; Bee et al., 1982; Bee, Hammond, Eyres, Barnard, & Synder, 1986; C. L. Booth, Lyons, & Barnard, 1984). Her multidisciplinary research includes the study of interventions for mothers in the mother–infant relationship (C. L. Booth, Barnard, Mitchell, & Spieker, 1987; C. L. Booth, Mitchell, Barnard, & Spieker, 1989).

Barnard's perspective was adapted from Bronfenbrenner and Ceci's (1994) ecological perspective of human development and research of parent–child interaction in the field of developmental psychology. She introduced a conceptualization of the ecology of young child health that includes behaviors of parent and child and environmental factors as critical determinants of a child's well-being (Bee et al., 1982; Booth, Mitchell, Barnard, & Spieker, 1989). Of significance is her finding that early parent–child interaction is a predictor of the later cognitive and language development of the child (Kelley, Morriset, Barnard, Hammond, & Booth, 1996; Morriset, Barnard, Greenberg, Booth, & Spieker, 1990). In addition to her multidisciplinary collaborations and publications, Kathryn Barnard translated her findings into practice knowledge for all health professions (Barnard, Wenner, et al., 1977) and created a multidisciplinary training program for health care workers worldwide known as the Nursing Child Assessment Training (NCAST) program (Barnard, Spietz, et al., 1977). NCAST is a major vehicle for scientific breakthrough. In 1979, NCAST was delivered via satellite to 19 western U.S. cities and 600 nurses. According to a review of "pathbreakers" in science and technology at the University of Washington:

By 1995 there are 394 certified and active NCAST trainers distributed in almost every American state and in eleven foreign countries. Nearly 14,000 health care professionals have received training in the use of the methods, which have been applied in many settings, including 40 Comprehensive Child Care Programs, the Memphis New Mothers Project, the Healthy Families America Movement, and projects promoted by the National Committee to Prevent Child Abuse. Thousands of nurses, physicians, psychologists, psychiatrists, nutritionists, occupational therapists, early childhood educators, and social workers now use Barnard's concept of parent–child interaction and assessment methods as a routine part of their practice. (Illman, 1996, p. 196)

Barnard continues her research, and NCAST has been established at the University of Washington, Seattle, as a self-sustaining, nonprofit program (Illman, 1996).

A second breakthrough in neonatal and young child development was made in the 1990s by pathfinders Barbara Medoff-Cooper and Susan

Gennaro. Medoff-Cooper and Gennaro's (1996) contribution is in the development and testing of a neonatal nutritive sucking behavioral tool to be used as a predictive measure of the 6-month developmental outcomes for very low birth weight infants (VLBWI).

Medoff-Cooper initiated this program of research in a scientific field with a long history of studies of neonatal sucking behaviors, nutritive and nonnutritive, as indicators of infant neurobehavioral development (Medoff-Cooper & Ray, 1996). Using an existing biomedical instrument, the Kron Nutritive Sucking Apparatus, Medoff-Cooper proceeded to develop a quantitative and clinically valid and reliable assessment tool to objectively measure sucking patterns, at first comparing sucking patterns of healthy full-term infants to those of preterm infants (Medoff-Cooper, Weininger, & Zukowsky, 1989). Medoff-Cooper also studied the physiologic correlates of the nutritive sucking patterns in VLBWI (Medoff-Cooper, Verklan, & Carlson, 1993), building in part on the earlier research by Paula Meier, who studied bottle and breast feeding of small preterm infants (Meier & Anderson, 1987).

The existing infant development assessment scales at the time of Medoff-Cooper's work included the well-established Bayley Scales of Infant Development Scales, intended for 6-month-old infants, and the newer Newborn Morbidity Scale, used for early assessment of the neonate in the intensive care unit. Using these scales and other measures of infant outcomes, Medoff-Cooper and Gennaro (1996) demonstrated that their measure of nutritive sucking behavior in the early neonatal period can be used to assess noninvasively the maturation and behavioral organization of VLBWI. Their nutritive sucking tool and measure is a better predictor of 6-month developmental outcome, assessed by the well-established Bayley Scales, than is the Neonatal Morbidity Scale (Medoff-Cooper & Gennaro, 1996). The nutritive sucking tool provides health professional and researchers with an objective and noninvasive tool that is predictive of developmental outcomes and that can be used to assess the effects of procedures and care of VLBWI during the beginning of their lives. This work is related to the breakthrough in site transitional care of Brooten, discussed later. Because of their emphasis on the health of VLBWI, pathfinders Medoff-Cooper and Genarro offer in their nutritive sucking tool a powerful research measure to guide studies of all aspects of care of VLBWI to assure that the VLBWI's future development is not compromised.

## Breakthrough in Research Utilization

At a time when nursing research was only in its initial phase of development, the mid-1970s, pathfinder JoAnne Horsley began an investigation called the Conduct and Utilization of Research in Nursing, known as the CURN project (Horsley, Crane, Crabtree, & Wood, 1983). In that era, nonnurse social scientists were exploring the translation of knowledge from research into practice; one was Donald C. Pelz of the Institute for Social Research at the University of Michigan (Ann Arbor), with whom Horsley collaborated (J. A. Horsley, personal communication, September 1998). The CURN project was the first of this type of investigation in nursing.

The CURN project "was designed to develop and test a method for stimulating the utilization of research-based knowledge in nursing practice. The methods employed by the project were based on a model that assumed that research and practice are inextricably linked" (personal communication, J. A. Horsley, Sept., 1998).

The CURN project was conducted in two parallel programs: the research utilization program directed by pathfinder Joyce Crane (Horsley, Crane, & Bingle, 1978) and the research conduct program, directed by pathfinder Maxine Loomis (1982). Research utilization was viewed as an organizational innovating process. The "subjects" in the quasi-experimental research design were departments of nursing in Michigan hospitals. Karen Haller and Margaret Reynolds were pathfinders participating in the study of the organization dynamics (Haller, Reynolds, & Horsley, 1979). As a part of the research utilization program that was initiated at test-group hospitals, 10 research-based protocols were introduced. The pathfinders were forward-thinking in that patient outcomes were included in these studies as measures of quality of care. The research conduct program provided seed money for five pilot research projects. According to Horsley (personal communication, September, 1998), the CURN project "served not only to illustrate the relationship between research and practice, but to stimulate others to pursue various means to achieve what is now referred to as evidence-based nursing practice and the use of patient outcomes to evaluate the success of nursing practice." This work also has served as the basis for practice guidelines development in nursing.

## Breakthroughs in Dementia Care

Scientific studies by nurse researchers in the area of dementia care did not begin until the early 1980s. This nursing research was initiated in the context of medical geriatric research that focused on the psychiatric diagnoses and biomedical disease underlying Alzheimer's disease and other types of dementia; a cause/cure model was prevalent, with studies focused on discovery of the pathological etiology of dementia and on pharmaceutical interventions to correct or diminish its signs and symptoms. Nurse research pathfinders conducted breakthrough studies in three new areas reflecting the nursing perspective: (a) autonomy and quality of life for the person with dementia, (b) new theoretical models and interventions for management of disruptive behavior, and (c) new approaches for preparing and supporting family caregivers. Taken together, the nursing scientific knowledge is the basis for dementia care management (Maas & Buckwalter, 1991).

Muriel Ryden, the first pathfinder in the field of dementia care, initiated a paradigm shift. Ryden's scientific research was the first to address the morale of cognitively impaired persons (Ryden, 1984; Ryden & Knopman, 1989). Ryden (1985) also introduced the concept of autonomy in a wellness mode for institutionalized elderly and related this to environmental support. She was influenced in her thinking by a book authored by Wolanin and Phillips (1981) that emphasized the importance of preserving dignity and respect in persons with dementia (M. Ryden, personal communication, October 1998).

Additional pathfinders bringing about the paradigm change and establishing the nursing realm of dementia care are Neville Strumpf and Lois Evans who, through philosophical debate and research studies, stimulated a multidisciplinary philosophical shift in thinking about care of elders from a view of the usefulness of physical restraints for safe care of elders to the acceptance of restraint-free environments as the approach for humane and individualized care of humans. Evans and Strumpf began their work in the mid-1980s, during a period of growing societal rebellion against the then prevalent custodial care of elders in the United States. According to Evans, "the larger social and political climate during the period of our work included congressional hearings, legislative mandates, legal and regulatory changes, shifting ethical perspectives, and alterations in practice standards. Our research helped to propel, and was propelled by those external forces" (L. Evans, personal communication, October 1998).

Pathfinders Strumpf and Evans (1988) published a research study of the subjective impact of physical restraints on the patient and the nurses' beliefs about the use of restraints, in which they documented the negative impact of restraints and the professional conflict ensuing from their use. Evans and Strumpf (1989) followed this research with two seminal review articles that summarized all of the studies of use of physical restraints and exposed all of the myths about elder restraint while advertising the success of restraint-free care of elders in other countries (Evans & Strumpf, 1990). This set the stage for their next clinical studies of the use of physical restraints (Capezuti, Evans, Strumpf, & Maislin, 1996; Capezuti, Strumpf, Evans, Grisso, & Maislin, 1998) and of falls and injuries in nursing home residents. The work of Evans and Strumpf has had a profound effect within and beyond nursing in bringing about, in the words of nonnurse researchers, "an alternative *philosophy,* and the practice that expresses this philosophy, that are the keys to restraint-free care and . . . individualized care . . . as the alternative to the task-driven, staff oriented care now practiced" (Williams & Finch, 1997, p. 774).

In addition to changing the thinking about dementia care across disciplines from that of custodial, or "safe," care structured for staff convenience to that of individualized care promoting patient autonomy, dignity, and independence, the nursing pathfinders in the field of dementia care also have developed middle-range theories to guide research and develop the field of dementia care management in the discipline of nursing.

A requisite for the restraint-free, individualized care called for by Strumpf and Evans (1992) and other researchers in other disciplines (Burger & Williams, 1996) is effective behavioral management or interventions, such as those developed by Ryden and other pathfinders in dementia care. Pathfinder Ryden identified disruptive behavior as a major phenomenon in dementia and developed an instrument to measure aggressive behavior that is now widely used in many disciplines, the Ryden Aggression Scale (Ryden, 1988). Using this tool, she determined that most aggressive behavior occurred during direct contact by nursing assistants (Ryden, Bossenmaier, & McLachlan, 1991); she then studied an educational intervention for nursing assistants that led to improved quality of their care (Feldt & Ryden, 1992).

Pathfinders Geri Hall and Kathleen Buckwalter proposed that Alzheimer's disease patients need a reduction in environmental demands to reduce stress and inappropriate behavior. Hall and Buckwalter developed the progressively lowered stress threshold (PLST) model as a part of their research (Hall & Buckwalter, 1987; Hall, Kirschling, & Todd, 1986). This model is widely used across disciplines, and Hall and Buckwalter's research findings as to the effectiveness of PLST have reversed the earlier thinking that Alzheimer's disease patients need increased environmental stimulation (Maas & Buckwalter, 1991).

Pathfinders Cornelia Beck and Patricia Heacock introduced a decision-making algorithm in which the cognitive deficit pattern of each elder is assessed, and this leads to specific care management strategies to improve the quality of life and interactions for the person with dementia and their caregivers (Beck, Heacock, Rapp, & Mercer, 1993). This work was based on earlier research by Beck (1988) in which she developed and studied what has become a very important assessment tool in the field: the Beck Dressing Performance Scale (BDPS). This tool measures the level of caregiver assistance provided during dressing and is the basis for the decision-making algorithm used in nursing assistant and staff training (Beck et al., 1997) and for family caregivers; thus, Beck has translated the knowledge into care management protocols through her research. Pathfinders Diane Algase and Ann Whall join the middle-range theory development group with their need-driven, dementia-comprised behavior model for explaining aggression, wandering, and disturbing vocalizations of patients with dementia (Algase et al., 1996; D. Booth, Bradley, & Whall, 1988; Roberts & Algase, 1988).

A third major content field in the realm of dementia care that was developed by nurse scientists is family caregiving. Prior work in this field focused on negative consequences, or burdens, of caregiving, primarily the psychological and social toll of caregiving on stress and coping and the mental health of the caregiver (Maas & Buckwalter, 1991). Nursing pathfinders introduced a new perspective, emphasizing family and family roles, caregiver career trajectories, and the positive aspects of caregiving.

Pathfinder Patricia Archbold offered the first conceptual model of family caregiving in research on the impact of parent caring on middle-aged offspring (Archbold, 1980) and women in particular (Archbold, 1983). Early pathfinders Beverly Baldwin (Baldwin, 1988; Baldwin, Klelman, Stevens, & Rasin, 1989), Barbara Given and Clare Collins (Given, King, Collins, & Givens, 1988; Given, Stommel, Collins, King, & Given, 1990), and Holly Wilson (1989) explored the stress and negative choices of family caregiving. This was consistent with the nonnursing research focus on burden and the mental health of individual caregivers (Given & Given, 1991).

Nurse researchers also sought to reframe family caregiving into a positive life experience. Pathfinder Carol Farran explored the meaning of caregiving in an alternate paradigm for Alzheimer's disease families (Farran, Keane-Haggerty, Salloway, Kupferer, & Wilken, 1991). Pathfinder Mary P. Quayhagen expanded the knowledge of the family aspects of caregiving by exploring correlates of caregiving satisfaction (Worcester & Quayhagen, 1983) and coping mechanisms used in the caregiving role and family-based strategies (Quayhagen & Quayhagen, 1988, 1989).

Caregiving was reconceptualized as a role with social worth and satisfaction, for which a family member could prepare. Pathfinder Karen Robinson (1988) demonstrated that a social skills training program for adult caregivers can decrease burden and increase quality of care and satisfaction. Pathfinders Pat Archbold and Barbara Stewart (Archbold, Stewart, Greenlick, & Harvath, 1990) and Karen Robinson (1988) are recognized for introducing the concept of preparedness. Pathfinder Farran studied a group intervention program for caregivers of persons with dementia and, along with pathfinder Buckwalter, recast caregiving as having a career trajectory (Farran & Keane-Haggerty, 1988). Pathfinder May Wykle expanded the nursing research focus and general scientific knowledge with her research addressing the needs of minority older adults (Wykle & Kaskel, 1991; Wykle & Morris, 1994). Thus, nurse scientists reconceptualized caregiving for persons with Alzheimer's disease as an individualized family care experience with a career trajectory.

Nurse scientists also developed the first interventions to assist family caregivers in preparing for and sustaining a positive experience in the caregiving role. Pathfinder Mary Quayhagen developed a model of cognitive stimulation that serves as the basis of improving function of the person with dementia and improves well being of the family caregiver (Corbeil, Quayhagen, & Quayhagen, 1999). She also developed a family-administered, home-based cognitive remediation therapy (Quayhagen, Quayhagen, Corbeil, Roth, Rodgers, 1995).

The new paradigm of individualized care for persons with dementia was advanced again by the research of pathfinder Ann Hurley. Hurley and her multidisciplinary team developed a means to assess discomfort in persons with advanced Alzheimer's disease (Hurley, Volicer, Hanrahan, Houde, & Volicer, 1992).

## Breakthrough in Site Transitional Care

Pathfinders Dorothy Brooten, Linda Brown, and Susan Bakewell-Sachs initiated the development and testing of a successful model of site transitional care with their study of nurse specialist–managed home follow-up services for VLBWI who were discharged early from the hospital (Brooten et al., 1986). Both quality of care, in terms of infant outcomes, and cost of the model care were compared to VLBWI who were not discharged early. The site transitional care model has been demonstrated to reduce costs while providing comparable quality to usual care for many patient groups (Brooten et al., 1988).

This transitional care model is different from that of Benoliel and McCorkle, discussed above (see Person and Family Health), in that the "transition" in site transitional care is from hospital to home, and the transitional care services provided by the advanced practice nurse specialist are intended to substitute for a portion of the hospital care that was lost due to early discharge. The site transitional care model was developed in response to the anticipated consequences of the prospective payment system enacted by the government in 1983; early hospital discharge was one type of cost-cutting measure employed to save health care dollars. Pathfinders Brooten, Brown, and Bakewell-Sachs recognized that early discharge of vulnerable patients, such as VLBWI, posed health risks for the infants and the potential for increased health care costs due to readmissions and complications. By demonstrating the cost-effectiveness and continuity of care for their comprehensive program of transitional home follow-up by nurse specialists, the pathfinders established a feasible model of care and a new role for master's-prepared advance practice nurses. This evidence-based practice model sets the standard, so any new models will have to be tested as to their ability to provide the same quality of care at equal or lower cost (Brooten et al., 1988).

The site transitional care model is also important as a framework for research. The research studies to test the model, using various types of patients and conditions, were conducted as randomized clinical trials. These studies provide data on patient outcomes, cost of care, and documentation of effectiveness of nursing interventions for patients with various conditions (Brooten et al., 1988). Pathfinders Susan Cohen and Lauren Arnold joined Brooten and Brown to study the scope and content of nursing practice encompassed by the model when used with VLBWI;

this generated a taxonomic classification of nursing interventions (Cohen, Arnold, Brown, & Brooten, 1991). Pathfinders Susan Gennaro and Ruth York also joined Brooten and Brown to study the model with VLBWI; this research demonstrated the usefulness of the model as a framework and source of data for research beyond the infant outcomes and cost of care. For example, the pathfinders studied the effects of clinical nurse specialist teaching roles and family variables related to VLBWI, such as patterns of parent communication during the period of infant hospitalization (Brooten, Gennaro, Knapp, Brown, & York, 1989; Brown, York, Jacobsen, Gennaro, & Brooten, 1989).

The site transitional care model also has been successfully tested and used as a multidisciplinary research framework for several other types of patients who are at health risk as a result of early discharge from the hospital. Pathfinders Dorothy Brooten, Marianne Roncoli, and Lauren Arnold used the model to study women after cesarean births (Brooten et al., 1994, 1996; Donahue et al., 1994; Miovech et al., 1992). Pathfinders Ruth York, Linda Brown, and Cynthia Armstrong Persily extended the study of the model to women with high-risk pregnancy (Persily, 1996; York et al., 1997). Pathfinders Andrea Hollingsworth and Susan Cohen used the site transitional care model to study women discharged from the hospital early after hysterectomy (Thomas, Graff, Hollingsworth, Cohen, & Rubin, 1997). The model also has been studied as a means for gaining understanding of the health needs of the elderly and for providing care to them. Pathfinders Mary Naylor, Dorothy Brooten, and Mathy Mzey have spearhead the study of elders (Naylor et al., 1994, 1999; Naylor & Shaid, 1991).

In summary, the site transitional care model is a breakthrough in nursing research that has been recognized by many health care disciplines. The knowledge from this sustained and broad program of research, has changed multidisciplinary thinking as to the value of nurse specialist care, or advanced practice nursing, in the management and provision of care across care sites for patients at risk for complications. This research-based knowledge also has resulted in classification of nursing interventions and of methods for determining cost and value of the nursing care.

## Breakthroughs in Health and Violence

Through the early to mid-1970s societal violence and violent and abusive behavior were not viewed in the context of human health. Rather, violent and abusive perpetrators were handled as criminals by the judicial system. Those subjected to their abuse were treated as victims within a health care system that focused on their illnesses, both mental and physical. In this paradigm the victim's response to violence-induced trauma was studied and treated as psychiatric pathology, physical injury, chronic pain and symptoms, and stress-related illness and morbidity, such as irritable bowel syndrome. The 1970s were also the era in which violence was just beginning to be recognized as a familial problem (Campbell, Anderson, Fulmer, Girovard, & McElmurry, 1993). Nursing research of the 1970s and 1980s was instrumental in changing the perspective on human violent behavior to that of interpersonal violence and family system dysfunction in the context of societal influences, with perpetrators of abuse viewed as persons in need of health care along with their victims (Campbell, 1981).

Against the backdrop of the 1970s, pathfinders Ann Burgess, Lynda Holstrom, and Maureen McCausland conducted the first research studies in nursing in the realm of health and violence. Burgess and Holstrom's (1974) study of rape and the rape trauma syndrome is considered a classic across disciplines. Burgess, Holstrom, and McCausland are early pathfinders in the study of child sexual assault, especially by a family member, and the child's emotional response to sexual abuse. These pathfinders challenged the prevailing ignorance of child and adolescent sexual abuse and of incest (Burgess, Groth, & McCausland, 1981; Burgess & Holstrom, 1975; Burgess, Holstrom, & McCausland, 1977; Groth & Burgess, 1977).

Pathfinder Barbara Parker, a contemporary of Burgess, Holstrom, and McCausland in the 1970s, conducted the first domestic violence research in nursing; this research identified and explored the battered wife syndrome and demonstrated the vertical transmission of the pattern from the nuclear family of origin. Pathfinder Parker demonstrated that frequently daughters of battered mothers became battered wives in this vertical transmission pattern (Parker & Schumacher, 1977). The significance of Parker's pathfinding research was recognized within and beyond nursing. The research offered new knowledge as to the response to women of battering and emphasized the significance of family roles and familial transmission of familial violence across generations (Parker & Schumaker, 1977).

The 1980s ushered in a new awareness of the role of the health care system in addressing violence as a health problem. The 1983 Department of Justice Task Force was followed by a Surgeon General's workshop to clarify the role of the health care system; nursing was represented by pathfinder Ann Burgess at the workshop (Campbell et al., 1993). The results of nursing research and the importance of nursing care in violence is evident in the U.S. Public Health Service *Healthy People 2000 Report* (Campbell et al., 1993).

The premier body of knowledge about physical abuse during pregnancy and the pattern of forced sex and partner/spousal battering is derived from nursing research. Pathfinder Ann Helton (1986) conducted one of the first studies documenting prevalence of abuse during pregnancy. Helton followed this contribution with her collaborative study with pathfinders Judith McFarlane and Elizabeth Anderson; together they documented the prevalence of abuse during pregnancy and demonstrated that this abuse is correlated with a higher prevalence of many complications of pregnancy (Helton, McFarlane, & Anderson, 1987). Pathfinders

McFarlane and Parker were joined by pathfinder Linda Bullock in contin-uing the research and the development of a tool for assessing abuse dur-ing pregnancy; this tool is used across disciplines (Bullock, McFarlane, Bateman, & Miller, 1989; McFarlane, Parker, Soeken, & Bullock, 1992). Parker and McFarlane (1991b) developed a research tool for identifying pregnant battered women that is also useful in clinical settings. To advance research across disciplines, Parker (Parker & Ulrich, 1990) devel-oped a protocol, now widely used across disciplines, to assure the safety of abused female subjects in studies of violence.

Pathfinders Bullock and McFarlane also initiated nursing research showing that battered pregnant women are more likely to deliver low birth weight infants than those not battered during pregnancy (Bullock & McFarlane, 1989). This is an interesting corollary to the research of pathfinder Dorothy Brooten and colleagues on VLBWI, discussed earlier (see site transitional care, in preceding section).

Pathfinder Jacquelyn Campbell opened a new area of violence research in the 1980s with her studies of domestic homicide; this research under-scores the social context and interpersonal relationship basis of abuse and the risk of homicide in domestic abuse (Campbell, 1981, 1986). Campbell (1989a, 1989b) also studied women's responses to battering in intimate relationships, developing knowledge for nursing assessments and inter-ventions for improvement of women's health. The seminal research of pathfinder Karen Landenburger (1989) offered an explanatory model and identification of the process by which women leave these abusive rela-tionships. Landenburger's model is used widely within nursing and has become the basis for clinical nursing interventions (Campbell, Kub, & Lewandowski, 1998). Pathfinder Sarah Torres opened the field of cultural difference in abuse of women; she studied the cultural differences in abuse for Hispanic and American cultures (Torres, 1987, 1991).

Among the most significant contributions of nursing research to the field of health and violence are the emergency room (ER) screening pro-tocols and staff training programs for identifying and assisting battered women. The pathfinders for this research are Virginia K. Drake, Virginia Tilden, and Patricia Shepherd (Drake, 1982; Tilden & Shepherd, 1987).

Another breakthrough was the introduction of elder abuse, which par-allels nursing's breakthrough in dementia care during the 1980s, as dis-cussed earlier. Pathfinder Linda Phillips (1983) opened the field of elder abuse in nursing research with her study of the frail elderly at home. She then engaged pathfinder Virginia Rempusheski, and together (Phillips & Rempusheski, 1985) they developed and studied a decision-making model for diagnosing and intervening in elder abuse and neglect. Pathfinders Terry Fulmer and Joanne Ashley (1986, 1988) extended this research by exploring the concept of neglect and developing instruments for assessing elder mistreatment (Fulmer, 1991). At the same time, pathfinder Margaret

Hudson (1989) was conducting an analysis of the concepts of elder mistreatment, abuse, and neglect as defined by clinicians.

Nursing research and pathfinders played a very important role in reconceptualizing health and violence as a family problem and in focusing on the family as a unit as well as in using a holistic perspective of the violent family and its members (Campbell et al., 1993). The family perspective of nursing research and care is summarized in a book by Campbell and Humphreys (1993) in which they emphasize the importance of studying and intervening in the family and improving family function. This is in contrast to addressing the batterer and the victim of abuse separately or in a subfamily dyad. The overriding desire for a family, albeit violent, was discovered by Campbell to be a major reason that battered women return to and remain in an abusive relationship. As one subject remarked in giving advice to caregivers trying to assist her in the cycle of love-abuse, "She doesn't need the abuse confirmed. She already knows that part. They may still be a family, so don't blow that fantasy for her, really all she's looking for desperately is a family" (Campbell, Pugh, Campbell, & Visscher, 1995, p. 221).

It is important to note that the pathfinders in health and violence used a feminist perspective and theory in the research related to abuse of women (Parker & McFarlane, 1991a). Angela B. McBride (1992) explicated feminism as an overarching theme in the research agenda for nursing in violence against women. This feminist perspective paralleled the breakthrough in women's health in nursing research discussed in the following section and reflected the national focus on women's health and issues (Campbell et al., 1993).

Following through on the family perspective, pathfinder Janice Humphreys (1991) studied the children of battered women to determine their worries about their mothers. Picking up this research theme, Campbell and Parker (1992) published the first major review of nursing research in health and violence, entitled "Battered Women and Their Children."

In summary, the pathfinders in health and violence have contributed significant scientific knowledge to the field. Their work serves as the basis for research in other disciplines and as the evidence for clinical detection and treatment or prevention of family violence.

## Breakthrough in Women's Health

The women's liberation movement that emerged nationally in the 1960s had an impact on nursing as a profession in that nurses were viewed as paradigmatic of women's issues in general. Nurses themselves were seen as victims of structural misogyny and as an oppressed group. A positive outcome for nursing as a result of the women's movement was that the profession responded by defining and developing careers for its members and advancing the significance of the perspective of nursing in terms of health care and the science (McBride, 1997).

By the 1980s, nurses were responding to the demands of women, as consumers of health care, to better understand their bodies and health, especially for self-help. Medicine continued its tradition of addressing the needs of women with specialists in obstetrics and gynecology. The focus of medical research and care for women through the 1980s was the biomedical function of female organs and systems, as they relate to reproduction and sexual function, and endocrine system balance. Outside this focus, disease and health were rarely studied by using female subjects; thus, much of the biomedical scientific knowledge used as the basis for health care related to men (McBride, 1998). Although the 1980s ushered in a new era of women's health and research with female subjects in medicine, the medical perspective has remained primarily that of disease: women's risk of and responses to disease and therapies for diseases of women (McBride, 1997). Normal events of biological transition, such as menopause, were seen as a disease by medicine and in need of medical therapy (MacPherson, 1981).

During the 1980s nurse scientists began to espouse feminist methodologies (MacPherson, 1983) that could potentially generate knowledge of women's lived experience of health over their life span (McBride, 1997; Stevenson & Woods, 1986). McBride called for demedicalization of women's health care by advocating a shift in perspective from gynecology to gyn-ecology, or women's health ecology (McBride, 1993, 1998; McBride & McBride, 1981).

One major branch of research in women's health was established, beginning in the early 1980s, by pathfinder Ann Voda. A strong proponent of feminist research methodology, Voda studied the normalcy of menopause and women's perimenopausal experiences (Voda, 1981; Voda, Imle, & Atwood, 1980). Her research findings are used across disciplines (Voda, 1980) and have prompted a nondisease view of menopause as a normal life transition of women, both biological and social (Voda & George, 1987).

Although other nurse researchers conducted studies in the 1980s in the general area of women's health (Woods, 1989), the establishment of the disciplinary scientific realm emanating from nursing's perspective and the acceptance of nursing knowledge by other disciplines is due to the early and sustained scientific research program of pathfinder Nancy Fugate Woods (Fogel & Woods, 1981; McBride, 1997; Woods, 1980, 1982, 1989; Woods & Longnecker, 1985). Woods collaborated with fellow pathfinders Gretchen K. Dery and Ada Most; together they conducted early studies of perimenstrual symptoms, studying their prevalence and relationship to stressful life events (Woods, Dery, & Most, 1982; Woods, Most, & Dery, 1982). Woods later collaborated with another pathfinder,

Joan Shaver, to explore biological dimensions of perimenstrual symptoms (Shaver & Woods, 1986).

What distinguishes the research of pathfinder Nancy Woods and her colleagues from that of other nurse researchers studying women is that she focused on women's personal experience, as affected by variables such as biology, cognition, and environment (social and physical), of a uniquely female process, menstruation. This is different from studying the impact of the same variables on women's roles or biological functions, such as ability to work, menstruate, maintain personal hygiene, engage in sexual intercourse, bear children, avoid conception, assume a parenting role, or remain disease-free (Woods, 1989). The theme of Woods's research is the social context of healthy women's lives and how this affects their health experience (Woods, personal communication, 1999).

Pathfinder Joan Shaver added another new dimension to women's health research in studying sleep patterns and stability in perimenopausal women. She was joined in this research by pathfinders Elizabeth Giblin, Martha Lentz, and Kathy Lee (Shaver, Giblin, Lentz, & Lee, 1988). Giblin was already engaged in sleep research, and her collaboration with Shaver moved this into the realm of women's health (Shaver, personal communications, October 1999). Shaver, Lee, and Giblin maintained the link to Woods's research by collaborating in a study of sleep patterns related to menstrual cycle phase and premenstrual affective symptoms (Lee, Shaver, Giblin, & Woods, 1990). Lee (1988) opened a new dimension of the women's health research realm by studying the circadian temperature rhythm of healthy women in relation to menstrual cycle phase.

Another pathfinder who joined Nancy Woods and Joan Shaver is Margaret M. Heitkemper, who has a long-standing research program in gastrointestinal (GI) function that began with her studies of enteral nutrition with Barbara Walike Hansen (Heitkemper, Hanson, Walike, 1977; Heitkemper, Martin, Hansen, Hanson, & Vanderburg, 1981). Heitkemper initiated a program of research in stress and GI tract function, using a rat model as a part of her dissertation work (Heitkemper & Marotta, 1983). She introduced this model into women's health by focusing on bowel patterns and functional bowel disorders, such as irritable bowel syndrome, across the menstrual cycle of women (Heitkemper, 1998). Pathfinder Ellen Mitchell joined Heitkemper, Shaver, and Woods in the early work on bowel patterns and menstrual cycle (Heitkemper, Shaver, & Mitchell, 1988).

Thus, what evolved from the above collaboration of many pathfinders who joined Nancy Woods, are three current teams of related researchers in women's health, led by Woods, Shaver, and Heitkemper. The National Institute of Nursing Research sponsors a center for women's health research at the University of Washington, Seattle, to support this work (McBride, 1998). This research utilizes a stress model that employs psychosocial and biological measures of stress to explore the relationship to the perimenstrual and menopausal symptoms and functional disturbances experienced most often by women; the emphasis is on the women's well-being, not disease (Shaver, personal communication, October 1999). This body of nursing knowledge is published in health literature within and beyond nursing, and pathfinder Woods presented the perspective and scientific knowledge to the Institute of Medicine, National Academy of Sciences, in 1992 (Woods, personal communication, October 1998).

## Breakthrough in Management of Stress Urinary Incontinence in Women

When nurse scientists began conducting research studies to improve the effectiveness and use of behavioral therapies for stress urinary incontinence (UI) in women, there was already a long history of medical research and medical therapy, tracing back to Kegel (1948), a physician who published the first intervention study for stress UI. Stress UI is the involuntary loss of urine associated with normal functions, such as coughing, laughing, sneezing, and minor postural changes or with certain sports, such as those involving high physical impact. The major contributing factor in women is weakness of the muscles of the pelvic floor; this weakness may occur as a result of disease, disuse atrophy, or trauma (e.g., childbirth). Kegel published the first studies of active exercise of pelvic floor muscles that demonstrated improvement of urine control in young and elderly women with stress UI (Jones & Kegal, 1952; Kegel, 1948, 1956). Kegel employed biofeedback in his exercise training program; he used a vaginal resistive device attached to a manometer (perinometer) so that the women could see the mercury level rise during contraction of their pelvic floor muscle. Other researchers in medicine have continued to study the use of Kegel exercises, or pelvic muscle exercise (PME), as a behavioral therapy for stress UI in women, replicating Kegel's early positive results and documenting the value of biofeedback for best results in terms of urine control and muscle training (Burgio, Robinson, & Engel, 1986).

Nurse researchers entered the field of stress UI by studying community-dwelling women; nursing research was initiated at a time when several national surveys had revealed that the prevalence rate of urinary incontinence was 30% for all older adults and 37.5% for women. Stress UI accounted for most of the incontinence in women (Diokno, Brock, Brown, & Herzog, 1986; White et al., 1985). Nurse researchers became aware through a review of the scientific literature in the area published by Wells (1990) that, despite the established clinical success of the Kegel exercise with biofeedback for stress UI, this safe behavioral treatment was not being used as the preferred therapy. Other medical therapies, such as reconstructive pelvic surgery and pharmacologic treatment, were being used instead. Pelvic muscle exercise had been shown in multiple studies over time to be roughly 70% effective for eliminating the symptoms of stress urinary incontinence in women of all ages, as shown in the original Kegel study (Kegel, 1948; Wells, 1990). The only new finding documented in Wells's review was that daily estrogen supplementation enhanced the outcomes of PME in postmenopausal women. Surgery was found to be no more effective than Kegel PME, nor were embellishments to PME, such as direct electrical stimulation of the perineum.

Possible problems with the acceptance of PME as a therapy were the wide variations in recommended protocols, the lack of standardized biofeedback equipment for clinical use, and the failure to demonstrate a relationship between changes in pelvic muscle strength due to PME and changes in urodynamics (uretheral pressure) measurements (Wells, 1990).

The conceptual framework for PME as a clinical therapy for stress UI attributed the effectiveness of PME to the increased strength and contraction of the pelvic floor muscle and, as a consequence, increased uretheral closing pressure. Wells (1990) postulated that failure to establish the relationship of improved pelvic muscle contraction and improved urodynamics in the earlier research studies caused the dissociation of the therapy from the perceived pathology, perhaps relegating PME into the category of a "lay" therapy, despite its clinical effectiveness for treating symptoms of stress UI in women. Nurse researchers were interested in using PME as a safe behavioral intervention that would allow self-care for stress UI as opposed to medicalization of the condition and the use of therapies such as surgery or pharmacologic agents.

Pathfinders Thelma Wells and Carol Brink collaborated with a physician colleague (Wells, Brink, & Diokno, 1987) to overcome the limitations of earlier survey prevalence and clinical evaluation studies; they conducted a comprehensive study of UI in 400 community-living women aged 55 years and older who described themselves as having uncontrolled loss of urine. Characteristics and etiology of UI were fully assessed for 200 of these women. The results showed that, for women 55–75 years of age, stress UI was the most prevalent form of incontinence and that most of the women with stress UI had not received treatment. Those who had received medical therapy usually reported some type of urinary bladder surgery (Wells, Brink, & Diokno, 1987). The concern of nurse scientists was that a large number of community-living women were experiencing social isolation (McCormick & Palmer, 1992) and alterations in their lives as a result of untreated stress UI, despite the known effectiveness and safety of PME, a form of self-care.

Nurse researchers used the nursing perspective and focused on improvement of the subjective symptom experience of the women with stress UI, rather than emphasizing a biological explanation in terms of reversal of pathology or altered biological function (i.e., urodynamics). Using the established parameters for successful PME, nurse scientists developed important research and clinical tools for the study and the clinical treatment of stress UI in women. Pathfinder Jean Wyman collaborated with investigators from medicine and other disciplines to demonstrate the reliability of a subject-recorded 1-week diary for assessing the frequency of voluntary micturition and involuntary urine loss (Wyman, Choi, Harkins, Wilson, & Fantl, 1988). The self-recorded diary, as opposed to history taken from one-time or episodic interviews, has become an important tool for all researchers in the field of incontinence.

Another very important research tool, the intravaginal balloon device (IVBD), was developed by pathfinder Molly Dougherty in the 1980s (Dougherty, Abrams, & McKey, 1986). The IVBD was shown to be a reliable, objective measure of pelvic floor muscle contraction. It measures muscle contraction as a pressure increase over time (i.e., pressure wave form), and it is superior to both the previous Kegel (1948) perinometer, which was not very sensitive, and pelvic floor electromyography (EMG) that measures recruitment of muscle cells rather than the actual force of contraction of pelvic floor muscle. Since the purpose of exercise training in PME is to increase the strength of contraction of pelvic muscle as a means of holding the urethera closed against increased intraabdominal/ intrabladder pressures, the best outcome measure for PME is force of contraction of pelvic muscle. Circumvaginal muscle (CVM), or pelvic floor muscle, contraction squeezes the outside of the IVBD, raising its internal pressure; thus, the IVBD pressure is a direct measure of the force, or strength, of pelvic muscle contraction (Dougherty et al., 1986; Dougherty, Bishop, Mooney, & Gimotty, 1989). Muscle contraction force can be increased by either increasing the number of fibers recruited to contract in unison, as measured by an electromyograph, or by increasing the strength of contraction of each fiber, or both. Measuring force as IVBD pressure captures both means of increasing force, whereas EMG would not detect a stronger contraction as a result of only stronger muscle fibers.

Dougherty was joined by pathfinder Ruth Mooney (Dougherty et al., 1989) in using the IVBD to study home training in exercise of CVM for normal women, to see if the CVM would hypertrophy, as expected in comparison to nonexercise control subjects. This was the first study demonstrating with quantitative data that the pelvic floor muscles actually increased their force of contraction in response to PME in normal women.

In the 1990s pathfinders Wells and Brink showed, in a multidisciplinary study, that PME is as effective as the usual pharmacologic agent phenylpropanolamine hydrochloride for alleviating symptoms of stress IU, in community-living women 55–90 years of age (Wells, Brink, Diokno, Wolfe, & Gillis, 1991). At the same time, pathfinder Pat Burns was studying, with a different multidisciplinary team, a group of older community-living women with stress UI in a randomized controlled trial that included 3- and 6-month follow-up evaluations (Burns, Pranikoff, Nochajski, Desotelle, &

Harwood, 1990; Burns et al., 1993). Burns and colleagues measured changes in urodynamic and EMG parameters as well as symptoms of stress UI in response to PME. Burns and colleagues (1993) found that the effectiveness of PME for treating stress UI was the same with or without biofeedback. Like earlier research by others (Wells, 1990), these studies confirmed that PME worked to alleviate stress UI symptoms but that PME did not change urodynamic measures. Unlike most previous work, this study assessed pelvic muscle strength as measured by EMG and showed no significant increase in the total EMG voltage as a result of PME. Only the peak magnitude of the EMG (millivolts) for quick pelvic muscle contractions was positively correlated, albeit weakly, with decreased symptoms of stress UI. The symptoms and EMG effects persisted for 6 months (Burns et al., 1993).

Pathfinder Carolyn Sampselle was interested in translating this knowledge of symptom effectiveness of PME into practice and so developed a stopwatch test of urine stream interruption, using a scientifically characterized uroflowmeter to validate the measure. The stopwatch test and uroflowmeter measurements of urine stream interruption were both highly correlated with a digital (intravaginal palpation) measure of pelvic muscle strength and measures of stress UI symptoms. The stopwatch measure offers an inexpensive, simple, validated tool for measuring the effectiveness of PME in any clinical setting (Sampselle, 1993). Sampselle then collaborated with Brink, Wells, and colleagues to validate the digital test of pelvic muscle strength against the vaginal EMG scores and to determine how these correlate with stress UI assessments (Brink, Wells, Sampselle, Taille, & Mayer, 1994). The digital test offers yet another inexpensive clinical tool for using PME as a clinical therapy for stress UI.

The group of Wells, Brink, and Sampselle was working independently of Dougherty's team, with different measures and tools. Both research groups were independently documenting the high variability between subjects as to measures of pelvic muscle contraction, the weak correlation between contraction strength (EMG voltage or IVBD pressure) and urine loss variables (Doughterty, Bishop, Mooney, Gimotty, & Williams, 1993), and the failure of PME to control symptoms of stress UI in more than 70% of women (Bishop, Dougherty, Mooney, Gimiotty, & Williams, 1992). Even more puzzling was the lack of correlation between urodynamic measures and indicators of incontinence severity; these observations were confirmed by Wyman and colleagues (Wyman, Elswick, Ory, Wilson, & Fantl, 1993). Clearly, the biological basis of stress UI is not reflected in the urodynamic measures. However, the nurse researchers understood that linkage of PME to some parameter of pelvic muscle contraction was needed in order for PME to be a more widely used therapy and to enhance the effectiveness of PME as a therapy for stress UI.

To this end, Dougherty enlisted the assistance of another nurse-scientist, pathfinder Christine E. Kasper, an expert in mammalian skeletal muscle contractile properties. Kasper was studying the differential contractile properties of the major skeletal muscle fiber (i.e., cell) types in rats, including their adaptation to exercise and recovery from atrophy and injury (Kasper, 1995; Kasper et al., 1990; Reiser, Kasper, Greaser, & Moss, 1988; Reiser, Kasper, & Moss, 1987). She was used to analyzing skeletal muscle contraction force–generation curves that look much like the IVBD pressure waveforms of Dougherty. She performed a post hoc analysis of Dougherty's circumvaginal muscle pressure tracings and made several important observations and discoveries. First, the high variability in the IVBD pressure curves between subjects appeared to be related to high variability in the mix of fiber types in their pelvic muscles. Second, the parameters of the IVBD pressure curves that were previously analyzed (peak magnitude, duration, area under the curve) were better measures of ability to hold urine, or endurance pelvic muscle contraction, under conditions of constant or slowly changing intraabdominal pressure (i.e., bladder filling), as opposed to the fast muscle contraction needed to stop urine flow during abrupt increase in intraabdominal pressure (e.g., during coughing, sneezing) associated with stress UI. The speed of PM contraction is best assessed by rate of rise of IVBD pressure or rate of rise of EMG voltage during a quick, forceful contraction. Finally, the PME protocols that were commonly used as the treatment or in training were uniform regimens and biased in favor of strengthening slow-twitch, or endurance-type, fibers that do not contract as quickly or forcefully as the fast-twitch fibers (Boyington, Dougherty, & Kasper, 1995). These nurse researchers changed the thinking in this field from standard PME training to individualized PME protocols designed for the woman's particular pelvic floor muscle composition and contractile behavior. The collaboration of pathfinders Boyington, Dougherty, and Kasper has led to a change in thinking about protocols of PME training for stress UI in women and about the analysis of pelvic muscle contractile properties. The new thinking about PME for stress UI in women that emerged from the nurse pathfinders' collaboration is clearly from the perspective of nursing, that of an individualized behavioral intervention based on the specific pelvic muscle status of each woman (Boyington et al., 1995).

## Breakthrough in Psychobiological Health

Researchers in nursing have traditionally been committed to a holistic view of humans as persons and to the study of human responses to and experiences of health and illness, as well as to the discovery of clinical interventions to improve the overall health status of individuals. However, nursing has only recently embarked on scientific inquiry into the mechanism through which psychosocial interventions may improve the biological health status of humans, including alleviation of distressing symptoms and prevention or limiting of disease processes. Most of the existing research knowledge in nursing at best correlates psychosocial and biological phenomena related to health without demonstrating the mechanisms linking the two sets of phenomena in a way that can serve as the basis for precise and controlled clinical interventions. However, nursing pathfinders are beginning to pioneer a new field, psychobiological health, that focuses on the factors and mechanisms that mediate psychological and biological systems in humans.

One subfield of psychobiological health is grounded in the scientific and theoretical framework of psychoneuroimmunology (PNI), which nurse researchers have adopted as the model for mind-body interactions (Post-White, 1998; Zeller, McCain & Swanson, 1996). As nurse pathfinders Janice Zeller, Nancy McCain, and Barbara Swanson note, "there remains a dearth of comprehensive research-based knowledge to explicate the relationships of behavioral factors to certain illness and to guide the use of biobehavioral approaches in health promotion, disease prevention and symptom management" (Zeller et al., 1996, p. 658). They advocate adoption and use of the PNI model for nursing research.

The relatively new nonnursing science of PNI emerged after centuries of observations that illnesses often occurred at the time of stressful life events (Holmes & Rahe, 1967; Locke, 1982). Cannon's (1926) discovery of the "fight or flight" response of intact organisms and Selye's (1946) general adaptation syndrome scientifically demonstrated that a mechanistic link between mind and body processes must exist. However, it wasn't until the 1960s that George Solomon proposed the new science of PNI to study systematically the interrelationships between psychological stressors, immune system alterations, and disease processes (Solomon & Moos, 1964). Ader and Cohen's (1975) discovery that immune responses can be conditioned by using classical methods and that the person's expectations rather than the actual stimulus can cause the immune response validated the PNI theoretical framework, or PNI model, and stimulated scientific growth of the field. PNI model research focuses on elucidation of the bidirectional interactions between the psyche and the neural, endocrine, and immune systems in humans. The immune system is viewed as the bidirectional modulator and mechanistic link between the neuroendocrine and behavioral systems and responses.

Scientific work in the field of PNI has established that environmental and psychosocial factors (i.e., stressors) can affect biological responses through postulated (PNI) pathways (Ader, 1996) and that biobehavioral strategies involving self-regulation (i.e., relaxation, imagery, biofeedback, stress management, conditioning, etc.) can be used to improve immune system status and disease state (Halley, 1991). Most of the research in the field of PNI has been directed toward establishing the nature and extent of bidirectional interactions between psyche and immune system. The characterization of environmental, social, and behavioral stressors is still rather rudimentary. Similarly, medical research using PNI model–based interventions to affect illness and disease state is only beginning to emerge (Halley, 1991). However, there is a significant background of research in PNI exploring psychological interventions as a means of modulating immunity (Kiecolt-Glaser & Glaser, 1992) and the relationship of stress and immunity in humans (Herbert & Cohen, 1993). Nurse researchers are expanding the PNI field by exploring the nature and characteristics of PNI–model stressors that influence the immune system and by studying clinical PNI model–based interventions that improve the symptom experience and disease status of humans.

Pathfinders Barbara Swanson, Diane Cronin-Stubbs, and Janice Zeller studied the bidirectionality of the PNI model in their multidisciplinary collaborative study of the effects of human immunodeficiency virus (HIV) infection and immune system changes in neuropsychological function of humans (Swanson, Cronin-Stubbs, Zeller, Kessler, & Bielauskas, 1993); this is the reverse of the more usual study of the effects of the mind on the immune system. Although they observed changes in neuropsychological function that progressed with changes in HIV disease state, they could not attribute them specifically to the immune system because of direct nervous system effects to the virus. However, this study represents a new approach to understanding effects of disease on mood and neuropsychological function, an underdeveloped knowledge area that is essential for guiding nursing therapeutics. Pathfinder Nancy McCain demonstrated in a study of men with HIV disease that positive life changes are associated with lower $CD4^+$ T-lymphocyte counts (McCain & Cella, 1995).

In another exploratory PNI-model study, pathfinder Donna McCarthy demonstrated that rats exposed to noise stress have altered biological function of macrophages and neutrophils in vitro. Even though she could not demonstrate whether the environmental noise stressor acted through the psyche or through nervous system auditory mechanisms, this work offers a means of understanding the negative effects of noise on wound healing and other health phenomena (McCarthy, Quimet, & Daun, 1992). Similarly, Swanson and Zeller produced new breakthrough knowledge in their study of the effects of the stress-related hormone cortisol on HIV p24 antigen production in cultured human monocyte-derived macrophages. Their finding that physiological concentrations of cortisol increase viral replication is a scientific first that lays the groundwork for clinical nursing studies of stress and environmental management as a means of improving immune system status and managing HIV disease (Swanson, Zeller, & Spear, 1998). The cell-culture cortisol study gives PNI-model mechanistic strength to the earlier research of McCain and Zeller, who demonstrated that stress management therapies may improve immune system status in persons with HIV disease (McCain, Zeller, Cella, Urbanski, & Noval, 1996).

Pathfinders Cathy Annie and Maureen Gröer made significant strides in their PNI-model study of childbirth stress and maternal salivary immunoglobulin A (IgA) levels. They found a significant drop in maternal salivary IgA at parturition and low maternal salivary IgA associated with increased incidence of postpartum complications and infant illness. This research demonstrates the relevance of the PNI framework for understanding and monitoring health risks during the normal life transitions such as childbirth (Annie & Gröer, 1991). Pathfinders Maureen Gröer, Sharron Humenick, and Pamela Hill studied secretory IgA and cortisol levels in human breast milk and found a negative correlation between cortisol and secretory IgA levels; they also noted that secretory IgA was significantly elevated in preterm versus term birth mother's milk, suggesting a protective effect in preterm births (Gröer, Humenick, & Hill, 1994).

Pathfinder Janice Post-White is pioneering the study of nursing interventions for persons with advanced-stage cancer. In contrast to early PNI-model studies by others that focused on stress and negative mood state as causes or enhancers of cancer, Post-White (1993) studied the effects of an intervention of guided imagery combined with social support as a means of improving emotional state, immune function, and cancer outcome in a controlled clinical trial of outpatient subjects receiving chemotherapy for advanced solid-tumor cancers. The nursing intervention is a self-management psychosocial strategy. When compared to control, the intervention group showed enhanced emotional coping responses, lymphokine-activated killer cell function, and monocyte cytotoxicity along with improved disease state; the 1 year mortality rate was also reduced in the treatment group. In a multidisciplinary follow-up study to differentiate the effectiveness of social support versus imagery as interventions, both were found to improve emotional, coping, and social responses as well as enhance some immune system parameters over those for the non-intervention control group (Richardson et al., 1997).

In summary, nurse pathfinders using the PNI model in their research are discovering health-related nondisease stressors that affect the immune system, such as environmental noise and childbirth; testing unique illness-related applications of the PNI model, such as bidirectionality in HIV disease; and testing its validity in clinical intervention trials. The intervention studies of Post-White (1993) that demonstrate a positive effect of a psychosocial intervention on disease state and short-term survival of patients with solid-tumor cancer receiving chemotherapy are a breakthrough for two reasons. First, the studies demonstrate the effectiveness of a nursing intervention in improving emotional state and disease outcomes; second, they test the limits of applicability of the PNI model as a conceptual framework for planning interventions to improve the health of humans. Although pathfinder Post-White found some immune system changes that are consistent with the PNI model, some were not. Natural killer (NK) cell cytotoxicity did not increase in the subjects who showed improved disease state. The PNI model predicts that NK cell cytotoxicity would be the basis for change in disease state with solid-tumor cancers. Post-White's (1998) finding of inconsistent immune parameter results is emerging in other human and clinical studies, and thus nursing research is stimulating the development of conceptualization that is broader than the PNI model to explain human mind-body interactions as applied to human clinical therapeutics.

The PNI model is not the only conceptual framework used by nurse pathfinders in the field of psychobiological health. Pathfinders Marie Cowan and Helen Nakagawa Kogan are pioneering a study of a psychosocial therapy grounded in a psychoneuroendocrine model for survivors of sudden cardiac arrest (SCA) that is intended to lower psychological distress and decrease mortality from a second SCA. In a randomized, controlled study they used a combination of cognitive behavioral strategies—biofeedback for physiological relaxation and health education as the psychosocial therapy. The mechanistic linkage between mind and body was conceptualized by using the known relationships of psychoneuroendocrinology and strategies from biological and behavioral sciences.

It is well documented that autogenic training in the form of conscious control of breathing and relaxation can alter the balance of parasympathetic versus sympathetic autonomic nervous system activity, thus influencing the heart rate (HR) and variability of HR over time, as well as stress and arousal state in general. Cowan and Kogan included these relaxation techniques with biofeedback for self-management, specifically to increase parasympathetic tone over time and to influence psychosocial distress. Interestingly, they found that survivors of SCA had decreased HR variability and that their intervention improved both psychological distress and HR variability in the survivors of SCA, demonstrating that a nursing psychobiological health therapy is capable of influencing two major factors associated with cardiac disease mortality (Cowan, 1997).

## Breakthroughs in Biobehavioral Health

Working in parallel with the nurse researchers in the field of psychobiological health is another group of scientists pursuing knowledge as to how intentional physical activities and nonsocial aspects of the environment can be altered to improve symptom management, physical function, and self-care. This realm is named biobehavioral health, and it is distinct from psychobiological health, discussed above, in which the interventions are psychosocial in nature and intended to affect function of selected physiological systems, such as the immune system or nervous system, as a means of counteracting disease effects or improving psychological well-being. Although presented previously in the section entitled Breakthrough in

Management of Stress Urinary Incontinence in Women, the clinical PME intervention studies are an example of biobehavioral health research because intentional physical exercise of pelvic muscle is used to reduce stress urinary incontinence. The term *biobehavioral* is often used in nursing to capture all scientific research that includes biological and behavioral variables; however, for purposes of this review the fields of psychobiological health and biobehavioral health are distinguished to reflect their two distinct types of interventions and different intended health outcomes.

A major subfield of biobehavioral health relates to nursing interventions that improve functional capacity and alleviate the perceived fatigue of patients that results from disease processes or medical therapies for disease. Early pathfinders in this subfield focused on interventions for cancer patients who experience hypokinetic conditions and physical deconditioning as a result of prolonged physical inactivity. Pathfinders Mary MacVicar and Maryl Winningham found, in early research studies, that exercise programs for patients with cancer receiving chemotherapy resulted in a decrease in perceived fatigue (MacVicar & Winningham, 1986) and nausea (Winningham & MacVicar, 1988).

Pathfinder Jennie L. Nickel joined them, and together these investigators conducted a study of an aerobic exercise intervention for women receiving adjuvant chemotherapy treatment for Stage II breast cancer to see if exercise would improve functional capacity (MacVicar, Winningham, & Nickel, 1989). This study was conducted at a time when rest and reduced physical activity were often prescribed for patients with cancer and prescribed specifically in response to their complaints of fatigue, even though exercise was prescribed for cardiac rehabilitation to prevent post-surgical complications and deconditioning effects of bed rest. The research of pathfinders MacVicar, Winningham, and Nickel led to an exercise intervention that was thus the opposite of what was typically prescribed clinically for patients with cancer who were experiencing fatigue. There were recommendations in the literature for exercise for persons with cancer to prevent the physiological sequelae of deconditioning, but no empirical data existed to support clinical use of an exercise regimen until the study by MacVicar, Winningham, and Nickel, which demonstrated the benefits of exercise over usual care. Their research was a breakthrough in this regard and also because they objectively quantified progressive exercise intensity and used a standard measure of maximum oxygen uptake for functional capacity; these standardized measures allow comparison between subjects and studies and for a given subject over time. Their scientific study used the perspective of nursing in that improvement in functional capacity was sought as a means of enhancing self-care activities and as a health-promoting behavior (MacVicar et al., 1989; Orem, 1980).

Building on this early work, Winningham joined pathfinders Victoria Mock and Paula Sheenan and a team of clinical oncology nurse specialists to conduct an intervention study using a more modest structured walking exercise program, with a support group for women on adjuvant chemotherapy for breast cancer; the experimental study was conducted at two medical centers. The intervention test group improved in physical performance and function over the usual-care group; in addition, a dose dependence of the effects exercise was demonstrated (Mock et al., 1994). The nursing conceptual model used in this study was the Roy adaptation model (Roy & Andrews, 1991). This clinical intervention study also demonstrated that perceived fatigue was a problematic symptom for both test and control subjects and that the exercise intervention alleviated fatigue for the test group (Mock et al., 1994), thus confirming the earlier observations of pathfinders MacVicar and Winningham (1986).

The fatigue or perceived fatigue reported by the cancer patients was emerging as different from the physiological fatigue resulting from impairment of neuromuscular motor unit function (Dalakis, Mock, & Hawkins, 1998; Kasper & Sarna, in press). Mechanisms underlying cancer fatigue are unclear, but nurse researchers have made progress in developing conceptualizations that incorporate the possible direct effects of tumor neurosis factor on skeletal muscle and the effectiveness of exercise to alleviate fatigue (St. Pierre, Kasper, & Lindsey, 1992). Pathfinders Kasper and Sarna (in press) found that skeletal muscle characteristics and performance patterns, such as physiological muscle strength and physiological fatigue, are different from the perceived fatigue of the women with breast cancer receiving adjuvant chemotherapy.

Mock joined pathfinders Karen Dow, Patricia Grimm, and Jacqueline Dienemann to study the effects of an exercise walking program for women with breast cancer receiving radiation therapy. This controlled clinical trial was conducted at two medical centers, and the intervention was managed by oncology nurse specialists. As with chemotherapy patients, the exercise intervention improved physical performance and function for the cancer-radiation subjects in the test group, compared to control group, and alleviated perceived fatigue selectively in the test group. The new findings were that the exercise intervention also significantly improved emotional distress and sleep. The combined results of the research of these nurse pathfinders are used across disciplines as the basis for exercise therapy for patients with cancer and serve as the basis for nursing assessments and clinical therapeutics (Mock et al., 1997).

Nurse researchers also have pursued activity restrictions and recovery from the physical deconditioning of bed rest as another subfield of biobehaviorial health. Pathfinder Christine Kasper conducted animal studies with a multidisciplinary team that demonstrated disuse atrophy of skeletal muscle resulting from non-weight bearing similar to the conditions of bed rest. Kasper's most significant finding for nursing was that the weight bearing and exercise that was intended for recovery actually damaged the atrophied rat muscles (Kasper, Maxwell, & White, 1996; Kasper, White, & Maxwell, 1990).

In a comprehensive review of the scientific literature, Maloni and Kasper (1991) documented that the common use of bed rest during pregnancy is not supported by scientific evidence; they found very few outcome studies documenting the positive or negative effects of bed rest during pregnancy on mother or infant. Furthermore, the physical deconditioning and negative psychosocial effects known to occur with bed rest in nonpregnant persons suggest that prolonged bed rest during pregnancy may be detrimental to maternal health. Pathfinder Maloni followed up by organizing a multidisciplinary research team to conduct breakthrough research in humans, comparing the physical and psychosocial effects of bed rest during pregnancy; subject comparison groups were assigned complete bed rest, partial bed rest, and no bed rest. Maloni and colleagues (1993) demonstrated that bed rest causes skeletal muscle dysfunction, weight loss, and dysphoria; the severity of these effects was directly related to the degree of activity restriction.

Exercise also has been used as an intervention for institutionalized, cognitively impaired elders as a part of the field of research in biobehavioral health. Pathfinder Mary Jirovec (1991) used a daily exercise regimen with this population and demonstrated that daily exercise improved the subjects' mobility and balance and also improved urine control. The effect of daily exercise on urinary incontinence in cognitively impaired elders was surprising, and it offers a low-cost intervention for alleviating urinary incontinence and improving self-care and independence.

In a completely different approach within the field of biobehavioral health pathfinder Donna Bliss explored an intervention for patients with chronic renal disease that stimulates gastrointestinal tract bacteria to metabolize urea and lower the blood urea nitrogen (BUN) level. At the time that pathfinder Bliss assembled a multidisciplinary team, it was already known that fecal bacteria were capable of using $NH_3$ for this purpose if the bacteria also had access to appropriate substrates, such as those in gum arabic fiber. However, no one had studied stimulating this mechanism of fecal metabolism in vivo to lower BUN in chronic renal patients. The accepted therapies at that time were decreased dietary protein intake to limit body urea production and dialysis to lower BUN. Bliss and colleagues (Bliss, Stein, Schleifer, & Settle, 1996) demonstrated that adding fermentable fiber, specifically gum arabic, to the low-protein diet of chronic renal failure patients causes an environmental change that increases human fecal bacterial mass and nitrogen excretion and lowers host BUN. In the unique use of gum arabic as part of a therapeutic diet, Bliss and her colleagues demonstrated a means of lowering BUN without dialysis; this was a scientific first. Bliss presented an unexpected view of fecal bacteria as a biological therapeutic agent that can be manipulated to serve the human host. This research represents an unusual perspective of the human biological environment and its influence on human function and health.

## SUMMARY OF BREAKTHROUGHS

### Pathfinding

In general, while the nursing pathfinders collaborated across disciplines, all of them focused their research by using the nursing perspective. The pathfinders attracted researchers from other disciplines to participate in the nursing research; this enhanced the generalizability and acceptance of the work and knowledge across disciplines. Pathfinders also disseminated their research widely. They published in nursing and premier research journals of other disciplines. In essence, the pathfinders demonstrated the general applicability of their research and findings. Another characteristic of pathfinders was significant to their identification; pathfinders attracted other nurse and nonnurse researchers into the realm they established. These recruited researchers then conducted studies independent of the pathfinder.

There are multiple patterns of pathfinding for the breakthroughs in research included in this review. Some nurse scientists collaborated more closely with nonnurse researchers than with nurse colleagues, such as Benoliel (patient and family health) in the 1960s, Johnson (pain management) and Barnard (parent and child health) in the 1970s, and Page and Miaskowski (pain) in the 1990s. It is of interest that these nurse researchers sought to change a prevailing paradigm in another discipline and perhaps this required their more direct participation with scientists in the nonnursing disciplines. Some pathfinders collaborated primarily with nursing colleagues in definable groups, either in one geographic site, such as Woods (women's health), Brooten (site transitional care), and Horsley (research utilization) and their colleagues, or in geographically distributed but intellectually coordinated teams, such as Burgess, Parker, McFarlane, and Campbell (violence and health) and Dougherty, Boyington, and Kasper (stress urinary incontinence). Pathfinders in dementia care are a cluster of geographically separate teams of researchers who track and reference each other's work but do not directly coordinate their research. In contrast, separate research teams in the area of stress urinary incontinence (Wells, Brink, and Samselle; Wyman; and Dougherty, Boyington, and Kasper) worked in parallel with different tools and measures. Researchers in the emerging realms of psychobiological health and biobehavioral health appear to follow the parallel path pattern.

What all pathfinders shared in common was a passion for challenging current thinking or existing paradigms and theories about significant human health phenomena. This assertive stance usually meant that they were expanding or revising the nursing perspective as well as that of other disciplines. As a result, the pathfinders experienced some degree of isolation within the discipline of nursing. Many of the pathfinders reported that their struggles for acceptance within nursing were the most difficult and that they persevered because of a commitment to patients and families who would benefit from the new knowledge more so than for recognition by nursing or advancement of the profession per se. Being a pathfinder clearly involved a willingness to continue despite isolation and, at times, rejection. Creative ideas and tremendous skill and dedication as a researcher were only part of what was needed to be a pathfinder. It is only when each breakthrough realm is viewed in its historical context that one can grasp the boldness of the ideas of the pathfinder and the obstacles that they had to overcome. This is important for future pathfinders to consider, in that celebrity and acceptance of one's current research is probably an indication that it is not breaking new ground.

## Opportunities for Future Research Breakthroughs

Several fields of nursing research are poised for significant scientific breakthroughs or for primary development by nurse researchers. Family health is a rich research domain for nursing, but nurse researchers in this field have not generated conceptualizations and sufficient knowledge to serve as the basis for clinical interventions or for shaping health care policy (Feetham, 1999). In reviewing the state of the science in nursing's field of family health, it appears that nursing is beginning to realign with the field opened by Benoliel (person and family health) in studying transitions of family units (Gillis & Knafl, 1999; McCubbin, 1999), but nurse researchers have yet to establish a definition of the family unit or a consistent conceptual framework for interventions studies for the family unit (Feetham, 1999; Feetham & Meister, 1999). Both of these are core to shaping knowledge in the discipline of nursing.

Nursing is the only health science discipline that addresses health care in all contexts, from disease prevention to promotion of the health of family units and persons in the context of their family (i.e., intimate social group) (S. K. Donaldson, 1999). For this reason it is essential that nurse researchers view their science and knowledge as coordinated with and linked to, although separate from, the nonhealth-science field of family social science. This stance of defining knowledge from the perspective of nursing as a corollary to related fields is characteristic of all of the breakthrough nursing research realms cited in this review; only nursing knowledge can serve as the basis for clinical nursing practice and shaping health care policy (Feetham & Meister, 1999). Feetham (1997) has specifically called for paradigm bridging the disciplines of public health and nursing in the area of health care policy. Policy is formed by using aggregate data and the epidemiologic methods of public health. Policy thus must be evaluated as to its impact on individuals and families, because these were not the units of analysis for policy formulation. Nursing should study the impact of health policy on persons and family units; this is the core of nursing as a discipline (S. K. Donaldson, 1999; Feetham, 1997).

Another opportunity for nursing and nursing researchers lies in combining the separate conceptualizations that have evolved within the discipline of nursing for the fields of psychobiological health and biobehavioral health. It would be of great value if nurse researchers in these separate realms combined models for a more comprehensive approach (Hinshaw, 1999); this would allow a more thorough testing of the bidirectional nature of mind-body interactions and the response of the person to social and physical environmental influences. It appears that nurse researchers are confining themselves to the limits of the theoretical and conceptual models of other disciplines (e.g., family social science, psychoneuroimmunology) rather than testing relevance of multiple models for informing nursing clinical therapeutics. A holistic conceptualization of humans as biopsychosocial persons is essential, as called for by Shaver (1985) and Cowan et al. (Cowan, Heinrich, Lucas, Sigmon, & Hinshaw, 1993), especially as this is seminal to the discipline and the perspective that has shaped nursing research breakthroughs.

As a field, human genetics and health care is in the beginning phases of research in many disciplines. There is an opportunity for nursing to integrate genetics into many of its disciplinary realms (S. K. Donaldson, 1999) and to use research-based knowledge to generate knowledge for individualized health care and lifestyle therapeutics. The latter type of knowledge development in genetics and health care is exemplified by two separate programs of research that are currently being conducted. One is the randomized, controlled clinical trial of a nursing biobehavioral multidisciplinary intervention for young urban Black males with hypertension (Hill, in press). As a part of this study, Hill and colleagues are tracking biological and genotype data for each subject so that patterns in their disease progression and responsiveness to the clinical intervention can be associated with their genotype and biologic phenotype. In a separate program of research, nurse researchers Strickland and Giger are studying coronary heart disease risk factors for African American women and testing, in a randomized, controlled clinical trial, a nurse-managed intervention. Giger and Strickland are tracking genotype and phenotype correlations in this population (Acton et al., 1997). These research programs will generate knowledge that can serve as the basis for the individualized health care of persons and that integrates the behavioral and biological nature of the person. This knowledge also can serve as the basis for self-management, health promotion, and disease prevention. Nursing is the health science discipline that is most prepared to generate this form of health care knowledge (S. K. Donaldson, 1997, 1999).

## Sources of New and Breakthrough Realms of Knowledge

The research breakthroughs cited in this review emanated from nurse researchers who used the person and family health perspective of nursing and who sought insights into or meanings for existing practices, knowledge, or naturally occurring phenomena. Thus, these behaviors on the part of nurse researchers are likely to be the basis of future research breakthroughs. The nurse pathfinders also were assertive and bold in proposing new conceptualizations and in recruiting collaborators from many disciplines to add a broad-based validity to the work and to ensure its dissemination. Thus, seeking cross-disciplinary collaboration and paradigm bridging are important means of creating additional breakthrough realms of nursing research and building nursing knowledge.

Another source of new breakthrough realms of nursing research and knowledge are predoctoral students and their dissertation projects. Doctoral students in nursing should be challenged to pursue research that is likely to change the thinking about a health care phenomenon rather than just to add new knowledge to the discipline of nursing. Encouraging students to learn this type of approach and to collaborate across disciplines by using bridging paradigms will serve them well as preparation to be future pathfinders. The education of doctoral students should include epistemology, patterns of pathfinding, and the context of innovation and research breakthroughs in nursing. In tracking the progress of nurse pathfinders in an existing field they can best identify successful strategies and opportunities for their own future breakthrough research.

The history of scientific breakthrough research is relatively short, but in the past quarter century the discipline of nursing has been greatly expanded and recognized by other disciplines as a source of knowledge for research and clinical practice. The breakthrough research of nurse scientist pathfinders, categorized into disciplinary realms and topics, is summarized in Table 10.1. Although this represents only a portion of nursing research—specifically, that which is scientific and has changed thinking within and beyond the discipline of nursing—the breakthrough research is significant in volume, scope, and innovation. Nursing and its pathfinders are to be commended for their accomplishments. There is also evidence of resources and opportunities for the growth of nursing research and future scientific breakthroughs.

**TABLE 10.1 Breakthroughs in Nursing Research**

| Research Realm | Decade | Topics in Realm | Pathfinders |
|---|---|---|---|
| Person and family health | 1960s | Women after mastectomy<br>Subjective experience<br>Longitudinal design (12 mo)<br>Patient experience<br>Negative impact of information control | |
| | | Family influence on adolescents with diabetes<br>Patient/family as partners<br>Grounded theory<br>Qualitative data | J. Q. Benoliel |
| | 1970s | Adaptive Stage Transitional Care<br>Patient/family adaptation to life-threatening illness<br>Assessments of loss and grief<br>Holistic approach to terminal illness | |
| | 1980s | Patient-centered outcomes as quality<br>Social dependence scale<br>Patient symptom distress scale<br>Family role in care | J. Q. Benoliel<br>R. McCorkle |
| Pain management | 1970s | Revised attribution theory for pain | |
| | | Anticipatory preparation<br>Physical sensations and sources of pain<br>Reduction of emotional response to pain | |

| Topic | Decade | Description | Author |
|---|---|---|---|
| | | Patient subjective rating<br>Physical intensity<br>Degree of distress | J. E. Johnson |
| | 1990s | Measurement scales | |
| | | Stress and surgical pain (animals)<br>Decrease natural killer cell cytotoxicity<br>Increase tumor metastases | G. G. Page |
| | | Pain Can Kill | |
| | | Human sex differences in biological analgesic effects | C. Miaskowski |
| Neonatal and young child development | 1970s | Identification and assessment of children at risk<br>Seriously ill newborns<br>Abused/neglected infants<br>Failure to thrive infants | |
| | 1980s | Ecology of young child health<br>Significance of family<br>Tool for assessment of behaviors of parent and child<br>Environmental factors critical to a child's well-being | |
| | | Parent-child interaction as predictor of cognitive and language development | |
| | | Nursing child assessment satellite training (NCAST) program (multidisciplinary) | K. Barnard |

**TABLE 10.1 Breakthroughs in Nursing Research (*Continued*)**

| Research Realm | Decade | Topics in Realm | Pathfinders |
|---|---|---|---|
| Neonatal and young child developmen (*cont.*) | 1990s | Nutritive sucking behavior<br>Index of infant status<br>Very low birth weight infant assessment<br>Quantitative pattern<br>Assessment of maturation, behavioral organization<br>Predictive outcomes | B. Medoff-Cooper<br>S. Gennaro |
| Research utilization | 1970s | Conduct and utilization of research in nursing<br>CURN Project<br>Development and testing of method for stimulating research-based practice in nursing<br><br>Research utilization program<br>Ten research-based protocols<br>Patient outcomes study<br>Research conduct program<br>Five pilot research projects<br>Evidence-based nursing practice | J. A. Horsley<br>J. Crane<br>M. E. Loomis |
| | 1980s | Practice guidelines development | K. B. Haller<br>M. A. Reynolds |

| Dementia care | 1980s | | |
|---|---|---|---|
| | | Paradigm change | M. Ryden |
| | | Morale of cognitively impaired | |
| | | Ethics of type of care | |
| | | Dignity and autonomy | |
| | | Wellness model | |
| | | Environment free of physical restraints | L. Evans |
| | | Individualized care | N. Strumpf |
| | | Behavioral interventions | |
| | | Conceptual model/middle range theories of care | |
| | | Ryden Aggression Scale | M. Ryden |
| | | Progressively lowered stress threshold model | G. Hall |
| | | | K. Buckwalter |
| | | Beck Dressing Performance Scale | C. K. Beck |
| | | Care assessment/decision making algorithm | P. Heacock |
| | | Disruptive behavior/patterns/management | M. Ryden |
| | | | K. Buckwalter |
| | | Need-driven, dementia Compromised model | D. Algase |
| | | | A. Whall |
| | | Family caregiving | |
| | | Conceptual Model | P. Archbold |
| | | Impact/Stress | P. Archbold |
| | | | B. Baldwin |
| | | | B. Given |
| | | | C. Collins |
| | | | H. Wilson |
| | | Positive aspects of family caregiving | |
| | | Meaning of family caregiving | C. Farran |
| | | Caregiving satisfaction | M. P. Quayhagen |

**TABLE 10.1 Breakthroughs in Nursing Research (*Continued*)**

| Research Realm | Decade | Topics in Realm | Pathfinders |
|---|---|---|---|
| Dementia care (*cont.*) | | Role preparedness/social worth | K. Robinson |
| | | | P. Archbold |
| | | | B. Stewart |
| | | Career trajectory of caregiving | C. Farran |
| | | | K. Buckwater |
| | | Minority populations | M. Wykle |
| | 1990s | Family interventions | |
| | | Cognitive stimulation | |
| | | Remedial therapy | M. P. Quayhagen |
| | | Experience of person with dementia | |
| | | Assessment of discomfort | |
| | | Advanced Alzheimer's disease | A. Hurley |
| Site transitional care | 1980s | Site transitional care model | |
| | | Research and care model | |
| | | Early discharge to home | |
| | | Comprehensive planning and home care follow-up | |
| | | Quality-cost model | |
| | | Nurse specialist model | |
| | | Patient outcomes | D. Brooten |
| | | Randomized clinical trails | L. Brown |
| | | | S. Bakewell-Sachs |
| | | Taxonomic classification of nursing interventions | S. Bakewell-Sachs |
| | | | L. Arnold |

|  |  | Model with very low birth weight infants (LBWI) | D. Brooten<br>L. Brown<br>S. Gennaro<br>R. York |
|---|---|---|---|
|  | 1990s | Model with cesarean births | D. Brooten<br>M. Roncoli<br>L. Arnold<br>R. York<br>L. Brown<br>C. Armstrong Persily |
|  |  | Model with high-risk pregancy | A. Hollingsworth<br>S. Cohen |
|  |  | Model with hysterectomy | M. Naylor<br>D. Brooten |
|  |  | Model with elderly | M. Mezey |
| Health and violence | 1970s | Sexual abuse<br>Rape and rape trauma syndrome<br>Child sexual assault by family member<br>Child's emotional response to sexual abuse | A. W. Burgess<br>L. L. Holstrum<br>M. P. McCausland |
|  |  | Domestic violence<br>Battered wife syndrome<br>Vertical transmission/nuclear family of origin | B. Parker |
|  | 1980s | Abuse during pregnancy<br>Patterns<br>Assessment screen | A. S. Helton<br>J. McFarlane<br>E. T. Anderson<br>B. Parker<br>L. Bullock |

**TABLE 10.1 Breakthroughs in Nursing Research (*Continued*)**

| Research Realm | Decade | Topics in Realm | Pathfinders |
|---|---|---|---|
| Health and violence (*cont.*) | | Battered women and low birth weight infants | L. Bullock<br>J. McFarlane |
| | | Social context of abuse<br>Domestic homicide/risk<br>Women's responses to battering over time/explanatory model<br>Nursing assessment<br>Women's health<br>Entrapment process<br>Cultural differences in abuse of women<br>Emergency room screening protocols and training | J. Campbell<br>K. Landenburger<br>S. Torres<br>V. K. Drake<br>V. P. Tilden<br>P. Shepherd |
| | | Elder abuse | L. R. Phillips<br>V. F. Rempusheski<br>T. L. Fulmer<br>J. Ashley<br>M. F. Hudson |
| | 1990s | Family/interpersonal violence as a health problem | J. Campbell<br>J. Humphreys |
| | | Concerns of children of battered women | J. Humphreys |
| Women's health | 1980s | Life and social context of perimenstrual symptoms | N. Fugate-Woods<br>G. K. Dery<br>A. Most |

| | | |
|---|---|---|
| | Menopause<br>Lived experience<br>Health and social construction | A. Voda |
| | Women's sleep science<br>Midlife women<br>Insomnia<br>Menstrual cycle sleep patterns | J. F. Shaver<br>E. Giblin<br>M. Lenz<br>K. A. Lee |
| 1990s | Gastrointestinal symptoms<br>Menstrual cycle and bowel patterns<br>Irritable bowel syndrome | M. Heitkemper<br>J. F. Shaver<br>E. Mitchell |
| 1980s | Women and urinary incontinence (UI)<br>Stress UI most prevalent type for community-living women<br>Stress UI untreated or treated with surgery | T .J. Wells<br>C. A. Brink |
| Management of stress urinary incontinence in women | Research tool development<br>One week self-recorded urinary diary<br>Intravaginal balloon device for measuring circumvaginal pelvic muscle (PM) | J. F. Wyman<br>M. C. Dougherty |

**TABLE 10.1 Breakthroughs in Nursing Research (*Continued*)**

| Research Realm | Decade | Topics in Realm | Pathfinders |
|---|---|---|---|
| Management of stress urinary incontinence in women (*cont.*) | | Behavioral intervention research | |
| | | Pelvic muscle exercise (PME) redux | |
| | | PME hypertrophies circumvaginal pelvic muscle in normals | M. C. Dougherty<br>R. Mooney |
| | | PME as effective as phenylpropanolamine HCL for stress UI in community of living women (55–90 yr) | T. J. Wells<br>C. A. Brink |
| | | Randomized controlled clinical trial of PME for women with stress UI | |
| | | Positive results related to peak PM electromyograph | |
| | | Positive results not related to urodynamic measurements | |
| | | PME effects persist for 6 months | P. A. Burns |
| | | Research-validated clinical assessment tools | |
| | | Stopwatch measure of urine stream interruption | C. M. Sampselle<br>T. J. Wells<br>C. A. Brink |
| | | Digital test for pelvic muscle (PM) strength | |
| | | Problems with PME as therapy for stress UI | C. M. Sampselle<br>T. J. Wells<br>C. A. Brink<br>M. C. Dougherty |
| | | PM strength highly variable between women | |
| | | PM strength and urine loss measures not correlated | |
| | | PME only 70% successful | |

| | | | |
|---|---|---|---|
| | | Post hoc analysis of pre/post PM contraction patterns | A. R. Boyington |
| | | PM predominant skeletal fiber type varies between subjects | C. E. Kasper |
| | | PME protocols build endurance, not speed | M. C. Dougherty |
| | | Individualized PME training protocols needed | |
| Psychobiological health | 1990s | Psychoneuroimmunology (PNI) model | |
| | | Neuropsychological function of persons with HIV/dementia | B. Swanson |
| | | | D. Cronin-Stubbs |
| | | | J. M. Zeller |
| | | Noise stress reduces rat neutrophil and macrophage function in vitro | D. O. McCarthy |
| | | Cortisol increases viral replication in macrophages in vitro | B. Swanson |
| | | | J. M. Zeller |
| | | Stress management therapy improves immune system status of person with HIV disease | N. McCain |
| | | Childbirth stress decreases maternal salivary IgA | C. Annie |
| | | Decreased maternal salivary IgA associated with postpartum complications and infant illness | M. Groër |
| | | Breast milk IgA higher after preterm than after term birth | M. Groër |
| | | | S. Humenick |
| | | | P. Hill |

**TABLE 10.1 Breakthroughs in Nursing Research (*Continued*)**

| Research Realm | Decade | Topics in Realm | Pathfinders |
|---|---|---|---|
| Psychobiological health (*cont.*) | | Psychosocial intervention for cancer/chemotherapy patients (guided imagery/support group) | |
| | | Alterations in emotional state, immune status, disease state, life span | |
| | | Self-management therapy | |
| | | Immune system variables do not all change according to PNI model | J. Post-White |
| | | Psychoneuroendocrine model | |
| | | Psychosocial (cognitive/behavioral) therapy with biofeedback for survivors of sudden cardiac arrest (SCA) | |
| | | Self-management therapy | |
| | | Cognitive/behavioral therapy to change autonomic nervous system responses and sympathetic arousal | |
| | | Alterations of psychological distress and heart rate variability | |
| | | Reduced mortality factors for survivors of SCA | M. J. Cowan |
| | | | H. N. Kogan |
| Biobehavioral health | 1980s | Exercise program for patients with cancer | M. G. MacVicar |
| | | Decreases perceived fatigue | M. L. Winningham |
| | | Decreases nausea | |

| 1990s | Aerobic interval training intervention for women with breast cancer on adjuvant chemotherapy<br>Increased physical functional capacity<br>Functional capacity as standardized quantitative measure of maximum oxygen uptake | M. G. MacVicar<br>M. L. Winningham<br>J. K. Nickel |
| | Structured walking exercise program for women with breast cancer on adjuvant chemotherapy<br>Oncology nurse specialist model<br>Improved physical performance and function<br>Perceived fatigue major symptom<br>Perceived fatigue reduced by exercise | V. Mock<br>P. Sheehan<br>M. L. Winningham |
| | Exercise walking program for women with breast cancer receiving radiation therapy<br>Oncology nurse specialist model<br>Improved physical performance and function<br>Exercise decreased perceived fatigue and emotional distress<br>Exercise improved sleep | V. Mock<br>K. H. Dow<br>P. Grimm<br>J. Dienemann |
| | Nonweight-bearing animal studies<br>Hindlimb suspension causes skeletal muscle atrophy<br>Atrophied muscles damaged during rehabilitation exercise and weight bearing | C. E. Kasper |

**TABLE 10.1 Breakthroughs in Nursing Research (*Continued*)**

| Research Realm | Decade | Topics in Realm | Pathfinders |
|---|---|---|---|
| Biobehavioral health (*cont.*) | | Bedrest during pregnancy in humans<br>Skeletal muscle dysfunction<br>Weight loss<br>Dysphoria<br>Severity of effects directly related to extent of bedrest | J. A. Maloni |
| | | Exercise for institutionalized, cognitively-impaired elders<br>Improved mobility and balance<br>Improved urine control | M. Jirovec |
| | | Fiber diet to feed fecal bacteria for chronic renal failure patients on low-protein intake<br>Gum arabic fiber fermented/metabolized by fecal bacteria<br>Increased fecal bacteria mass<br>Increased fecal nitrogen excretion<br>Decreased blood urea nitrogen in host | D. Z. Bliss |

# REFERENCES

Acton, R. T., Bell, D. S., Collins, J., Giger, J. N., Go, R. C., Harrison, R., McDonald, R., Rivers, C., Roseman, J. M., Taylor, H. A., Jr., & Vanichanan, C. (1997). Genes within and flanking the major histocompatibility region are risk factors for diabetes, insulin resistance, hypertension, and microalbuminuria in African-American women. *Transplantation Proceedings, 29*(8), 3710–3712.

Ader, R. (1996). On teaching of psychoneuroimmunology [Commentary]. *Brain, Behavior, and Immunity, 10,* 315–323.

Ader, R., & Cohen, N. (1975). Behaviorally conditioned immunosuppression. *Psychosomatic Medicine, 37,* 333–340.

Algase, D. L., Beck, C., Kolanowski, A, Whall, A., Berent, S., Richards, K., & Beattie, E. (1996). Need-driven dementia-compromised behavior: An alternative view of disruptive behavior. *American Journal of Alzheimer's Disease, 11*(6), 10–19.

Annie, C. L., & Gröer, M. (1991). Childbirth stress: An immunologic study. *Journal of Obstetric, Gynecologic, and Neonatal Nursing, 20,* 391–397.

Archbold, P. G. (1980). Impact of parent caring on middle-aged offspring. *Journal of Gerontological Nursing, 6*(2), 78–85.

Archbold, P. G. (1983). Impact of parent-caring on women. *Family Relations, 32,* 39–45.

Archbold, P., Stewart, B., Greenlick, M., & Harvath, T. (1990). Mutuality and preparedness as predictors of caregiver role strain. *Research in Nursing and Health, 13,* 375–384.

Baldwin, B. A. (1988). The stress of caring: Issues confronting mid-life caregivers. *Caring, 7,* 16–18, 66.

Baldwin, B., Klelman, K., Stevens, G., & Rasin, J. (1989). Family caregiver stress: Clinical assessment and management. *International Psychogeriatrics, 1,* 185–194.

Barnard, K. E. (1973). The effects of stimulation on the sleep behavior of the premature infant. In M. Batey (Ed.), *Communicating nursing research* (Vol. 6, pp. 12–33). Boulder, CO: WICHE.

Barnard, K. E. (1976). The state of the art: Nursing and early intervention with handicapped infants. In T. Tjossem (Ed.), *Proceedings of 1974 President's Committee on Mental Retardation.* Baltimore: University Park Press.

Barnard, K. E. (1979). How focusing on the family changes the health care system. In T. B. Brazelton & V. C. Vaughan (Eds.), *The family: Setting priorities* (pp. 181–191). New York: Science and Medicine Publishing Co.

Barnard, K. E., & Bee, H. L. (1983). The impact of temporally patterned stimulation on the development of preterm infants. *Child Development, 54,* 1156–1167.

Barnard, K. E., Bee, H. L., & Hammond, M. A. (1984). Developmental changes in maternal interactions with term and preterm infants. *Infant Behavior and Development, 7,* 101–113.

Barnard, K. E., & Collar, B. S. (1973). Early diagnosis, interpretation, and intervention: A commentary on the nurse's role. *Annals of the New York Academy of Sciences, 205,* 373–382.

Barnard, K. E., Spietz, A. L. Snyder, C., Douglas, H. B., Eyres, S. J., & Hill, V. (1977). *The nursing child assessment satellite training study guide.* Unpublished manuscript. University of Washington, Seattle.

Barnard, K. E., Wenner, W., Weber, B., Gray, C., & Peterson, A. (1977). Premature infant refocus. In P. Miller (Ed.), *Research to practice in mental retardation: Vol. 3. Biomedical aspects.* Baltimore: University Park Press.

Beck, C. (1988). Measurement of dressing performance in persons with dementia. *American Journal of Alzheimer's Care and Related Disorders and Research, 3*(3), 21–25.

Beck, C., Heacock, P., Mercer, S. O., Walls, R., Rapp, C. G., & Vogelpohl, T. S. (1997). Improving dressing behavior in cognitively impaired nursing home residents. *Nursing Research, 46,* 126–132.

Beck, C., Heacock, P., Rapp, C. G., & Mercer, S. (1993). Assisting cognitively impaired elders with activities of daily living. *American Journal of Alzheimer's Care and Related Disorders and Research, 8*(6), 11–20.

Bee, H. L., Barnard, K. E., Eyres, S. J., Gray, C. A., Hammond, M. A., Spietz, A. L., Snyder, C., & Clark, B. (1982). Prediction of IQ and language skill from perinatal status, child performance, family characteristics, and mother-infant interaction. *Child Development, 53,* 1134–1156.

Bee, H. L., Hammond, M. A., Eyres, S. J., Barnard, K. E., & Snyder, C. (1986). The impact of parental life change on the early development of children. *Research in Nursing and Health, 9,* 65–74.

Beecher, H. K. (1959). *Measurement of subjective response: Quantitative effects of drugs.* New York: Oxford University.

Benoliel, J. D., & McCorkle, R. (1978). A holistic approach to terminal illness. *Cancer Nursing, 2,* 143–149.

Benoliel, J. Q., & McCorkle, R. (1983). Symptom distress, current concerns and mood disturbance after diagnosis of life-threatening disease. *Social Science and Medicine, 17,* 431–438.

Bishop, K. R., Dougherty, M., Mooney, R., Gimotty, P., & Williams, B. (1992). Effects of age, parity, and adherence on pelvic muscle response to exercise. *Journal of Obstetric, Gynecologic and Neonatal Nursing, 21*(5), 401–6.

Bliss, D. Z., Stein, T. P., Schleifer, C. R., & Settle, R. G. (1996). Supplementation with gum arabic fiber increases fecal nitrogen excretion and lowers serum urea nitrogen concentration in chronic renal failure patients consuming a low protein diet. *American Journal of Clinical Nutrition, 63,* 392–398.

Booth, C. L., Barnard, K. E., Mitchell, S. K., & Spieker, S. J. (1987). Successful intervention with multiproblem mothers: Effects on the mother-infant relationship. *Infant Mental Health Journal, 9,* 288–306.

Booth, C. L., Lyons, N. B., & Barnard, K. E. (1984). Synchrony in mother-infant interaction: A comparison of measurement methods. *Child Study Journal, 14,* 95–114.

Booth, C. L., Mitchell, S. K., Barnard, K. E., & Spieker, S. J. (1989). Development of maternal social skills in multiproblem families: Effect on the mother-child relationship. *Developmental Psychology, 25*(3), 403–412.

Booth, D., Bradley, W., & Whall, A. (1988). Description of early and late functional changes in persons with Alzheimer's disease. *Journal of Nursing Science and Practice, 1*(3), 9–16.

Boyington, A. R., Dougherty, M. C., & Kasper, C. E. (1995). Pelvic muscle profile types in response to pelvic muscle exercise. *International Urogynecology Journal, 6,* 68–72.

Brink, C., Wells, T., Sampselle, C., Taille, E., & Mayer, R. (1994). A digital test for pelvic muscle strength in women with urinary incontinence. *Nursing Research, 43*(6), 352–356.

Brodie, B. (1997). Mothers and pediatric nursing's changing values 1880–1960. *Reflections, 23*(3), 33–35.

Bronfenbrenour, U. & Ceci, S. J. (1994). Nature–nurture reconceptualized in developmental perspective: A biological model. *Psychological Review, 101,* 568–586.

Brooten, D., Brown, L. P., Munro, B. H., York, R., Cohen, S., Roncoli, M., & Hollingsworth, A. (1988). Early discharge and specialist transitional care. *Image: Journal of Nursing Scholarship, 20,* 64–68.

Brooten, D., Gennaro, S., Knapp, H., Brown, L., & York, R. (1989). Clinical specialist pre- and post-discharge teaching of parents of very low birthweight infants. *Journal of Obstetric, Gynecologic and Neonatal Nursing, 18*(4), 316–322.

Brooten, D., Knapp, H., Borucki, L., Jacobsen, B., Finkler, S., Arnold, L., & Mennuti, M. (1996). Early discharge and home care after unplanned cesarean birth: Nursing care time. *Journal of Obstetric, Gynecologic and Neonatal Nursing, 25,* 595–600.

Brooten, D., Kumar, S., Brown, L., Butts, P., Finkler, S., Bakewell-Sachs, S., Gibbons, S., & Delivoria-Papdopoulos, M. (1986). A randomized clinical trial of early hospital discharge and home follow-up of very low birth weight infants. *New England Journal of Medicine, 315,* 934–939.

Brooten, D., Roncoli, M., Finkler, S., Arnold, L., Cohen, A., & Mennuti, M. (1994). A randomized trial of early hospital discharge and home follow-up of women having cesarean birth. *Obstetrics and Gynecology, 84,* 832–838.

Brown, L., York, R., Jacobsen, B., Gennaro, S., & Brooten, D. (1989). Very low birthweight infants: Parental visiting and telephoning during initial infant hospitalization. *Nursing Research, 38*(4), 233–236.

Bullock, L., & McFarlane, J. (1989). Higher prevalence of low birth weight infants born to battered women. *American Journal of Nursing, 9,* 1153–1155.

Bullock, L., McFarlane, J., Bateman, L., & Miller, V. (1989). The prevalence and characteristics of battered women in a primary care setting. *Nurse Practitioner, 14,* 47–56.

Burger, S. G., & Williams, C. C. (1996). Individualized care [Editorial]. *Journal of Gerontological Nursing, 22*(3), 5.

Burgess, A. W., Groth, A. N., & McCausland, M. P. (1981). Child sex initiation rings. *American Journal of Orthopsychiatry, 51,* 110–119.

Burgess, A. W., & Holstrom, L. L. (1974). Rape trauma syndrome. *American Journal of Psychiatry, 131,* 981–986.

Burgess, A. W., & Holstrom, L. L. (1975). Sexual trauma of children and adolescents. *Nursing Clinics of North America, 10,* 551–563.

Burgess, A. W., Holstrom, L. L., & McCausland, M. P. (1977). Child sexual assault by a family member: Decisions following disclosure. *Victimology, 2,* 236–250.

Burgio, K. L., Robinson, J. C., & Engel, B. T. (1986). The role of biofeedback in Kegel exercise training for stress urinary incontinence. *American Journal of Obstetrics and Gynecology, 154,* 58–64.

Burns, P., Pranikoff, K., Nochajski, T., Desotelle, P., & Harwood, K. (1990). Treatment of stress incontinence with pelvic muscle exercises and biofeedback. *Journal of the American Geriatrics Society, 38*(3), 341–344.

Burns, P., Pranikoff, K., Nochajski, T., Hadley, E., Levy, K., & Ory, M. (1993). A comparison of effectiveness of biofeedback and pelvic muscle exercise treatment of stress incontinence in older community-dwelling women. *Journal of Gerontology, 48*(4), M167–M174.

Campbell, J. (1981). Misogyny and homicide of women. *Advances in Nursing Science, 3,* 67–85.

Campbell, J. C. (1986). Nursing assessment for risk of homicide with battered women. *Advances in Nursing Science, 8*(4), 36–51.

Campbell, J. C. (1989a). A test of two exploratory models of women's responses to battering. *Nursing Research, 38,* 18–24.

Campbell, J. C. (1989b). Women's responses to sexual abuse in intimate relationships. *Women's Health Care International, 8,* 335–347.

Campbell, J. C., Anderson, E., Fulmer, T. L., Girouard, S., & McElmurry, B. (1993). Violence as a nursing priority: Policy implications. *Nursing Outlook, 41*(2), 83–92.

Campbell, J., & Humphreys, J. (Eds.). (1993). *Nursing Care of Victims of Family Violence.* Reston, VA: Reston Publishing Co.

Campbell, J. C., Kub, J. & Lewandowski, L. (1998). Violence as a nursing area of inquiry. In J. J. Fitzpatrick (Ed.), *Encyclopedia of nursing research* (pp. 584–587). New York: Springer Publishing Co.

Campbell, J., & Parker, B. (1992). Battered women and their children. In J. Fitzpatrick (Ed.), *Annual review of nursing research* (Vol. 10, pp. 77–94). New York: Springer Publishing Co.

Campbell, J. C., Pugh, L. C., Campbell, D., & Visscher, M. (1995). The influence of abuse on pregnancy intention. *Women's Health Issues, 5*(4), 214–223.

Cannon, W. B. (1926). The emergency function of the adrenal medulla in pain and the major emotions. *American Journal of Physiology, 33,* 356–372.

Capezuti, E., Evans, L., Strumpf, N., & Maislin, G. (1996). Physical restraint use and falls in nursing home residents. *Journal of the American Gerontological Society, 44,* 627–633.

Capezuti, E., Strumpf, N. E., Evans, L. K., Grisso, J. A., & Maislin, G. (1998). The relationship between physical restraint removal and falls and injuries among nursing home residents. *Journal of Gerontology: Medical Sciences, 53A*(1), M47–M52.

Casey, K. L., & Melzack, R. (1967). Neural mechanisms of pain, a conceptual model. In E. Leong Way (Eds.), *New concepts in pain and its clinical management* (pp. 13–31). Philadelphia: F. A. Davis.

Cohen, S., Arnold, L., Brown, L., & Brooten, D. (1991). Taxonomic classification of transitional follow-up care nursing interventions with low birthweight infants. *Clinical Nurse Specialist, 5,* 31–36.

Corbeil, R. R., Quayhagen, M. P., & Quayhagen, M. (1999). Intervention effects on dementia caregiving interaction: A stress-adaptation modeling approach. *Journal of Aging and Health, 11,* 79–95.

Cousins, M. J. (1991). Prevention of postoperative pain. In M. R. Bond, J. E. Charlton, & C. J. Woolf (Eds.), *Pain research and clinical management* (Vol. 4, pp. 41–52). Amsterdam: Elsevier.

Cowan, M. J. (1997). Innovative approaches: A psychosocial therapy for sudden cardiac arrest survivors. In S. B. Dunbar, K. A. Ellenbogen, & A. E. Epstein

(Eds.), *Sudden cardiac death: Past, present, and future* (pp. 371–386). Armonk, NY: Futura Publishing Co.

Cowan, M. J., Heinrich, J., Lucas, M., Sigmon, H., & Hinshaw, A. S. (1993). Integration of biological and nursing sciences: A 10 year plan to enhance research and training. *Research in Nursing and Health, 16*(1), 3–9.

Dalakis, M. C., Mock, V., & Hawkins, M. J. (1998). Fatigue: Definitions, mechanisms, and paradigms for study. *Seminars in Oncology, 25*(Suppl. 1), 48–53.

Diokno, C. A., Brock, B. M., Brown, M. B., & Herzog, A. R. (1986). Prevalence of urinary incontinence and other urologic symptoms in the non-institutionalized elderly. *Journal of Urology, 135,* 1022.

Donaldson, G., McCorkle, R., Georgialou, F., & Benoliel, J. Q. (1986). Distress, dependency, and threat in newly diagnosed cancer and heart disease patients. *Multivariate Behavioral Research, 21,* 267–298.

Donaldson, S. K. (1997). Future of nursing scholarship. *Image, 29*(2), 117–121.

Donaldson, S. K. (1999). Genetic research and knowledge in the discipline of nursing. *Biological Research in Nursing, 1*(2), 90–99.

Donaldson, S. K., & Crowley, D. M. (1978). The discipline of nursing. *Nursing Outlook, 26,* 113–120.

Donohue, D., Brooten, D., Roncoli, M., Arnold, L., Knapp, H., Borucki, L., & Cohen, A. (1994). Acute care visits and re-hospitalization in women and infants after cesarean birth. *Journal of Perinatology, 14*(1), 36–40.

Dougherty, M., Abrams, R., & McKey, L. (1986). An instrument to assess the dynamic characteristics of the circumvaginal musculature. *Nursing Research, 35*(4), 202–206.

Dougherty, M., Bishop, K., Mooney, R., & Gimotty, P. (1989). The effect of circum-vaginal muscle (CVM) exercise. *Nursing Research, 38*(6), 331–335.

Dougherty, M., Bishop, K., Mooney, R., Gimotty, P., & Williams, B. (1993). Graded pelvic muscle exercise. *Journal of Reproductive Medicine, 38*(9), 684–691.

Drake, V. K. (1982). Battered women: A health care problem in disguise. *Image, 14,* 40–47.

Evans, L. K., & Strumpf, N. E. (1989). Tying down the elderly. *Journal of the American Geriatrics Society, 37,* 65–74.

Evans, L. K., & Strumpf, N. E. (1990). Myths about elder restraint. *Image: Journal of Nursing Scholarship, 22*(2), 124–128.

Fairman, J. (1997). Thinking about patients: Nursing science in the 1950's. *Reflections, 23*(3), 30–32.

Farran, C. J., & Keane-Haggerty, M. A. (1988). A group intervention program for caregivers of persons with dementia. In K. C. Buckwalter (Eds.), *Intervention strategies for maintaining control throughout the caregiving trajectory* (pp. 14–19). Iowa City: Iowa Geriatric Education Center, Interdisciplinary Monograph Series.

Farran, C. J., Keane-Haggerty, E., Salloway, S., Kupferer, S., & Wilken, C. S. (1991). Finding meaning: An alternate paradigm for Alzheimer's disease family caregivers. *Gerontologist, 31*(4), 483–489.

Feetham, S. (1997). The genetics revolution: Outcomes and recommendations. In F. E. Lashley (Ed.), *The genetics revolution: Implications for nursing* (pp. 35–39). Washington, DC: American Academy of Nursing.

Feetham, S. L. (1999). Families in health, illness, and life transitions. In A. S.

Hinshaw, S. L. Feetham, & J. L. Shaver (Eds.), *Handbook of clinical nursing research* (pp. 199–200). Thousand Oaks, CA: Sage Publications.

Feetham, S. L., & Meister, S. B. (1999). Nursing research of families: State of the science and correspondence with policy. In A. S. Hinshaw, S. L. Feetham, & J. L. Shaver (Eds.), *Handbook of clinical nursing research* (pp. 251–271). Thousand Oaks, CA: Sage Publications.

Feldt, K., & Ryden M. B. (1992). Aggressive behavior: Educating nursing assistants. *Journal of Gerontological Nursing, 18*(5), 3–12.

Fillingim, R. B., & Maixner, W. (1995). Gender differences in the response to noxious stimuli. *Pain Forum, 4,* 209–221.

Fogell, C., & Woods, N. (Eds.). (1981). *Health care of women: A nursing perspective.* St. Louis: C. V. Mosby.

Fulmer, T. (1991). Elder mistreatment: Progress in community detection and intervention. *Family Community Health, 14*(2), 26–34.

Fulmer, T., & Ashley, J. (1986). Neglect: What part of abuse? *Pride Institute Journal, 5*(4), 18–24.

Fulmer, T., & Ashley, J. (1988). Toward the development of a social policy statement on elder abuse. *Oasis, 5*(3), 1–3.

Gear, R. W., Gordon, N. C., Heller, P. H., Paul, S. M., Miaskowski, C., & Levine, J. D. (1996). Gender difference in analgesic response to the kappa-opioid pentazocine. *Neuroscience Letters, 205,* 207–209.

Gear, R. W., Miaskowski, C., Gordon, N. C., Paul, S. M., Heller, P. H., & Levine, J. D. (1996). Kappa-opioids produce significantly greater analgesia in women than in men. *Nature Medicine, 2*(11), 1248–1250.

Gillis, C. L., & Knafl, K. A. (1999). Nursing care of families in non-normative transitions. In A. S. Hinshaw, S. L. Feetham, & J. L. Shaver (Eds.), *Handbook of clinical nursing research* (pp. 231–249). Thousand Oaks, CA: Sage.

Given, B. A., & Given, C. W. (1991). Family caregiving for the elderly. In J. Fitzpatrick (Ed.), *Annual review of nursing research* (Vol. 10, pp. 77–101). New York: Springer Publishing Co.

Given, B., King, S., Collins, C., & Given C. W. (1988). Family caregivers of the elderly: Involvement and reactions to care. *Archives of Psychiatric Nursing, 2,* 281–288.

Given, B., Stommel, M., Collins, C., King, S., & Given, C. W. (1990). Responses of elderly spouse caregivers. *Research in Nursing and Health, 13*(2), 77–85.

Gröer, M. W., Humenick, S., & Hill, P. D. (1994). Characterizations and psychoneuroimmunological implications of secretory immunoglobulin A and cortisol in preterm and term breast milk. *Journal of Perinatal and Neonatal Nursing, 7*(4), 42–51.

Groth, A. N., & Burgess, A. W. (1977). Motivational intent in the sexual assault of children. *Criminal Justice and Behavior, 4,* 253–264.

Haber, L. C. (1998). Family theory and research. In J. J. Fitzpatrick (Ed.), *Encyclopedia of nursing research* (pp. 196–197). New York: Springer Publishing Co.

Hall, G., & Buckwalter, K. (1987). Progressively lowered stress threshold: A conceptual model for care of adults with Alzheimer's disease. *Archives of Psychiatric Nursing, 1,* 309–406.

Hall, G., Kirschling, V., & Todd, S. (1986). Sheltered freedom: An Alzheimer's unit in an ICF. *Geriatric Nursing, 7,* 132–137.

Haller, K. B., Reynolds, M. A., & Horsley, J. A. (1979). Developing research-based innovation protocols: Process, criteria, and issues. *Research in Nursing and Health, 2,* 45–51.

Halley, F. M. (1991). Self-regulation of the immune system through biobehavioral strategies. *Biofeedback and Self-Regulation, 16,* 55–74.

Hammer, S. L., & Barnard, K. E. (1966). The mentally retarded adolescent: A review of the characteristics and problems of 44 non-institutionalized adolescent retardates. *Pediatrics, 38,* 845–857.

Heitkemper, M. (1998). A biopsychosocial model of irritable bowel syndrome. *Communicating Nursing Research, 31,* 73–79.

Heitkemper, M. M., Hanson, R., & Walike, B. C. (1977). Effects of rate and volume of tube feeding. In M. V. Batey (Ed.), *Communicating nursing research* (Vol. 10, pp. 71–89). Boulder, CO: WICHE.

Heitkemper, M. M., & Marotta, S. F. (1983). Development and neurotransmitter enzyme activity. *American Journal of Physiology, 244,* G58–G64.

Heitkemper, M. M., Martin, D. L., Hansen, B. C., Hanson, R., & Vanderburg, V. (1981). Rate and volume of intermittent feeding administration. *Journal of Parenteral and Enteral Nutrition, 5,* 125–130.

Heitkemper, M., Shaver, J., & Mitchell, E. (1988). Gastrointestinal symptoms and bowel patterns across the menstrual cycle in dymenorrheic and nondysmenorrheic women. *Nursing Research, 37,* 108–113.

Helton, A. S. (1986). The pregnant battered woman. *Response, 9*(1), 22–23.

Helton, A. S., McFarlane, J., & Anderson, E. (1987). Battered and pregnant: A prevalence study. *American Journal of Public Health, 77,* 1337–1339.

Herbert, T. B., & Cohen, S. (1993). Stress and immunity in humans: A meta-analytic review. *Psychosomatic Medicine, 55,* 364–379.

Hill, M. N. (in press). Comprehensive hypertension care in young urban black men: An example of a program of nursing research that bridges genetic science, clinical interventions, and the potential to improve patient outcomes. *Nursing Clinics of North America.*

Hinshaw, A. S. (1999). Evolving nursing research traditions. In A. S. Hinshaw, S. L. Feetham, & J. L. Shaver (Eds.), *Handbook of clinical nursing research* (pp. 19–30). Thousand Oaks, CA: Sage Publications.

Holmes, T. H., & Rahe, R. H. (1967). The social readjustment rating scale. *Journal of Psychosomatic Research, 11,* 213–218.

Horsley, J. A., Crane, J., & Bingle, J. (1978). Research utilization: An organizational process. *Journal of Nursing Administration, 8*(7), 4–6.

Horsley, J. A., Crane, J., Crabtree, M. K., & Wood, D. J. (1983). *Using research to improve nursing practice: A guide.* New York: Grune & Stratton.

Hudson, M. F. (1989). An analysis of the concepts of elder mistreatment, abuse, and neglect. *Journal of Abuse and Neglect, 1,* 5–25.

Humphreys, J. (1991). Children of battered women: Worries about their mothers. *Pediatric Nursing, 17*(4), 342–345.

Hurley, A., Volicer, B., Hanrahan, P., Houde, S., & Volicer, L. (1992). Assessment of discomfort in advanced Alzheimer patients. *Research in Nursing and Health, 15,* 367–377.

Illman, D. (1996). 1979: Parent-child interaction. In A. L. Kwiram (Ed.), *Pathbreakers: A century of excellence in science technology at the University of Washington* (pp. 195–196). Seattle: University of Washington, Office of Research.

Jirovec, M. M. (1991). The impact of daily exercise on the mobility, balance, and urine control of cognitively impaired nursing home residents. *International Journal of Nursing Studies, 28*(2), 145–151.

Johnson, J. E. (1973). Effects of accurate expectations about sensations on the sensory and distress components of pain. *Journal of Personality and Social Psychology, 27,* 261–265.

Johnson, J. E., & Rice, V. H. (1974). Sensory and distress components of pain Implication for the study of clinical pain. *Nursing Research, 23,* 203–209.

Johnson, J. E., Rice, V. H., Fuller, S. S., & Endress, M. P. (1978). Sensory information, instruction in coping strategy and recovery from surgery. *Research in Nursing and Health, 1,* 4–17.

Jones, E. G., & Kegel, A. H. (1952). Treatment of urinary stress incontinence. *Surgery of Gynecology and Obstetrics, 94,* 179–188.

Kasper, C. E. (1995). Sarcolemmal disruption in reloaded atrophic skeletal muscle. *Journal of Applied Physiology, 79,* 607–614.

Kasper, C. E., Maxwell, L. C., & White, T. P. (1996). Alterations in skeletal muscle related to short-term impaired physical mobility. *Research in Nursing and Health, 19*(2), 133–142.

Kasper, C. E., & Sarna, L. P. (in press). Influence of adjuvant chemotherapy on skeletal muscle and fatigue in women with breast cancer. *Nursing Research.*

Kasper, C. E., White, T. P., & Maxwell, L. C. (1990). Running during recovery from hind-limb suspension induces transient muscle injury. *Journal of Applied Physiology, 68*(2), 533–539.

Kegel, A. H. (1948). Progressive resistance exercise in the functional restoration of the perineal muscles. *American Journal of Obstetrics and Gynecology, 56,* 242–245.

Kegel, A. H. (1956). Stress incontinence of urine in women: Physiologic treatment. *Journal of International College of Surgeons, 25,* 487–499.

Keller, S. E., Weiss, J. M., Schleifer, S. J., Miller, N. E., & Stein, M. (1981). Suppression of immunity by stress: Effect of a graded series of stressors on lymphocyte stimulation in the rat. *Science, 213,* 1397–1400.

Kelley, J. F., Morrisset, C. E., Barnard, K. E., Hammond, M. A., & Booth, C. L. (1996). The influence of early mother-child interaction on preschool cognitive/linguistic outcomes in a high social risk group. *Infant Mental Health Journal, 17*(4), 310–321.

Kiecolt-Glaser, J. K., & Glaser, R. (1992). Psychoneuroimmunology: Can psychological interventions modulate immunity? *Journal of Consulting and Clinical Psychology, 60,* 569–575.

Kiecolt-Glaser, J. K., Page, G. G., Marucha, P. T., MacCallum, R. C., & Glaser, R. (1998). Psychological influences on surgical recovery. *American Psychologist, 53*(11), 1209–1218.

Landenburger, K. (1989). A process of entrapment in and recovery from an abusive relationship. *Issues in Mental Health Nursing, 10,* 209–227.

Laudenslager, M. L., Ryan, S. M., Drugan, R. C., Hyson, R. L., & Maier, S. F. (1983). Coping and immunosuppression: Inescapable but not escapable shock suppresses lymphocyte proliferation. *Science, 221,* 568–570.

Lee, K. A. (1988). Circadian temperature rhythms in relation to menstrual cycle phase. *Journal of Biological Rhythms, 3,* 255–263.

Lee, K. A., Shaver, J. F., Giblin E. C., & Woods, N. F. (1990). Sleep patterns related to menstrual cycle phase and premenstrual affective symptoms. *Sleep, 13*(5), 403–409.

Lewis, J. W., Shavit, Y., Terman, G. W., Gale, R. P., & Liebeskind, J. C. (1983/84). Stress and morphine affect survival of rats challenged with a mammary ascites tumor (MAT 13762B). *Natural Immunity and Cell Growth Regulation, 3,* 43–50.

Locke, S. E. (1982). Stress, adaptation, and immunity: Studies in humans. *General Hospital Psychiatry, 4,* 49–58.

Loomis, M. E. (1982). Resources for collaborative research. *Western Journal of Nursing Research, 4,* 65–74.

Maas, M., & Buckwalter, K. C. (1991). Alzheimer's disease. In J. Fitzpatrick (Ed.), *Annual review of nursing research* (Vol. 9, pp. 19–55). New York: Springer Publishing, Co.

MacPherson, K. I. (1981). Menopause as disease: The social construction of a metaphor. *Advances in Nursing Science, 3,* 95–113.

MacPherson, K. I. (1983). Feminist methods: A new paradigm for nursing research. *Advances in Nursing Science, 5,* 17–25.

MacVicar, M. G., & Winningham, M. L. (1986). Promoting the functional capacity of cancer patients. *Cancer Bulletin, 38,* 235–238.

MacVicar, M. G., Winningham, M. L., & Nickel, J. L. (1989). Effects of aerobic interval training on cancer patient's functional capacity. *Nursing Research, 38*(6), 348–351.

Maloni, J. A., Chance, B., Zhang, C., Cohen, A. W., Betts, D., & Gange, S. J. (1993). Physical and psychosocial side effects of antepartum hospital bed rest. *Nursing Research, 42*(4), 197–203.

Maloni, J. A., & Kasper, C. E. (1991). Physical and psychosocial effects of antepartum hospital bed rest: A review of the literature. *Image, 23*(3), 187–192.

McBride, A. B. (1992). Violence against women: Overarching themes and nursing's research agenda. In C. M. Samselle (Eds.), *Violence Against Women* (pp. 83–89). New York: Hemisphere.

McBride, A. B. (1993). From gynecology to gynecology: Developing a practice-research agenda for women's health. *Health Care for Women International, 14,* 316–325.

McBride, A. B. (1997). Nursing and the women's movement. *Reflections, 23*(3), 39–41.

McBride, A. B. (1998). Women's health research. In J. J. Fitzpatrick (Ed.), *Encyclopedia of nursing research* (pp. 598–601). New York: Springer Publishing Co.

McBride, A. B., & McBride, W. L. (1981). Theoretical underpinnings for women's health. *Women and Health, 6,* 37–55.

McCain, N. L., & Cella, D. F. (1995). Correlates of stress in HIV disease. *Western Journal of Nursing Research, 17,* 141–155.

McCain, N. L., Zeller, J. M., Cella, D. F., Urbanski, P. A., & Noval, R. M. (1996). The influence of stress management training in HIV disease. *Nursing Research, 45,* 246–253.

McCarthy, D. O., Quimet, M. E., & Daun, J. M. (1992). The effects of noise stress on leukocyte function in rats. *Research in Nursing and Health, 15,* 131–137.

McCorkle, R., Quint-Benoliel, J., & Young, K. (1980). Development of a social dependency scale. *Research in Nursing and Health, 3,* 3–10.

McCormick, K. A., & Palmer, M. H. (1992). Urinary incontinence in older adults. *Annual Review of Nursing Research, 10,* 25–53.

McCubbin, M. (1999). Normative family transitions and health outcomes. In A. S. Hinshaw, S. L. Feetham, & J. L. Shaver (Eds.), *Handbook of clinical nursing research* (pp. 201–230). Thousand Oaks, CA: Sage.

McFarlane, J., Parker, B., Soeken, K., & Bullock, L. (1992). Assessing for abuse during pregnancy. *Journal of the American Medical Association, 267*(23), 3176–3178.

Medoff-Cooper, B., & Gennaro, S. (1996). The correlation of sucking behaviors and Bayley Scales of infant development at six months of age in very-low-birth-weight infants. *Nursing Research, 45,* 291–296.

Medoff-Cooper, B., & Ray, W. (1996). Neonatal sucking behaviors. *Image: Journal of Nursing Scholarship, 27,* 195–199.

Medoff-Cooper, B., Verklan, T., & Carlson, S. (1993). The development of sucking patterns and physiologic correlates in very-low-birth-weight infants. *Nursing Research, 44,* 100–105.

Medoff-Cooper, B., Weininger, S., & Zukowsky, K. (1989). Neonatal sucking as a clinical assessment tool: Preliminary findings. *Nursing Research, 38,* 162–165.

Meier, P., & Anderson, G. (1987). Responses of small preterm infants to bottle- and breastfeeding. *MCN: American Journal of Maternal and Child Nursing, 12,* 97–105.

Melzack, R., & Wall, P. D. (1965). Pain mechanisms: A new theory. *Science, 150,* 971–979.

Miaskowski, C. (1997). Pain management in women. In B. J. McElmurry & R. S. Parker (Eds.), *Annual review of women's health* (Vol. 3, pp. 245–255). New York: National League for Nursing Press.

Miovech, S., Knapp, H., Borucki, R., Roncoli, M., Arnold, L., & Brooten, D. (1992). Major concerns of women after cesarean delivery. *Journal of Obstetric, Gynecologic and Neonatal Nursing, 23,* 53–59.

Mock, V., Burke, M. B., Sheehan, P., Creaton, E. M., Winningham, M. L., McKenney-Ledder, S., Schwager, L. P., & Liebman, M. (1994). A nursing rehabilitation program for women with breast cancer receiving adjuvant chemotherapy. *Oncology Nursing Forum, 21,* 899–907.

Mock, V., Dow, K. H., Meares, C. J., Grimm, P. M., Dienemann, J. A., Haisfield-Wolfe, M. E., Quitasol, S. M., Chakravarthy, A., & Gage, I. (1997). Effects of exercise on fatigue, physical functioning, and emotional distress during radiation therapy for breast cancer. *Oncology Nursing Forum, 24*(6), 991–1000.

Morriset, C. E., Barnard, K. E., Greenberg, M. T., Booth, C. L., & Spieker, S. J. (1990). Environmental influences on early language development: The context of social risk. *Development and Psychopathology, 2,* 127–149.

Naylor, M. D., Brooten, D., Campbell, R., Jacobsen, B. S., Mezey, M. D., Pauly, M. V., & Schwartz, J. S. (1999). Comprehensive discharge planning and home follow-up of hospitalized elders. *Journal of the American Medical Association, 281,* 613–620.

Naylor, M., Brooten, D., Jones, R., Lavizzo-Mourey, R., Mezey, M., & Pauly, M. (1994). Comprehensive discharge planning for the hospitalized elderly. *Annals of Internal Medicine, 120,* 999–1006.

Naylor, M. D., & Shaid, E. C. (1991). Content analyses of pre- and post-discharge topics taught to hospitalized elderly by clinical nurse specialists. *Clinical Nurse Specialist, 5*(2), 111–116.

Nisbett, R. E., & Schachter, S. (1966). Cognitive manipulation of pain. *Journal of Experimental Social Psychology, 12,* 279–288.

Orem, D. E. (1980). *Nursing: Concepts of practice* (2nd ed.). New York: McGraw Hill.

Page, G. G., & Ben-Eliyahu, S. (1998). Pain kills: Animal models and neuroimmunological links. In R. Payne, R. B. Pott, & C. S. Hill (Eds.), *Assessment and treatment of cancer pain: Progress in pain research and management* (Vol. 1, pp. 135–143). Seattle: IASP Press

Page, G. G., Ben-Eliyahu, S., & Liebeskind, J. C. (1994). The role of LGL/NK cells in surgery-induced promotion of metastases and its attenuation by morphine. *Brain, Behavior, and Immunity, 8,* 241–250.

Page, G. G., Ben-Eliayhu, S., & McDonald, J. S. (1997). The attenuating effects of morphine on the metastatic and hormonal sequelae of surgery in rats. In T. S. Jensen, J. A. Turner, & Z. Wisenfeld-Hallin (Eds.), *Proceedings of the 8th World Congress on Pain: Progress in pain research and management* (Vol. 8, pp. 815–823). Seattle: IASP Press.

Page, G. G., Ben-Eliyahu, S., Yirmiya, R., & Liebeskind, J. C. (1993). Morphine attenuates surgery-induced enhancement of metastatic colonization in rats. *Pain, 54,* 21–28.

Page, G. G., McDonald, J. S., & Ben-Eliyahu, S. (1998). Pre-operative versus post-operative administration of morphine: Impact on the neuroendocrine, behavioral and metastatic enhancing effects of surgery. *British Journal of Anesthesia, 81,* 216–223.

Parker, B., & McFarlane, J. (1991a). Feminist theory and nursing: An empowerment model for research. *Advances in Nursing Science, 13*(3), 59–67.

Parker, B., & McFarlane, J. (1991b). Identifying and helping pregnant battered women. *Maternal Child Nursing, 16*(3), 161–164.

Parker, B., & Schumacher, D. N. (1977). The battered wife syndrome and violence in the nuclear family of origin: A controlled pilot study. *American Journal of Public Health, 67*(6), 760–761.

Parker, B., & Ulrich, Y. (1990). A protocol of safety: Research on abuse of women. *Nursing Research, 39*(4), 248–250.

Persily, C. A. (1996). Relationships between the perceived impact of gestational diabetes mellitus and treatment adherence. *Journal of Obstetric, Gynecologic and Neonatal Nursing, 25,* 602–607.

Phillips, L. R. (1983). Abuse/neglect of the frail elderly at home: An exploration of theoretical relationships. *Journal of Advanced Nursing, 8,* 379–392.

Phillips, L. R., & Rempusheski, V. F. (1985). A decision making model for diagnosing and intervening in elder abuse and neglect. *Nursing Research, 34,* 134–139.

Post-White, J. (1993). The effects of mental imagery on emotions, immune function, and cancer outcome. *Midwest Nursing Research Society: Mainlines Research Brief, 14*(1), 18–20.

Post-White, J. (1998). Psychoneuroimmunology: The mind-body connection. In R. M. Carroll-Johnson, L. M. Gorman, & N. J. Bush (Eds.), *Psychosocial care along the cancer continuum* (pp. 349–364). Pittsburgh, PA: Oncology Nursing Press.

Quayhagen, M. P., Quayhagen, M. M., Corbeil, R. R., Roth, P. A., & Rodgers, J. A. (1995). A dyadic remediation program for care-recipients with dementia. *Nursing Research, 44,* 153–159.

Quayhagen, M. P., & Quayhagen, M. (1988). Alzheimer's stress: Coping with the caregiving role. *Gerontologist, 28,* 391–396.

Quayhagen, M. P., & Quayhagen, M. (1989). Differential effects of family-based strategies on Alzheimer's disease. *Gerontologist, 29,* 150–155.

Quint, J. C. (1962). Delineation of qualitative aspects of nursing care. *Nursing Research, 11,* 204–206.

Quint, J. C. (1963). The impact of mastectomy. *American Journal of Nursing, 63,* 88–91.

Quint, J. C. (1965). Institutionalized practices of information control. *Psychiatry, 28,* 119–132.

Quint, J. C. (1966). Communication problems affecting patient care in hospitals. *Journal of American Medical Association, 195,* 36–37.

Quint, J. C. (1970). The developing diabetic identity: A study in family influence. In Marjorie Batey (Ed.), *Communicating nursing research: Methodological issues in research* (Vol. 3, pp. 14–32). Boulder, CO: WICHE.

Quint, J. C. (1972a). The impact of mastectomy. In L. H. Schwartz and J. L. Schwartz (Eds.), *The psychodynamics of patient care* (pp. 256–266). Englewood Cliffs, NJ: Prentice-Hall.

Quint, J. C. (1972b). Institutionalized practices of information control. In E. Freidson & J. Lorber (Eds.), *Medical men and their work* (pp. 220–238). Chicago: Aldine-Atherton.

Quint, J. C. (1977). Role of the family in managing young diabetics. *Diabetes Educator, 3,* 5–8.

Quint, J., Strauss, A., & Glaser, B. (1964). The nonaccountability of terminal care. *Hospitals: Journal of the American Hospital Association, 38,* 73–78.

Reiser, P. J., Kasper, C. E., Greaser, M. L., & Moss, R. L. (1988). Functional significance of myosin transitions in single fibers of developing soleus muscle. *American Journal of Physiology, 254 (Cell Physiology 23),* C605–C613.

Reiser, P. J., Kasper, C. E., & Moss, R. L. (1987). Myosin subunits and contractile properties of single fibers from hypokinetic rat muscles. *Journal of Applied Physiology, 63,* 2293–2300.

Richardson, M. A., Post-White, J., Grimm, E., Moye, L. A., Singletary, S. E., & Justice, B. (1997). Coping, life attitudes, and immune responses to imagery and group support after breast cancer. *Alternative Therapies in Health and Medicine, 3*(5), 62–70.

Roberts, B. L., & Algase, D. L. (1988). Victims of Alzheimer's disease and the environment. *Nursing Clinics of North America, 35*(2), 113–118.

Robinson, K. M. (1988). A social skills training program for adult caregivers. *Advances in Nursing Science, 10*(2), 59–72.

Roy, C., & Andrews, H. A. (1991). *The Roy Adaptation Model: The definitive statement.* Norwalk, CT: Appleton & Lange.

Ryden, M. B. (1984). Morale and perceived control in institutionalized elderly. *Nursing Research, 33*(3), 130–135.

Ryden, M. B. (1985). Environmental support for autonomy in institutionalized elderly. *Research in Nursing and Health, 8,* 363–371.

Ryden, M. B. (1988). Aggressive behavior in persons with dementia who live in the community. *Alzheimer's Disease and Associated Disorders: An International Journal, 2*(4), 342–355.

Ryden, M. B., Bossenmaier, M., & McLachlan, C. (1991). Aggressive behavior in cognitively impaired nursing home residents. *Research in Nursing and Health, 14*(2), 87–95.

Ryden, M. B., & Knopman, D. (1989). Assess not assume: Measurement of morale in the cognitively impaired. *Journal of Gerontologic Nursing, 15*(11), 27–32.

Sampselle, C. (1993). Using a stopwatch to assess pelvic muscle strength in the urine stream interruption test. *Nursing Practice, 18*(1), 14–20.

Schacter, S., & Singer J. E. (1962). Cognitive, social, and physiological determinants of emotional state. *Psychological Review, 69,* 379–399.

Selye, H. (1946). The general adaptation syndrome and the diseases of adaptation. *Journal of Clinical Endocrinology, 6,* 117–230.

Shaver, J. F. (1985). A biopsychosocial view of human health. *Nursing Outlook, 33*(4), 186–191.

Shaver, J. L. F., Giblin, E., Lentz, M., & Lee, K. (1988). Sleep patterns and stability in perimenopausal women. *Sleep, 11,* 556–561.

Shaver, J., & Woods, N. F. (1986). Consistency of perimenstrual symptoms across two cycles. *Research in Nursing and Health, 8,* 313–319.

Sklar, L. S., & Anisman, H. (1979). Stress and coping factors influence tumor growth. *Science, 205,* 513–515.

Solomon, G. F., & Moos, R. H. (1964). Emotions, immunity and disease: A speculative theoretical integration. *Archives of General Psychiatry, 11,* 657–674.

St. Pierre, B. A., Kasper, C. E., & Lindsey, A. M. (1992). Fatigue mechanisms in patients with cancer: Effects of tumor neurosis factor and exercise on skeletal muscle. *Oncology Nursing Forum, 19*(3), 420–425.

Stevenson, J., & Woods, N. (1986). Nursing science and contemporary science: Emerging paradigms. In G. Sorensen (Ed.), *Setting up the agenda for the year 2000: Knowledge development in nursing* (pp. 6–20). Kansas City, MO: American Academy of Nursing.

Strumpf, N. E., & Evans, L. K. (1988). Physical restraint of the hospitalized elderly: Perceptions of patients and nurses. *Nursing Research, 37,* 132–137.

Strumpf, N., & Evans, L. (1992). Alternatives to physical restraints [Editorial]. *Journal of Gerontological Nursing, 18*(11), 4.

Swanson, B., Cronin-Stubbs, D., Zeller, J. M., Kessler, H. A., & Bielauskas, L. A. (1993). Characterizing the neuropsychological functioning of persons with human immunodeficiency virus infection: Part 2. Neuropsychological functioning of persons at different stages of HIV infection. *Archives of Psychiatric Nursing, 7,* 82–90.

Swanson, B., Zeller, J. M., & Spear, G. (1998). Cortisol upregulates HIV p24 antigen in cultured human monocyte-derived macrophages. *Journal of the Association of Nurses in AIDS Care, 9,* 78–83.

Thomas, J., Graff, B., Hollingsworth, A., Cohen, S., & Rubin, M. (1997). Home visiting for a post-hysterectomy population. *Home-Health Care Nurse, 10*(3), 47–52.

Tilden, V. P., & Shepherd, P. (1987). Increasing the rate of identification of battered women in an emergency department: Use of a nursing protocol. *Research in Nursing and Health, 10,* 209–215.

Tønnesen, E. (1989). Immunological aspects of anesthesia and surgery. *Danish Medical Bulletin, 36,* 263–281.

Torres, S. (1987). Hispanic-American battered women: Why consider cultural differences? *Response, 10*(3), 20–21.

Torres, S. (1991). A comparison of wife abuse between two cultures: Perceptions, attitudes, nature and extent. *Issues in Mental Health Nursing, 12,* 113–131.

Unruh, A. M. (1996). Gender variations in clinical pain experience. *Pain, 65,* 123–157.

Visintainer, M. A., Volpicelli, J. R., & Seligman, M. E. P. (1982). Tumor rejection in rats after inescapable or escapable shock. *Science, 216,* 437–439.

Voda, A. (1980). Pattern of progesterone and aldosterone in ovulating women during the menstrual cycle. In A. Dan, E. Graham, & C. Bucher (Eds.), *The menstrual cycle: Vol. 1. A synthesis of interdisciplinary research* (pp. 223–236). New York: Springer Publishing Co.

Voda, A. M. (1981). Climacteric hot flash. *Maturities, 3,* 73–90.

Voda, A. M., & George, T. (1987). Menopause. In J. Fitzpatrick (Ed.), *Annual review of nursing research* (Vol. 5, pp. 55–75). New York: Springer Publishing Co.

Voda, A., Imle, M., & Atwood, J. (1980). Quantification of self-report data from two-dimensional body diagrams. *Western Journal of Nursing Research, 2,* 707–729.

Wells, T. J. (1990). Pelvic (floor) muscle exercise. *Journal of the American Geriatrics Society, 38,* 333–337.

Wells, T., Brink, C., & Diokno, A. (1987). Urinary incontinence in elderly women: Clinical findings. *Journal of the American Geriatrics Society, 35,* 933–939.

Wells, T. J., Brink, C. A., Diokno, A. C., Wolfe, R., & Gillis, G. G. (1991). Pelvic muscle exercise for stress urinary incontinence in elderly women. *Journal of the American Geriatrics Society, 39,* 785–791.

White, L. R., Kahout, F., Evans, A., Cornoni-Huntley, J., & Ostfield, A. M. (1985). Related health problems. In J. Cornoni-Huntley, & D. B. Brock (Eds.), *Established populations for epidemiologic studies of the elderly: Resource data book.* Washington, DC: U.S. Department of Health and Human Services, National Institute on Aging.

Williams, C. C., & Finch, C. E. (1997). Physical restraint: Not fit for woman, man, or beast. *Journal of the American Geriatrics Society, 45,* 773–775.

Wilson, H. S. (1989). Family caregiving for a relative with Alzheimer's dementia: Coping with negative choices. *Nursing Research, 38,* 94–98.

Winningham, M. L., & MacVicar, M. G. (1988). The effects of aerobic exercise on patient reports of nausea. *Oncology Nursing Forum, 15,* 447–450.

Wolanin, M., & Phillips L. (1981). *Confusion: Prevention and care.* St. Louis: C. V. Mosby.

Woods, N. A., & Longnecker, G. D. (1985). Major life events, daily stressors, and perimenstrual symptoms. *Nursing Research, 34,* 263–267.

Woods, N. F. (1980). Women's role and illness episodes: a prospective study. *Research Nursing Health, 3,* 137–145.

Woods, N. F. (1982). Women's health perspectives for nursing research. *Nursing Clinics of North America, 17*(1), 113–119.

Woods, N. F. (1989). Women's health. *Annual Review of Nursing Research, 7,* 209–237.

Woods, N. F., Dery, G. K., & Most, A. (1982). Stressful life events and perimenstrual symptoms. *Journal of Human Stress, 8,* 23–31.

Woods, N. F., Most, A., & Dery, G. K. (1982). Prevalence of perimenstrual symptoms. *American Journal of Public Health, 72,* 1257–1264.

Worcester, M. I., & Quayhagen, M. P. (1983). Correlates of caregiving satisfaction: Prerequisites to elder home care. *Research in Nursing and Health, 6*(2), 61–67.

Wykle, M., & Kaskel, B. (1991). Increasing the longevity of minority older adults through improved health status. In United States Administration on Aging (Ed.), *Minority elders: Longevity, economics, and health—building a public policy base* (pp. 24–31). Washington, DC: Gerontological Society of America.

Wykle, M. L., & Morris, D. L. (1994). Nursing care in Alzheimer's disease. *Clinics in Geriatric Medicine, 10*(2), 351–365.

Wyman, J. F., Choi, S. C., Harkins, S. W., Wilson, M. S., & Fantl, J. A. (1988). The urinary diary in evaluation of urinary incontinence in women: A test retest analysis. *Obstetrics and Gynecology, 71*, 812–817.

Wyman, J., Elswick, R., Ory, M., Wilson, M., & Fantl, A. (1993). Influence of functional, urological and environmental characteristics on urinary incontinence in community-dwelling older women. *Nursing Research, 42*(5), 270–275.

York, R., Brown, L., Samuels, P., Finkler, S. A., Jacobsen, B., Persily, C. A., Swank, A., & Robbins, D. (1997). A randomized trial of early discharge and nurse specialist transitional follow-up care of high risk childbearing women. *Nursing Research, 46*, 254–261.

Zeller, J. M., McCain, N. L., & Swanson, B. (1996). Psychoneuroimmunology: An emerging framework for nursing research. *Journal of Advanced Nursing, 23*, 657–664.

# Index

# Contents of Previous Volumes

## VOLUME II

# ORDER FORM

Save 10% on Volume 19 with this coupon.

_____ Check here to order the *Annual Review of Nursing Research,* Volume 19, 2001 at a 10% discount. You will receive an invoice requesting prepayment.

Save 10% on all future volumes with a continuation order.

_____ Check here to place your continuation order for the *Annual Review of Nursing Research.* You will receive a prepayment invoice with a 10% discount upon publication of each new volume, beginning with Volume 19, 2001. You may pay for prompt shipment or cancel with no obligation.

Name _____

Institution _____

Address _____

City/State/Zip _____

Examination copies for possible adoption are available to instructors "on approval" only. Write on institutional letterhead, noting course, level, present text, and expected enrollment (include $3.50 for postage and handling). Prices slightly higher overseas. Prices subject to change.

Mail this coupon to:
SPRINGER PUBLISHING COMPANY
536 Broadway
New York, NY 10012-3955

# Geriatric Nursing Research Digest

*New*

**Joyce J. Fitzpatrick,** PhD, RN, FAAN
**Terry Fulmer,** PhD, RN, FAAN, Editors
**Meredith Wallace,** PhDc, RN, CS-ANP,
Associate Editor
**Ellen Flaherty,** PhDc, RN, CS-GNP,
Assistant Editor

GERIATRIC NURSING
RESEARCH DIGEST

JOYCE J. FITZPATRICK
TERRY FULMER
EDITORS

$ SPRINGER PUBLISHING COMPANY

This unique synopsis of geriatric nursing research represents an important resource for the care of the elderly. Written by leading experts in the forefront of the field, each entry describes the most significant research in a selected area and illuminates the relevance of this research to clinical practice.

For nurse researchers, geriatric nurses, and beginning to advanced nursing students.

**Contents:**
• Health Promotion and Risk Reduction
• Normal Aging Through the Lifespan
• Environments of Care
• Emotional Health
• Pathological Conditions
• Neurobehavioral and Cognitive Changes of Aging
• References

*2000   400pp.   0-8261-1332-X   hardcover*
*www.springerpub.com*

536 Broadway, New York, NY 10012-3955 • (212) 431-4370 • Fax (212) 941-7842